Mental Retardation:
The Changing Outlook

Mental Retardation

The Changing Outlook

Robert P. Ingalls
New York State Department of Mental Hygiene

John Wiley & Sons
New York / Santa Barbara / Chichester / Brisbane / Toronto

Chapter Opener Photo Credits

Chapter 2 Opener: Pierre Pittet/WHO.

Chapter 3 Opener: Courtesy of Albany County Chapter of the Association of Retarded Children. Photo by Leonard Smoke.

Chapter 6 Opener: William M. Wakefield.

Chapter 7 Opener: Susan Erber.

Chapter 8 Opener: Susan Erber.

Chapter 9 Opener: Susan Erber.

Chapter 11 Opener: Courtesy of Albany County Chapter of the Association of Retarded Children. Photo by Leonard Smoke.

Chapter 12 Opener: Susan Erber.

Chapter 13 Opener: Bruce Roberts/Rapho-Photo Researchers

Chapter 14 Opener: Susan Erber.

Chapter 15 Opener: Susan Erber.

Chapter 16 Opener: Susan Erber.

Chapter 17 Opener: Courtesy of Albany County Chapter of the Association of Retarded Children. Photo by Leonard Smoke.

Chapter 18 Opener: Bruce Roberts/Rapho-Php Researchers.

Library of Congress Cataloging in Publication Data

Ingalls, Robert P 1945–
Mental retardation.

Bibliography: p.
Includes index.
1. Mental deficiency—Etiology. 2. Mentally handicapped—Care and treatment. 3. Mentally handicapped children—Education. 4. Intelligence tests. I. Title.
[DNLM: 1. Mental retardation. 2. Education of mentally retarded. WM300 I44m]
RC570.I4 616.8′588 77-23359
ISBN 0-471-42716-0

Printed in the United States of America

10 9 8 7 6 5 4 3 2 1

Preface

Different cultures value different kinds of abilities. A society of warriors may value bravery above all and heap its greatest honors on its bravest members. A society centered around religion might value most the strength of an individual's faith or their virtue. In modern Western societies, tremendous value is placed on the ability to think clearly and rationally, a process often referred to as intelligence. Examples of this are easy to find. Our economic system is theoretically designed to reward those people who demonstrate their mental abilities either by getting a good deal of education or by solving society's problems. Parents are quick to boast about the bright things that their children say and do. Intelligence is held in such high esteem by some segments of the population that numerous different tests and other screening devices have been developed to distinguish the more intelligent from the less intelligent, and performance on such tests can frequently determine whether individuals can be trained in the career of their choice or get a job with the government.

As a result of the value that is usually placed on intellectual competence, perhaps the most serious accusation that can be leveled against someone is that they are deficient in intelligence. This book discusses those individuals who are most deficient of all in intellectual abilities—those people who have been labeled mentally retarded. These people have traditionally suffered some of the worst degradations that society can heap on people, and even today, in these supposedly enlightened times, prejudice against the mentally retarded is still widespread. Witness the resistance that many communities have against having group homes for the retarded in their neighborhood. This prejudice is not limited to the relatively uninformed but can also be found even among highly educated people including many psychologists, psychiatrists and other physicians, social workers, and teachers who view work with the mentally retarded as unrewarding and uninteresting and, in private, refer to the mentally retarded in derogatory terms.

However, such prejudices and stereotyped thinking have greatly diminished in the past few years, and mental retardation is far more in the public eye today than it was just a few years ago. This book reviews this progress in public attitudes toward and understanding of the mentally retarded. The approach is, to some extent, historical in nature, comparing current attitudes and understanding with different attitudes that characterized earlier decades.

An underlying theme of this book is its denial of a specific psychology of the mentally retarded. People labeled mentally retarded are such a diverse group of people that it is practically impossible to make any meaningful generalizations about them. Except for those individuals at the very low end of the intelligence scale, who make up only a tiny minority of those people considered retarded, most mentally retarded people do not differ in important ways from other people in society who are not considered mentally retarded. While virtually all retarded people have difficulty in school (as do many people not considered mentally retarded) extensive research has failed to discover any unique learning characteristics or deficits that characterize their mental processes, and there are no instructional techniques that have been shown to work better for retarded children than with nonretarded children. As with any large group of people, some get in trouble with the law or do other antisocial things, but the majority do not. Hopefully, this book will help to abolish the myth that the mentally retarded are a unique group of people different from everyone else.

There were several people who helped prepare the manuscript. The entire staff at John Wiley & Sons, editor Deborah Wiley in particular, were invaluable. Laird Heal, Peter O'Connor, and Allan Ross, who reviewed the manuscript, provided numerous useful suggestions and comments. Ora Schongar, who typed the final manuscript, deserves special recognition for effort beyond the call of duty. Finally, my wife Naomi deserves a special tribute for putting up with me during the years that I was writing.

Robert P. Ingalls

Contents

Mental Retardation:
The Changing Outlook

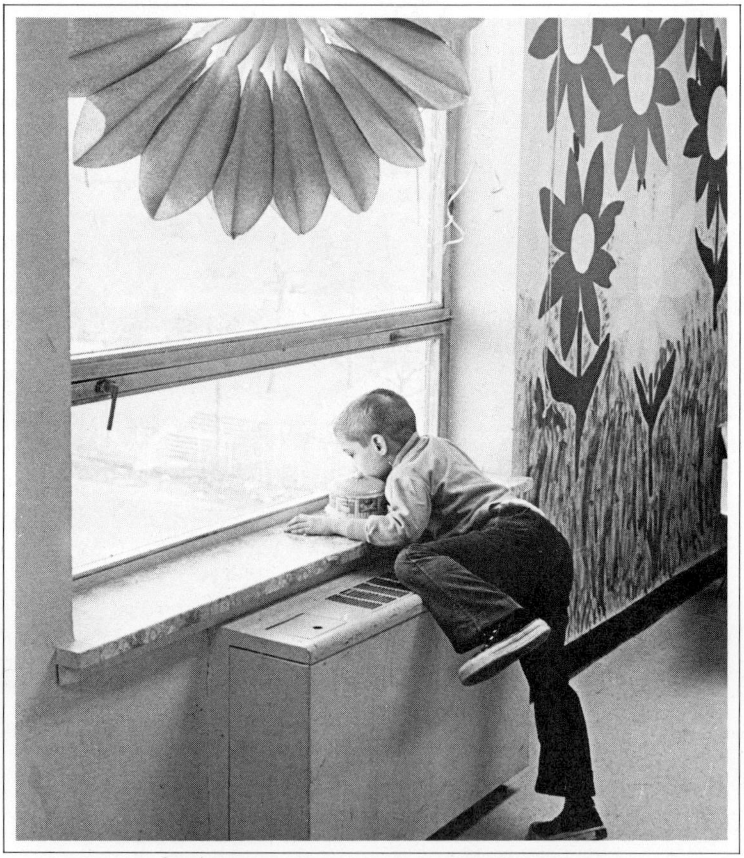

1

Labels, Labeling, and the Mentally Retarded

Dividing people into different categories, labeling them, and then determining how the people who have been labeled differ from the general population is a common activity in any discipline that deals with people. A sociologist might label a certain group of people as disadvantaged, a physician might label someone schizophrenic, a psychologist might label some people extroverts, and an educator might label certain children as gifted. Labels can be positive, neutral, or negative, but they all distinguish a certain group of people from the rest of humanity.

Most such labeling activity is undoubtedly necessary, but labels can easily lead to misunderstandings. A label tends to divide people into two mutually exclusive, homogeneous populations; that is, a person is either disadvantaged or not disadvantaged, either schizophrenic or not schizophrenic, either gifted or not gifted, and all those people who have been given one of these labels are thought of as being similar to each other and different in important ways from the normal population. In reality, the line separating the labeled from the unlabeled is almost always blurry; there is usually a grey area made up of people who show some characteristics of the labeled group but not enough to be reliably labeled. A great many people will at some point in their life manifest the bizarre behavior of the schizophrenic. Nearly half the population of the United States probably meets some of the criteria of social disadvantage. Another problem with labeling is that it becomes very easy to assume that all of the people who are assigned a particular label are quite similar to each other. This leads to stereotyped thinking such as "all blacks are disadvantaged." or "schizophrenics are dangerous." In fact, the kinds of people who have been assigned a label, such as extroverted or disadvantaged or schizophrenic or gifted, often have little in common besides their labels.

The Mentally Retarded Label

This book is about a group of people who have been labeled mentally retarded. All of the problems associated with labeling apply particularly well to this group. Most people who have not worked closely with retarded people tend to think of this label as being a very distinct category; an individual is or is not mentally retarded, and retarded people are all similar to each other and quite different from those people who are not retarded. In fact, exactly the opposite is the case. Mental retardation is on a continuum with normalcy, and where the line is drawn that separates the retarded from the nonretarded is entirely arbitrary. Most retarded people do not differ qualitatively from nonretarded people. More importantly, there is a good deal of overlap in abilities between those people who are labeled mentally retarded and those who are not. Some children who are in special classes for the retarded are functioning better intellectually, academically, and socially than some children in regular classes who have never been labeled mentally retarded. Many people who have been labeled retarded are able to lead independent, productive lives as adults while many "normal" people are completely unable to hold a job.

This overlap may be obvious, but all too many parents and teachers seem to think of mental retardation and normalcy as being two distinct categories. Many parents have asked their pediatrician "Is my child retarded?" If the physician answers "No," the parents breath a sigh of relief because this means that the child is normal. If the answer is "Yes," the parents panic because in their minds mental retardation always means hopeless incompetence and lifelong dependency. Similarly, teachers may refer one of their pupils to the school psychologist for testing to find out if the pupil is retarded or not. If the psychologist decides that the child is not retarded, the teacher will gladly keep the child in class, but if the evaluation determines that the child is retarded, then the teacher will push to have the child placed in a special class because the child is unable to profit from regular class placement.

There is no way that a book about mental retardation can completely avoid reinforcing this type of thinking. The very fact that a book has been written about retarded people implies that they differ in important ways from other people and that they have some characteristics in common that are worth talking about. For example, it will frequently be necessary to refer to research in which a group of retarded people is compared to a group of nonretarded people on some characteristic, say learning speed. Such an experiment cannot avoid the implication that the retarded are in some way a homogeneous group different from normal people even though this is not the intent of the book at all. If there is one point which this book is trying to make above all else, it is that the mentally retarded do not constitute a homogeneous and unique group, and, for the most part, they do not differ to any great extent from those people who are not considered mentally retarded. There is no such thing as a psychology of the mentally retarded any more than there is a psychology of people named Harry. There are very few educational practices that are unique to retarded people, and, in fact, there are very few therapeutic procedures of any kind that apply to retarded people but not to other kinds of people. It is difficult to make many statements that are true of all or even of most retarded people. The range of intellectual abilities among the retarded is as great or greater than it is in the range of people labeled normal, and the kinds of problems that confront the retarded are just as diverse as the problems facing any group of normal individuals. It is unfortunate that the very writing of a book on mental retardation must suggest the opposite.

However, it is also important not to go to the opposite extreme of assuming that those people who are labeled retarded are no different from everyone else. Simply because it is impossible to clearly distinguish the retarded from the nonretarded does not mean that they are exactly the same as other people. While almost any generalization about the retarded is apt to be misleading, the label mentally retarded is not assigned to people on an entirely capricious basis. While there is a good deal of diversity among the retarded and a good deal of overlap in abilities between those people labeled retarded and those who are not so labeled, on the average, retarded people are clearly different from the general population.

It seems to be difficult for people to avoid these two extremes. While the first type of error, thinking of retarded people as being qualitatively different from other people, is certainly more common, it is easy to find writers who go too far in the opposite direction and suggest (although no one explicitly states) that most retarded people are *no* different from everyone else (e.g., Braginsky and Braginsky, 1974).

In addition to the general problems associated with any kind of labeling, there are some specific problems that are associated with labels that refer to disabilities, handicaps, or deficiencies of character. There is no way that a label such as mentally retarded can avoid being a severe blow to the self-esteem of an individual. Our society places tremendous value on the capacity to think clearly and rationally, a process sometimes referred to as intelligence, and the label mentally retarded implies that people so labeled have so little competence in these areas that they require special instruction and are likely to require assistance throughout life. The term *stigma* refers to any characteristic that devalues individuals and makes them less worthy in the eyes of others (Goffman, 1963). Almost any handicap or disability is stigmatizing, but, in a sense, the label mentally retarded is the ultimate stigma. While blindness or amputation are defects of the body, mental retardation implies a far more fundamental type of deficit, a deficit of the mind, and for this reason, it has been widely shunned and otherwise dealt with irrationally both by the general public and by professionals. It is surrounded by the myths and half truths that come about through ignorance. For example, it is almost universally assumed that mental retardation is a hopeless condition. As a result, retarded children and adults have traditionally been far more likely than other handicapped people to be put away in institutions isolated from the rest of society or deprived of services normally guaranteed to everyone, such as proper schooling. Many psychologists and psychiatrists refuse to deal with retarded clients assuming, as the general public does, that the diagnosis of retardation implies hopelessness. Teachers freely express the feeling that they don't want retarded children in their classrooms because the children cannot learn. As recently as the 1960s, many pediatricians advised parents of retarded children to institutionalize the unfortunate creatures and forget about them.

Fortunately, these attitudes are changing, and, if present trends continue, it may not be necessary to begin future books on mental retardation with such a discouraging note. Courses in mental retardation, once a rarity on college campuses, are now widespread, not only in schools of education, but also in psychology departments, medical schools, social work programs, and human services programs in community colleges. The various levels of government have at last realized their obligation to provide *every* citizen with the opportunity to live a fulfilling life even if this means providing special services to those citizens less well endowed. Universal public education is finally becoming truly universal, and more and more states are passing legislation that guarantees all children, even the most severely handicapped, the right to an educational program appropriate to their needs. Federally funded research on mental retardation, virtually nonexistent in the 1950s, is now common. Almost all kinds of programs for the retarded—special education, vocational training, speech therapy, and recreational programs to name a few—have expanded geometrically throughout the 1960s and 1970s. The large state residential institutions, the ultimate symbol of dehumanizing treatment for the retarded, are being rapidly phased out in favor of more homelike living arrangements for those people who are unable to live independently.

Mental retardation has always been recognized as a multidisciplinary problem, but the disciplines that have traditionally been involved with the retarded—medicine and education—have increasingly been supplemented by a variety of other areas of knowledge. Psychologists have done research on the nature of learning and memory in the retarded and have developed new training methods. Speech therapists and physical therapists are now found at most facilities providing service to the retarded. Retardation is being recognized more and more as a social problem, something that affects not only individuals, but also their families and communities. There is a realization that the diagnosis, and in many cases the etiology (cause), of mental retardation are social in that a person may be considered retarded in some societies but not in others. As a result, sociologists, social workers, and even anthropologists have begun to take an interest in retardation. Architects have become involved in designing buildings that are better suited to the needs of the retarded and other handicapped people. Lawyers have begun to take an interest in the civil rights of retarded citizens. In the recent past, many retarded people were locked up against their will, denied access to treatment, and even forced to work essentially as slaves in institutions, but a number of recent lawsuits have guaranteed that a retarded or insane person can only be institutionalized according to due process and that they are entitled to proper treatment. The courts have even assured the right of a retarded person to vote.

Nomenclature

The condition of low intelligence has been given numerous different labels; mental retardation, mental deficiency, mentally defective, mentally handicapped, feeblemindedness, mental subnormality, amentia, and oligophrenia, among others. Throughout this book, the first term—mental retardation—will generally be used. This is consistent with current practice in the United States. The other terms are all essentially synonymous, with occasional differences in connotation. For example, the term feebleminded, while being largely abandoned in this country because of its objectionable overtones, is still occasionally used in England to refer to the group labeled educable mentally retarded in this country. Mental deficiency is sometimes distinguished from retardation, referring to those whose mental capacities are diminished as a result of organic pathology rather than from environmental causes. Mental subnormality is the English equivalent to the American term mentally retarded. Amentia is an old term, distinguishing the retarded or amented from the mentally ill or demented. The distinction is important, but the terms are obsolete. Oligophrenia is the accepted term for mental retardation in some European countries.

There is a trend toward the use of less stigmatizing labels for all sorts of disabilities. Many educators and other professionals now refer to exceptional children or atypical children or children with developmental disabilities rather than using more specific labels. There are several reasons for this. First, labels such as mentally retarded are not at all precise. Not only do they refer to a variety of different kinds of people, but there is frequently considerable disagreement about whether a given child ought to be labeled retarded or learning disabled, retarded or emotionally disturbed, retarded or brain damaged, retarded or autistic. In most cases, the specific diagnostic label is not important in the treatment or education of the child, and thus it is often expedient to refer to all such children with a general term. Second, there is increasing awareness of the damaging effects that a label such as mentally retarded can have on children. Teachers may expect less of them, other children may tease them, parents may feel guilty or ashamed. It is certainly easier for some parents to talk about their exceptional child rather than their retarded child. This trend is admirable in many ways, but terms such as exceptional child are too general for some purposes, since they refer not only to the mentally retarded, but also to the physically handicapped, the emotionally disturbed, the blind or hearing impaired, and even the gifted. While it may be damaging to label a particular child as retarded, the category is still needed for administrative and research purposes.

Some Examples of Retarded People

One of the best ways to demonstrate the diversity of the kinds of people who are labeled mentally retarded is to describe a number of cases. Case studies are instructive because they emphasize the human aspects of the problem of mental retardation, and they help to reduce stereotypes and preconceived notions about what mentally retarded people are like. Each of the five cases described below was at one time in his or her life diagnosed as being mentally retarded, and each typifies certain kinds of retarded people, but obviously each is unique in many ways.

Mary

Mary was the sixth child, third daughter, of a lower-middle-class family living in a large Eastern city. Her father had come to this country from Italy when he was five and had gone to school through seventh grade. Then he had gone to work in various odd jobs. At the time of Mary's birth, he was working in a bakery owned by an uncle where he earned an income barely enough to support his large family. Mary's mother had gone to school through ninth grade and then had worked briefly as a waitress before marrying. The family lived in a four-room apartment in an older building. It was poorly furnished, and there were no books except the Bible, but it was always kept spotless. Mary's prenatal development and birth were uneventful, and there was nothing unusual about her preschool development. Her mother didn't have much time to spend with her, but there were lots of older brothers and sisters to look after her. The other children were progressing normally in school, although none was doing very well academically. Mary entered first grade when she was six. Her academic performance was quite poor. She was a quiet, shy, and passive girl who never caused any trouble, but she was completely unable to read at the end of the first grade. She received a social promotion to the second grade where the teacher was a family friend. This teacher took an unusual interest in Mary, and at the end of the second grade, Mary could recognize all of the letters of the alphabet and read a few simple words. However, in the third grade, more was expected of her, and her deficits, not only in reading but also in arithmetic and other academic skills, became more apparent. Her teacher did not have the time to give Mary the individual attention that she needed, and, although she was recommended for remedial help, the reading specialist was too overworked to fit Mary in. At the end of that year, Mary was so far behind that she was held back. At the end of her second year in the third grade, when she was almost 11 years old, she was still reading at the first-grade level, and the other children had begun to tease her about this. She was referred to the school psychologist for evaluation. He determined that Mary was functioning intellectually at the level of the average seven and a half year old and he recommended that she be placed in a special class for the mentally retarded. Mary spent the next three years attending a special class in her local elementary school, and at the end of that time, her reading and arithmetic skills were almost to the third-grade level.

Mary's parents knew that she was attending a special class, but they were not overly concerned about this because they did not worry about the academic progress of their daughters. Her family did not perceive her as exceptional in any way although they were worried about her shyness and lack of friends. Her mother taught her how to cook, sew, and clean the apartment, and she had little unusual difficulty learning how to be an adequate housekeeper.

Mary spent the next two years attending an experimental program for special children at the high school, where she received instruction in grooming, health, home economics, and the like. She dropped out of school when she was 16 and went to work in a laundry owned by her brother-in-law. She worked there for two years until she met Mark, a neighborhood boy who had just returned from the Army. She and Mark were married three months later, and Mary quit her job to become a full-time housewife and, shortly afterward, a mother. She was a reasonably competent housekeeper although she had no interests other than her family, and her social life was limited to visiting with relatives.

Comment. It is important to remember that there is often considerable disagreement concerning whether a given individual is mentally retarded or not, and Mary is a case whom some people, such as the school psychologist, would consider mentally retarded while other people would not. She is in some ways typical of the kind of person who would be labeled borderline mentally retarded, or perhaps high-level mildly retarded or educable mentally retarded (the specific meaning of these terms will be discussed in a later chapter). She certainly had a good deal of difficulty in school, but her adjustment to nonacademic situations was at worst only slightly impaired, and after she left school she lived a relatively normal, independent existence.

It is also important to notice that Mary had nothing medically wrong with her, and the cause of her diminished mental capacities was completely unknown. Contrary to widespread belief, most children who are mentally retarded do not have obvious brain damage or other organic conditions, and the diagnosis of mental retardation is made on the basis of poor school performance rather than by a medical doctor.

Roy

Roy was the second of two boys born to a black family in New York City's Harlem. His father deserted his mother when he was two years old, and so Roy doesn't really remember his father at all. After her husband left, Roy's mother went on welfare, and the family remained on public assistance throughout Roy's childhood except for a brief period when his mother took a job as a cleaning woman. During his preschool years, Roy usually had enough to eat, but, in order to make ends meet, his mother had to feed the two boys a lot of inexpensive, starchy food. The family moved three times before Roy started school, once because the building they lived in was being torn down, once when they were evicted because of nonpayment of rent, and once they moved voluntarily because the landlord refused to provide enough heat during a cold winter. There was nothing unusual about Roy's early physical development. His mother was a hostile and authoritarian woman who was continually yelling at her children and who would beat them with a hairbrush at the slightest provocation. As a result, Roy spent as little time as possible at home even when he was very young. In the first grade, Roy did not like his teacher, and she did not like him. She complained that she couldn't understand much of what he said because he slurred his words and that he was frequently dirty and smelled of urine. Roy spent most of his schooltime trying to avoid work rather than trying to learn. He had a great deal of difficulty sitting still for any length of time, and his constant wandering around further aggravated his teacher. When he was promoted to second grade, he was placed in a special section for slow learners where he continued to avoid learning. With special remediation he was able to learn all of his letters and could read a few simple words, in spite of the fact that he really had no interest in schoolwork. None of his friends were doing much better, and they teased the few children who actually were doing their work. In the third grade, he was suspended for three days for fighting. He started to skip school with increasing regularity and hang around with his older brother and his friends. A year later, he was arrested for shoplifting, but was released with a warning. After his third suspension from school in the fifth grade, he was given a thorough examination by the school psychologist, who administered a standard intelligence test to him and determined that Roy's IQ was 63. As a result, he was placed in a special class. Here there were fewer students, and the teacher could give him more individual attention. Roy began to apply himself and by the end of the year was reading at the second-grade level. By this time, however, his older friends were getting into bigger trouble. The next year, he was arrested for stealing money from a cash register and again released with only a warning. A short time later however, he and his brother were arrested again for stealing a car and taking it on a joy ride, and this time he was referred to a private residential school for delinquent boys upstate. There he received intensive counseling and some special tutoring. A year later, he was returned to his mother. After that, Roy managed to stay out of trouble for a while and even attended school regularly because he liked to work in the machine shop in the high school. However, he still could not read very well and didn't put much effort into his English, history, and math courses. When he was 16, he quit school. He could not find a job, and a few months later, he was arrested for the armed robbery of a liquor store. He was sent to prison for six months and then was let out on parole. The parole board found him a job in a gas station. His boss taught him a good deal about fixing cars, and Roy became a fair mechanic. He got married a year later and settled down. Most of his former friends were in prison, and it was easy for him to stay out of trouble if there was no one to encourage him to transgress. He is still working at the gas station and spends most of his spare time fixing cars, watching television, or drinking beer at the local bar.

Comment. This is a case in which mental retardation results from the social and psychological environment of the child. Any child needs intellectual stimulation and emotional support for proper development, and Roy's mother was too overwhelmed with her own problems to provide these. It is important to realize that an inadequate environment can produce mental deficits just as serious as those produced by organic conditions.

As with Mary, there would be considerable debate among professionals regarding whether Roy should be considered mentally retarded. Many people would argue that he was simply a product of a different culture, and that his family and his friends had taught him to achieve success in ways other than by academic achievement. The reason why he did so poorly in school and on intelligence tests was because they were based on white middle-class values and ideas, and if Roy had been tested in black dialect on concepts important for survival in the black culture, he would have done very well.

Fred

Fred was born the first of four children to a carpenter and his wife. He was born somewhat prematurely, but the physician assured his parents that nothing was wrong. From the day they brought him home from the hospital, he was a difficult child; he wouldn't eat, he was continually crying, and he seemed to sleep about half as much as other babies. He started walking when he was only a year old, and the problems became worse. Fred was always getting into everything, and he couldn't be left alone for a minute without getting into some kind of trouble. Because he was a firstborn child, his parents had no other children to compare him to, and as a result, they were not too concerned about his difficult behavior, being convinced that he would grow out of it. When he started first grade, he was completely unable to sit still for more than a few minutes, and he was unable to learn anything. In second grade, his behavior became even worse; Fred was continually running around and bothering the other children. His teacher referred him to the school psychologist, who gave him an IQ test. Fred was given a diagnosis of minimal brain dysfunction with possible retardation. The diagnosis of retardation could not be confirmed because he would not sit still long enough to do anything. Under considerable pressure from his teacher, he was placed in a special class for exceptional children. Things began to get worse at home. Fred was continually running around the house, breaking things, and otherwise getting into trouble. He did not respond to increasingly severe punishment, and the rest of the family was having more and more difficulty coping with him. His father was spending less time at home, and his mother, with two smaller children and a third on the way, was at the end of her rope. After another year of this, his teacher was firmly convinced that Fred was retarded, and she communicated this to his parents. They inquired about placing him in a state institution, but they were told that there was little possibility of this because there was a waiting list and children functioning as well as Fred were not usually admitted. Fred's tested IQ was

60. Two months later, Fred's mother had a nervous breakdown and was admitted to a state mental hospital. The children were taken by her sister, and Fred's father again inquired about institutionalization. This time, because of the severity of the situation, Fred was admitted. At first, he was totally unmanageable. He was placed on heavy dosages of drugs and largely ignored. His parents came to visit him every month or so, his mother having recovered after Fred had left. Fred was sent to school on the training school grounds, where he was eventually taught to read at about the third-grade level. His behavior gradually improved over the next few years, and he was given jobs of increasing complexity, first working in the laundry room, then in the dining hall, and finally helping to maintain the grounds. His mother died when Fred was 16, and his father stopped coming to visit. Two years later, Fred was released with a job working in the kitchen of a nursing home. His social worker got him a small apartment. He worked for about six months but became increasingly lax about promptness and cooperation and was laid off. When he couldn't find another job, he was returned to the institution. Shortly afterward, he was released again, this time to a job in the cafeteria of a college dormitory. He worked there for about a year, and then was fired abruptly when he was charged with exposing himself to a coed. Again he was returned to the institution where he was given counseling about his problems. He was eventually released for a third time to another kitchen job in a nursing home, and he has kept this job for three years now. He is quite contented with his life although he is making little money, lives in the poorest section of town, and has few interests other than watching television.

Comment. Many people who have been diagnosed as mentally retarded have other behavioral and emotional problems as well. In Fred's case, these secondary problems proved to be more of an obstacle to successful adjustment than was the problem of mental retardation per se. He lost his jobs not because he was unable to do the work but because he had little impulse control, and this is a very common pattern.

One of the somewhat atypical features of Fred's case is that he was institutionalized even though he was not severely retarded. Only a small minority of those people labeled mentally retarded are ever institutionalized, and these are almost always either the most severely retarded or those with unusual management problems such as Fred. Fewer and fewer retarded people are being institutionalized today as other alternatives are developed.

Fred's retardation may well have had an organic cause, perhaps due to his premature birth, but there is no way of knowing for sure. In fact, determining the cause is not really important, since this knowledge would probably not contribute to his treatment or management.

Karen

Karen was born the last of three children to an accountant and his wife. Both her parents were college graduates, and they lived in a middle-class suburb. The two older children did well in school. She was diagnosed at birth as having Down's syndrome or mongolism, a disorder that is associated with mental retardation. Her parents were horrified when the physician told them that their child would be retarded, but they accepted the fact and tried to raise her as they would any other child. Her mother started reading about mental retardation, and she joined the local association for retarded children. Because of her interest, she was elected an officer. Karen's development was quite slow. She didn't sit up until she was a year old, and didn't walk until she was nearly two years old. Her mother, after a good deal of effort, had her completely toilet trained by the time she was five, but the local school system had no facilities for a child as severely retarded as Karen, and so she was excluded. She stayed at home with her mother for another year and a half, and her mother conscientiously taught her proper self-help skills such as dressing and table manners, and Karen was able to talk in short sentences, although she was hard to understand. Karen started to attend a private nursery for retarded children. A year later, the school system initiated a classroom for trainable level children, and Karen was a charter member. In school, she continued to learn social and self-help skills, and an attempt was made to teach her to read, write, and count. She attended school until she was 17, and then was given a certificate of attendance. At this time, she was able to count, although she had little idea of what numbers meant. She could write her name, but she had no functional reading skills. A psychologist determined that she was functioning at the level of the average six year old, and she told Karen's parents that her IQ was 40. After Karen left school, her parents became increasingly concerned about her future. She would always need some sort of supervision, but they were totally opposed to institutionalizing her. They had visited the state training school and were horrified by what they saw. They could not afford to place her in a private facility, and so she just stayed at home with them. She became a burden to her mother because she was frequently bored, and she would tag after her mother wherever she went. She had no friends, and the only socializing that she did was attending a dance once a week sponsored by the community association for the retarded. After several years of doing nothing, they were finally able to enroll Karen in a sheltered workshop where she was given jobs of assembling simple parts for a local factory and stuffing envelopes. Karen loved her work, and the knowledge that she was being paid made her very proud, although she had no idea how much she made. Karen is still at the workshop. Her father recently had a heart attack, and her parents are now more concerned than ever about Karen's future since they know that they will be too old to care for her much longer. Her older brother and sister are married and refuse to have much to do with her. Her sister will occasionally take Karen for a weekend while her parents are away, but she has children of her own and can't take care of Karen for more than a few days.

Comment. Down's syndrome is the most common of the organic syndromes of mental retardation. It does not generally run in families and is found more often among older mothers. Karen was fortunate in that her parents were able to accept her retardation and did not react by overprotecting her or by denying her limitations as some parents do. Because of her healthy home life, she was relatively free of secondary emotional problems.

The chief difficulty that Karen and her parents encountered was inadequate services. For a while, there was no public school program for her, and after she left school there was little in the way of community programming for the retarded. This is a very common problem, although in the decade of the 1970s vast strides were made toward filling these gaps. Most states now have education-for-all legislation that stipulates that even the most handicapped children must be provided with an appropriate educational program, and many communities now have coordinated programs of vocational training and recreation for the adult retarded. The problem of humane residential facilities is also being solved with the establishment of group homes and the like so that it is likely that Karen will have a place to go when her parents are no longer able to care for her.

Richard

Richard was born the fourth of five children to a machinist. His prenatal development and birth were normal, but he was diagnosed as having cerebral palsy by the family doctor when he was eight months old. His mother had suspected that something was wrong for some time before that because he was so inactive and wouldn't reach for anything. His physical development was very slow. He did not sit up until he was more than a year old, and he never learned to walk at all. When he was 14 months old, he had a series of epileptic seizures. The doctor put Richard on anticonvulsant medication and the seizures ceased. As he grew older, he became an increasing problem to his family. He began to say a few words when he was three, but his control over his articulators was so poor that no one could understand him except his immediate family. His oldest sister, a sophomore in high school, was quite embarrassed by her younger brother, who at five was still not toilet trained, was confined to a wheel chair, and drooled almost continually. He couldn't even feed himself. She refused to have friends over, which greatly inhibited her budding social life. Richard's parents tried to get him admitted to public school, but he was refused because he was not toilet trained and because there was no class appropriate for him. A year later, they found a privately run nursery for cerebral palsied children and enrolled him. Here he received some physical therapy and speech training as well as training in self-help skills, but he didn't learn very much. It seemed like he had just stopped developing. A psychologist gave him an estimated IQ of only 30. He attended this class for the next four years, then was dropped to make room for others who showed more promise. Richard still could not even take care of his most basic needs, and his parents began to look for a more permanent placement for him. He was finally admitted to a state institution for the retarded. His psychological evaluation on admission determined that Richard was functioning at the level of the average three year old mentally. Immediately after he was admitted, he began having violent seizures again, which subsided only gradually as the doctors experimented with various medications. At the institution, the staff eventually taught him to signal his toileting needs so that he could be brought to the bathroom, and a speech therapist devoted considerable time to improving his language, but with little success. He is still unable to walk or dress himself, and there is little hope that he will improve very much or ever be released except to some other total care facility.

Comment. Richard has multiple handicaps. Not only is he severely mentally retarded, but he also has cerebral palsy and epilepsy. Such cases used to be routinely institutionalized and forgotten, and only in the past few years have there been any attempts to provide systematic programming for the severely retarded and the mutliply handicapped. Today, cases such as Richard are less likely to be completely excluded from the public schools and less likely to be institutionalized, although they will certainly always require custodial care. Fortunately, individuals as severely handicapped as Richard comprise only a small minority of retarded people.

The main point of these cases is to demonstrate that the mentally retarded are a heterogeneous group of people; some retarded people, such as Mary, seem to have few adjustment problems other than poor school performance. Others, such as Roy, seem to be in continual conflict with society, although this conflict is not always directly related to low intelligence. Some people, such as Fred, are characterized by severe behavioral and emotional problems, while others, such as Karen, have no more emotional instability than anyone else. Many retarded people, such as Richard, have other handicaps as well, such as epilepsy, cerebral palsy, or sensory impairment, while others have no physical problems at all. Just as it is difficult to make generalizations about these five people, it is difficult to make general statements about the estimated six million retarded people in the United States.

Summary

It is easy to think of the mentally retarded as being very different sorts of people from those who are considered normal, and the most important point to keep in mind as one reads this book is that this is not entirely true. Even though it will sometimes be necessary to discuss how retarded people differ from those people who are not retarded, in most characteristics most retarded people do not differ in important ways from everyone else. Mental retardation, rather than being a condition qualitatively different from normalcy, is on a continuum with it, and whether a given individual is labeled mentally retarded or not is often somewhat arbitrary.

A second point of the chapter is that mental retardation is not a unitary condition; it is not a single disease or disorder but refers to a very general category of people with little in common beyond the fact that they do poorly on intelligence tests and in school. There is disagreement not only on the subject of who is mentally retarded and who is not, but also on the very definition of mental retardation and even on whether the concept of mental retardation is a useful one.

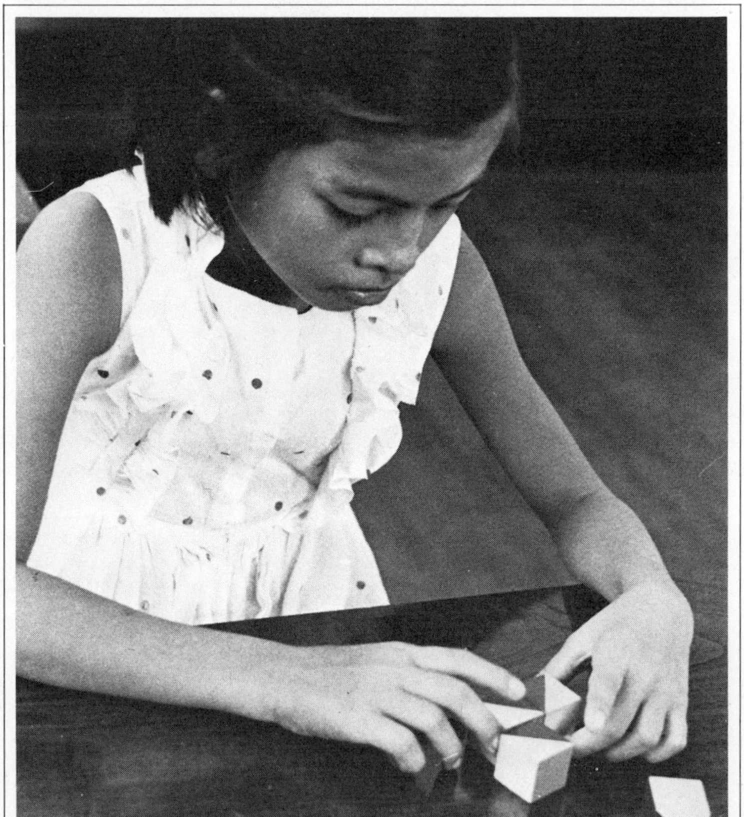

2
Intelligence and Intelligence Tests

It would normally be appropriate to provide a working definition of mental retardation at this point, but this would be difficult without first discussing the concept of intelligence. The concept of mental retardation and the concept of intelligence are so intimately related that it is virtually impossible to talk about one without also making a statement about the other. Mental retardation is usually considered to be fundamentally a defect in intelligence, and thus one's beliefs about the nature of intelligence must necessarily have an effect on one's views about the nature of mental retardation. As a result, the task of providing a precise definition of mental retardation will be deferred for a chapter in order to provide some background on the psychology of intelligence.

Defining Intelligence

It is probably impossible to completely define any word that is in common usage and still retain all of the various denotations and connotations of the word, and one of the major problems in defining and conceptualizing intelligence is that there is a folk meaning of the term. Almost everyone, even a small child, seems to have some feeling about the nature of intelligence. Virtually everybody at some point in their life must have remarked that so-and-so is pretty smart or that someone is pretty stupid. These are statements about intelligence, and the fact that these statements are made implies that people have some idea about what intelligence is. However, as soon as one begins to think seriously about exactly what it means to say that someone is intelligent, an issue that used to be simple and obvious becomes obscure and perplexing as certain contradictions become apparent. For example, many people consider intelligence to be the same as judgment or common sense, yet one frequently hears remarks that someone isn't very intelligent but has a lot of common sense. The terms gifted and genius are used to refer either to someone who is highly intelligent or to someone who is very creative, suggesting that these two faculties must be similar. Yet, it is generally agreed that creativity and intelligence are two separate processes. Intelligence usually refers to something innate or at least constitutional, unaffected by an individual's upbringing or education. Yet toys are sold that promise to raise the user's intelligence and improvements in intelligence test scores are used to determine the effectiveness of certain nursery and compensatory education programs. Another issue concerns whether intelligence is a single process or whether it can be broken down into several relatively independent abilities. The folk meaning treats intelligence as a single, unitary process, yet people see no contradiction in saying that a child has high mathematical intelligence but low verbal intelligence. For the most part, attempts to measure intelligence have tried to measure this folk meaning, despite its vagueness and its apparent contradictions. This situation has produced many of the problems that have surrounded the study of intelligence.

Some Traditional Definitions

Attempting to define intelligence has been a popular endeavor among psychologists. For example, in 1921 the *Journal of Educational Psychology* invited a number of leading psychologists of the time to submit their definitions for a symposium. Unfortunately, there was little that the participants could agree on at that time, and little progress has been made since in producing a definition that has wide popular support. A satisfactory definition should have at least two features; it should not grossly violate the folk use of the word, and it should be objective or operational rather than simply being a list of synonyms as is customary in most dictionary definitions. Among the basic approaches to defining intelligence are the following:

1. *Intelligence is the ability to learn.* Superficially, such an approach to defining intelligence makes sense. The more people are able to learn, the smarter they probably are. The faster people can learn, the more they can learn by a given age, and thus the better they can score on intelligence tests. However, there are certain difficulties with such an approach. First, learning ability does not appear to be a unitary phenome-

non. There are many different kinds of learning, and individuals who do well on some kinds of learning do not necessarily do well on others. Guilford (1967) reviewed a number of experiments addressed to this question. The general approach of such research is to determine the rate of learning in several different kinds of learning tasks for a number of subjects. If there is such a thing as general learning ability, then those subjects who do the best on some learning tasks ought to do well on others also, but this was not the case. Almost universally, correlations between learning rates for various tasks were quite small.

A second problem is that learning ability does not seem to be related in any direct way to the more complex sorts of problems found on many intelligence tests. Zeaman and House (1966) have reviewed the research on the relationship between learning and intelligence (as measured by performance on standard intelligence tests), and they conclude that as long as the learning task is simple enough, subjects of low intelligence are not poorer learners than subjects of higher intelligence, although the results are far from clear. An important exception to this generalization is school learning. Numerous studies report a high relationship between school grades (presumably a measure of learning) and intelligence test performance (e.g., Bond, 1940).

2. *Intelligence is what has been learned.* An example of this approach is Wesman's (1968) definition, "Intelligence is a summation of learning experiences." This definition implies that intelligence tests are not measuring an ability or potential as much as they are measuring achievement. In a sense, they are measuring our knowledge. One difficulty with such an approach is that it does not fit in with popular notions of what intelligence is. Most people feel that an intelligence test should be something other than an achievement test, reflecting not so much what a person has learned so far but rather measuring some sort of potential for future achievement. It is easy to imagine an individual who through dint of hard work has learned a great deal but who is not particularly intelligent. It is generally felt that such factors as hard work or motivation should not be included as part of intelligence while they are certainly directly related to how much one has learned.

3. *Intelligence is the ability to adapt to the environment, particularly to new situations in the environment.* For example, Stern (1914) the developer of the concept of IQ, defined intelligence as "general adaptability to the new problems and conditions of life." The difficulty with this definition is that it is difficult or impossible to define "adapt." There are some people whom it is generally agreed are not very intelligent and who do not do very well on intelligence tests, yet they adapt very well to their environ-

ment. They have well-paid, secure jobs and manage to cope with all of life's adversities. Other people, who score very well on intelligence tests and are generally agreed to be quite gifted, effect a very poor adjustment to their environment. An example would be an artist or musician who is not quite talented enough to make a living with his talent and who is continually unhappy because he is unwilling to cope with the everyday problems of living. Certainly what is a successful adjustment for one individual would be a poor adjustment for someone else, since different people have different goals and aspirations. This problem is magnified when a variety of different cultures are considered, since each culture reinforces different skills and talents. It has been suggested that intelligence is a culture specific ability, but this is not consistent with popular usage.

4. *Intelligence is the ability to carry on abstract thinking.* Terman (1921), the developer of the Stanford-Binet Intelligence Test, defined intelligence in this way. As a result, there are a number of items on his test directly measuring the capacity to think abstractly. Research on the relationship between learning and intelligence shows little relationship between simple learning and IQ, but when the material to be learned is complex or abstract, high IQ subjects perform better than low IQ subjects. Such a definition is not as general as the others mentioned since it limits intelligence to one mental ability rather than attempting to encompass all mental functioning. Recently, Jensen (1970) has proposed two kinds of intelligence, Level I and Level II. Level I refers to basic associative abilities and would be best measured by a test such as digit span (e.g., remembering a phone number) while Level II refers to abstract problem solving, and thus corresponds closely to the capacity for abstract thought.

5. *Global definitions.* A number of people have defined intelligence in very global terms rather than in terms of a specific ability. Two examples follow: "Intelligence is the aggregate or global capacity of the individual to act purposefully, to think rationally, and to deal effectively with his environment" (Wechsler, 1944, p. 3) and "Intelligence is the ability to undertake activities that are characterized by (1) difficulty, (2) complexity, (3) abstractness, (4) economy, (5) adaptiveness to a goal, (6) social value, and (7) the emergence of originals, and to maintain such activities under conditions that demand a concentration of energy and a resistance to emotional forces" (Stoddard, 1943, p. 4).

These definitions represent the best attempt to capture the popular usage of the word. The principal difficulty with them is that many of the terms used are so vague that the definitions have little meaning. It would be extremely difficult to demonstrate that any given intelligence test is actually measuring "the global capacity to act purposefully, to think rationally, and to deal effectively with the environment."

The Current View of Intelligence

In recent years, psychologists have been less interested in defining intelligence, recognizing that developing a definition that can be agreed on by more than a handful of people is probably a fruitless task. Thus it appears that psychologists have gotten themselves into the awkward situation of having a vast literature on the subject of intelligence without any generally accepted idea of what it is. The usual solution to this contradiction is the recognition that intelligence is not a thing, or even a process. The word is appropriate for use as a chapter title, but it does not describe a psychological entity or operation. Since this is the case, intelligence or terms related to it cannot be used as an explanation of behavior. If a teacher asks a psychologist why a particular student isn't learning how to read, the reply "Because the student has low intelligence" explains nothing. Such an answer would only be acceptable if intelligence were a specifiable process, which it is not. Intelligence is only a word describing certain kinds of behaviors, of which not learning how to read is one example. Two other examples may clarify this point. Whenever four-year-old Susy is around strangers, she blushes, refuses to talk, and hides behind her mother. It might be correct to say that she is shy, but this statement does not explain the behavior, it is only labeling it. Bill has refused to get a job since he graduated from high school; he just lives with his parents and does as little housework as possible. The statement that Bill does not like to work because he is lazy makes no sense. Laziness is not an explanation of his behavior, it is merely a label. Intelligence, like laziness and shyness, is not an explanation, it is merely a word used to describe certain patterns of behavior.

This conclusion has some extremely important implications for the study of mental retardation. The label mentally retarded, like the labels shy or lazy, should not be used as an explanation of behavior. It is merely a descriptive term to describe certain kinds of behavior.

Intelligence Testing

One of the most important characteristics of the concept of intelligence is that people differ in it. These differences can at least in theory be measured and quantified; hence the development of the intelligence test. The first modern intelligence test was developed around the turn of the century, and within a few decades these tests became widely used in virtually all school systems in this country, Britain, and many other Western nations. They have been used to place children in appropriate classes in school, they have been used to determine the effectiveness of school curricula and other training programs, they have been used as a screening device for hiring in a wide variety of occupations, and intelligence test scores have been either the dependent or the independent variable in thousands of research projects and experiments. Despite their wide use the basic philosophical questions surrounding intelligence testing are still unanswered. Not only is there little agreement concerning the proper definition of intelligence, but people disagree on just what it is that intelligence tests are measuring, the question of what determines success on these tests, and whether they are measuring one ability or many. In fact, it is somewhat remarkable that intelligence tests have received such widespread use despite our ignorance about what they can in fact be used for.

History of Mental Testing

Although people have been aware of individual differences in mental abilities for thousands of years, and references can be found to this effect in the writings of ancient Greeks and Romans, it was not until the late nineteenth century that the intellectual climate was such that questions regarding the mind, behavior, or intellect of man could be studied rationally or scientifically. Prior to this time, it was assumed that scientific methods, which had proved to be so productive in such fields as physics and chemistry, were inappropriate for the study of human nature because the human mind did not follow natural or scientific laws.

The first attempts to measure what we now call intelligence tested simple sensory functions such as the ability to discriminate weights or the ability to detect a high-pitched whistle or tests of reaction time. These tests were considered failures because not only did these tests correlate poorly with each other (those people who did well on some items did not necessarily do well on others) but there was little relationship between performance on such tests and other supposed measures of intellectual ability such as teacher ratings or success in life. In other words, these early tests were invalid.

A much more successful intelligence test was developed by the French experimental psychologist Binet in 1905. Binet had been commissioned by the Minister of Public Education in Paris to develop a test that would detect at a young age those children who were too dull to benefit from regular schooling. Binet's first attempt, developed with his colleague Simon, was called the Measuring Scale of Intelligence, and it contained 30 items. Their approach to mental testing was very different from earlier attempts since they selected items that measured such functions as memory, comprehension, and vocabulary rather than simple sensory abilities. For example, their 1905 test contained such items as recognition of food (discriminating between a piece of chocolate and a piece of wood), naming pictured objects, repeating three digits, repetition of a 15-word sentence, drawing geometric designs from memory, stating the similarity of common objects, and distinguishing between pairs of abstract words. Unlike earlier attempts to measure mental abilities, Binet's test proved to be a fairly good predictor of later school achievement.

In 1908, Binet and Simon published a revised version of their test with many improvements. The total number of items was increased from 30 to 59. The test was standardized on 203 Paris school children. To standardize a test means to administer it to a large number of children of different ages (modern intelligence tests are standardized on several thousand children) in order to collect norms concerning what the average child of each age will be able to do. The items of the test were grouped by age level as a result of the standardization. An item was said to be at a given age level if two-thirds to three-fourths of the children at that age level were able to pass it. It can be assumed that if an item is at, say, the six-year level, about two-thirds of six year olds will be able to pass it, a somewhat smaller proportion of five year olds will pass it, and a somewhat larger proportion of seven year olds will pass it. Because of the standardization, the revised test was useful not only in discriminating retardates from normals, but also in detecting differences in levels of normal intelligence.

This test was based on the assumption that children increase in intellectual ability as they get older. From this idea comes the concept of mental age. A mental age is synonymous with a given performance on a test. To say that a child has a mental age of seven years means that the child performed as well as the average seven year old in the standardization group. In other words it is a measure of the child's intellectual functioning independent of chronological age. However, to say that a child has a mental age of seven years does not mean that the child passed all of the items up to the seven year level and none above that. The child may have failed items at the five- and six-year levels (items that most five and six year olds pass) and passed items at the eight- and nine-year levels, but got the same total number of items correct as the average seven year old.

Tests based on the Binet model dominated intelligence testing for many years, and there have been numerous translations, imitations, and revisions. The basic idea behind all such tests is to produce a number of items that seem to be measures of intelligence. Then these items are administered to a large number of children of different ages. An item is eliminated if it does not meet several criteria. First, a larger number of older children than younger children should be able to pass it. Second, performance on each item should correlate positively with overall performance on the test; in other words, those who do better on the test should be more likely to get the item correct than those who do poorly. Third, the item ought not to favor one sex over the other. That is, there are some items that males are more likely to pass then females and others on which females do better than males. These items are either eliminated from the test or else systematically counterbalanced so that one sex will not be favored over the other. For this reason, standard intelligence tests are not good instruments for investigating differences in intellectual abilities between the sexes.

Note that there is no real theory of intelligence underlying the test. Binet himself never actually defined intelligence. Items are selected solely on the criterion that they appear to measure the common sense notion of intelligence, vague as it is. An attempt is made to include as wide a variety of different items as possible—from vocabulary to memory, from copying designs to abstract reasoning. There is an implicit assumption that intelligence is a unitary trait, that is, that all of these diverse items are measuring essentially the same thing.

The next major theoretical development was the concept of intelligence quotient or IQ proposed by Stern in 1912 and quickly adopted almost universally. Binet and Simon had suggested that children be labeled retarded if their mental age were more than two years behind their chronological age. Stern pointed out that a two-year lag was much more serious for a 4-year-old than for a 14-year-old, and he proposed that deficiency be determined by a ratio rather than by simply subtracting mental age from chronological age. The formula that he proposed was

$$\text{Intelligence quotient (IQ)} = \frac{\text{mental age (MA)}}{\text{chronological age (CA)}} \times 100$$

For example, a 5-year-old child with a mental age of 5 years would have an IQ of 100. This means that the child is doing as well on the test (and presumably as well on mental development) as the average 5-year-old. Another 5-year-old might achieve a mental age of 6 years on the test, so that child's IQ would be 120. A third 5 year old might have a mental age of only 4 years, so that child's IQ is 80. Thus, an IQ of 100 means that a subject's performance is average for his or her age group. The higher a child's IQ is above 100, the better the child is doing relative to his or her age mates, and similarly the lower a child's IQ is below 100, the worse that child is doing on the test relative to his or her age mates.

Let's assume that three years later these three children are tested again. Normally, all would have improved on the test and so all would have higher mental ages. Our subjects now have a chronological age of 8 years, and so in order for the first one's IQ to remain the same at 100, his or her mental age would now have to be 8 years. The second child, in order to achieve the same IQ of 120, would have to achieve a mental age of 9.6 years. In other words, the second child would have to improve 3.6 years in mental development over a three-year period. Notice that a one-year difference in mental age between two children means a larger difference in IQ at younger ages than at older ages. A one-year difference in mental age at age 5 means a difference of 20 IQ points, but a one-year difference in mental age at 8 years means an IQ difference of only 12½ points.

Thus, an IQ score is a measure of how well an individual is performing on an intelligence test relative to others of the same age. Notice that children's IQs do not normally increase as they get older. To the extent that subjects retain their same relative positions in mental ability during development their IQs will remain the same. If a child's IQ happens to rise during development, this means that he or she has improved relative to his or her peers. In other words, the child has gained more in mental ability than did the average child of the same IQ.

Another way of viewing the IQ is as a measure of the rate of development. Those children who are developing faster have higher IQs. A child whose rate of development is only 80 percent of average would have an IQ of 80. Similarly, an IQ of 120 means that that child has developed 120 percent as fast as average.

There is one difficulty in computing IQ in this manner. In general, a subject's performance on the test, in other words, the mental age, will increase with some regularity until the subject is in the late teens, but after that the increase is much more gradual. Most individuals cannot be expected to do much better on an IQ test at 25 than they did at 20. Thus, it is assumed that the average adult has a mental age of 16 to 18 years. If no correction is made for this in the formula, then the average 32 year old would have an IQ of about 50 ($16/32 \times 100 = 50$). Therefore, in the traditional IQ formula the divisor for anyone older than 16 is 16 (or 18 in some tests).

The Stanford-Binet

The American descendant of the original Binet tests is the 1960 revision of the Stanford-Binet. This revision is based on two earlier tests developed by Terman and Merrill at Stanford. The test has a total of 120 items, 6 at each half-year level from ages two to five, and 6 at each year level after age five up through several adult levels. Thus, passing each item below the 5-year level adds one month to mental age, and passing each item above the 5-year level adds two months to mental age. The test is similar in many ways to the original tests developed by Binet, and, in fact, many of the items are identical to or similar to Binet's original questions. Some of the items at the 3-year level include stringing beads, naming pictures of everyday objects, and copying a circle. Examples of items at the 6-year level include defining everyday words, telling the difference between such things as a car and a boat,[1] saying what is missing from a picture, and tracing mazes. Items at the 9-year level include verbal absurdities (A man had two heart attacks; he died from the first one but fully recovered from the second. What's foolish about that?), copying a geometric design from memory, several problems involving making change, and repeating four digits reversed. The 12-year items include defining abstract words such as pity, repeating five digits reversed, and filling in the missing word in sentences such as the following: "The picnic was called off __?__ there had been a heavy rain." Examples of items at the average adult level include explaining the difference between abstract words such as laziness and idleness, giving the meaning of simple proverbs such as "Mighty oaks from little acorns grow," defining abstract words such as generosity, and orientation problems such as "Which direction would you have to face so that your right hand is toward the north?." The test was standardized on more than 4000 children between the ages of 2 and 18 who were selected to reflect the population of the United States.

The Wechsler Tests

Recently, a series of intelligence tests developed by David Wechsler have begun to replace the Stanford-Binet as the most popular individual tests of general intelligence. There are three Wechsler tests currently in use: the Wechsler Preschool and Primary Scale (WPPSI), published in 1967; the Welchsler Intelligence Scale for Children (WISC), revised in 1974; and the Wechsler Adult Intelligence Scale (WAIS) published in 1955. The first is appropriate for children from 4 to 6, the second for children from 6 to 16, and the last is appropriate for adults over 15.

There are two major design differences between the Wechsler Tests and the Stanford-Binet, and both differences are generally regarded as improvements. First, unlike the Stanford-Binet, each of the Wechsler tests is divided into a number of subscales. In addition to an overall measure of intelligence, the Wechsler tests also yield a measure of verbal intelligence, a measure of nonverbal intelligence called performance, and a number of subtest scores. For example, the subtests of the revised WISC are as follows.

Verbal Subtests

1. *Information.* This is a test of general information to which most people in this culture would have been exposed. It is primarily a test of specific

[1] These examples are similar to but not identical to the items on the test. Test publishers do not like to have their test questions published in general textbooks.

learned facts. For example, "How many fingers do you have?" [2] "In what continent is India?" "Where does sugar come from?"

2. *Similarities.* All these questions are of the form "In what way are ______ and ______ alike?" This subtest requires reasoning, judgment, and awareness of relationships. Examples are "In what way are an orange and a pear alike?" or "In what way are a fork and a spoon alike?"
3. *Arithmetic.* This is a test of general arithmetic and mathematical skills, but nothing advanced enough to require a pencil and paper. The items are timed, and bonus points are given for rapid solution of the more difficult ones. The items range from simple counting through multiplication and division problems like "Five boys have a total of 55 pieces of candy, and they divide this candy up equally among them. How many pieces does each boy get?"
4. *Vocabulary.* This test involves defining words. Performance on this test is largely a function of how well subjects can express their ideas, although it is also a measure of their exposure to verbal material.
5. *Comprehension.* This is a test not so much of factual information but of how well the subject understands why things are the way they are. It is very much a test of reasoning power and judgment. Sample questions include "Why do we have judges?" and "Why does the government license airplane pilots?"
6. *Digit Span.* This is a supplementary test, which means that administering it is optional and a full-scale IQ can be determined without it. It involves reading a list of numbers of progressively longer length that the subject must repeat back. A second part of the test involves repeating a string of digits backwards. The former test is a relatively pure test of short-term memory, while the latter also involves organizational and concentration powers.

Performance Tests

1. *Picture Completion.* This subtest involves showing the subject a series of pictures, each with a part missing, and the subject must indicate which part is missing. Examples are a dog with a leg missing and a bicycle with no seat.
2. *Picture Arrangement.* This subtest consists of a series of sets of pictures. In each set, the pictures can be put together to make a story, and the subject must put them in the correct order. This is a test of visual com-

[2] As with the Stanford-Binet, these items are similar to but not identical to the items on the test.

prehension skills and requires the ability to pick out essential cues from irrelevant ones.

3. *Block Design.* The subject is given nine blocks, each with red, white, and red and white sides. The subject must copy certain designs with the blocks within a specified time. This is a good test of nonverbal spatial abilities.

4. *Object Assembly.* A disassembled object is presented to the subject and he must put the pieces together. This is a timed test.

5. *Coding.* This is a timed test in which the subject must write a coded symbol for each of a long series of numbers. It does not require any real reasoning power since the code is right in front of the subject, but it is a test of short-term associate memory and manual dexterity.

6. *Mazes.* This is a supplementary test that involves having the subject trace mazes of varying complexity. It tests impulsiveness, forethought, and general spatial relations as well as manual dexterity.

The second difference between the Wechsler Scales and the Stanford-Binet is that the former does not use the concept of mental age. Raw scores on the test are converted directly into IQ scores. Since mental age is not used, the Wechsler IQ is computed somewhat differently from the ratio formula, and in a sense, IQ is a misnomer since the Wechsler IQ is not a quotient. However, even though IQs are computed differently for the two tests, they can be interpreted in much the same way, and, in fact, most people will achieve similar IQs regardless of which method is used to determine it. The Wechsler IQ is called a deviation IQ and is based on the assumption that intelligence is normally distributed; this means that the distribution of intelligence test scores will form the familiar bell shaped curve shown in Figure 2-1. This means that there are more people with an IQ on the average (arbitrarily designated to be 100) than any other single score. There are relatively more people with IQs close to the average than there are with IQs far away; for example, there are more people with an IQ of 105 or 93 than there are people with IQs of 115 or 80. The unit of variance or deviation from an average is called the standard deviation. The closer most scores are to the average, the smaller the standard deviation will be. For example, suppose a large number of people are timed in running 100 yards and in running a half mile. The times for the running of the 100 yards will all be relatively close to each other. The times for the fastest and the slowest runners would only differ by a few seconds. Thus, the scores have a relatively small standard deviation. The times for the half mile would be far more scattered; the difference between the times of the fastest and slowest runners might be as

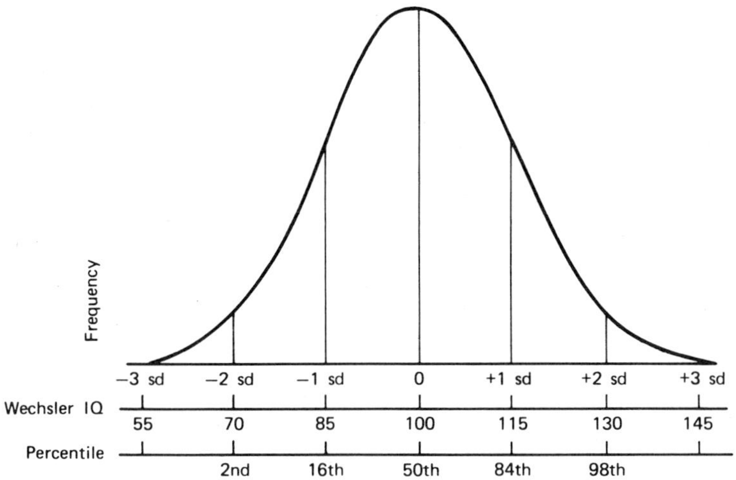

Figure 2-1 The theoretical distribution of intelligence.

much as a minute. These times would have a relatively larger standard deviation because most of the scores are farther from the average.

When IQs are calculated by the formula MA/CA × 100, the standard deviation of IQ tends to be smaller at younger age groups than for older children and adults. A disadvantage of this variable standard deviation is that the same IQ represents different percentiles at different ages. A percentile indicates the percentage of scores that were below a given score. If an individual scores at the 85th percentile on a test, this means that 85 percent of those people who took the test scored below him. Notice that a percentile has nothing to do with the total number of correct answers. A score at the 85th percentile does not mean that the individual got 85 percent of the items correct.

When Wechsler developed his tests, he wanted the same IQ to have the same meaning regardless of age; in other words, he wanted a given IQ to represent the same percentile at each age. He accomplished this by arbitrarily designating the standard deviation of IQ to be 15 for all age groups. Statistics tell us that if a variable is normally distributed, then 34 percent of the population will fall between the average and one standard deviation below the average. Another 34 percent will fall between the average and one standard deviation above the average. Thus, 34 percent of any age group has an IQ between 100 and 115. Similarly, 34 percent of a given age group has an IQ between 85 and 100. Fourteen percent of a set of normally distributed scores lie between one and two standard deviations from the average. Thus, in theory, 14 percent of an age group has IQs between 115 and 130, 14 percent have IQs between 70 and 85, and thus, 96 percent of a population has IQs between 70 and 130 with 2 percent being above 130 and 2 percent being below 70.

An example of how IQs are actually determined will clarify this method. The WAIS (or any other intelligence test) is standardized by administering it to a large number of individuals selected to represent the general population. The WAIS was administered to a total of 1700 people to standardize it—200 between the ages of 16 and 17, 200 between the ages of 18 and 19, 200 between the ages of 20 and 24, and so on. Consider the age group 20 to 24. Of these 200 people, the median scaled score (a modification of the raw score to insure that all 11 subtests will be equally weighted) for the entire test was 94. Thus, for this age group, a scaled score of 94 is designated to represent an IQ of 100. The standard deviation of the scaled scores for this age group was computed to be 9. Because the standard deviation of IQ scores is arbitrarily designated to be 15, this means that a score of 103 (94 + 9) is assigned the IQ of 115. Similarly, if a subject achieves a scaled score of 85 (94 − 9), he or she would be assigned the IQ of 85 (the fact that the scaled score and the IQ are the same is just a coincidence). In similar fashion, each scaled score can be assigned an IQ.

However, for the age group 35 to 44, the average scaled score of the standardization group was 106 with a standard deviation of 25. Notice that the average is somewhat higher, and the standard deviation is considerably larger. The larger standard deviation means that the scores were not as closely bunched as they were in the younger group. This means that a person in this age group would have to achieve a scaled score of 131 in order to receive an IQ of 115. In each age group, an IQ of 115 means that a person is in approximately the 84th percentile relative to others of similar age, but in the younger group an IQ of 115 meant a scaled score of 103 while in the older age group an IQ of 115 meant a scaled score of 131. Virtually all modern intelligence tests now compute IQs using deviation score methods as described above. The latest edition of the Stanford-Binet includes tables for converting MA scores to deviation IQ scores, but in this case the standard deviation of the IQ scores is 16 rather than 15. The main advantage of this method is the fact that a given IQ can be easily translated to a percentile score regardless of the age of the subject.

Specialized Intelligence Tests

The Stanford-Binet and the Wechsler tests are by far the most widely used individual tests of intelligence, but there are many people for whom these tests will not produce a valid score for reasons such as low mental age or any one of a number of sensory or motor handicaps. As a result, other intelligence tests have been developed to measure the intellectual capabilities of specialized populations.

A number of people have attempted to devise tests to measure the intelligence of young infants. The Stanford-Binet is only appropriate for individuals functioning at the two-year level or above, and occasionally there is a need to assess the abilities of a younger or less capable child. Such tests are frequently used with the mentally retarded. One of the best tests of this type is the Bayley Scales of Infant Development (1969). This is actually three different tests designed to assess the development of infants from birth to 30 months. The first test is a mental scale that measures sensory and perceptual abilities, discriminations, language development, problem-solving abilities, and learning skills. Typical items include following a light with the eyes, picking up blocks, playing appropriately with various toys such as a bell or toy car, placing forms in formboards, and various kinds of expressive and receptive vocabulary items. The second test is a motor scale designed to assess gross motor development using such items as turning the head from one side to the other, rolling over, sitting and standing without help, standing on one foot, and hopping. Each of these tests produces a separate score; the mental scale yields a mental development quotient that corresponds closely to a deviation IQ, and the motor test yields a psychomotor development quotient. The correlation between the two varies between .5 and.6 depending on age. The third test is a personality test assessing emotional development. It does not produce an overall score but yields a description of the child's personality.

There are a number of other tests of infant intelligence which, although they were developed many years ago, are still occasionally used. Psyche Cattell (1947) developed a downward extension of the 1937 Stanford-Binet called the Cattell Infant Intelligence Scale. It has items grouped by age level and is similar to the mental scale of the Bayley. Tests such as the Merrill-Palmer and Arthur Point Scale involve fewer verbal items and are thus occasionally still used for nonverbal subjects, although they are considered obsolete for most purposes. The difficulty with all of the infant mental ability tests is that they correlate poorly with ability at older ages. They do not do a very good job of predicting future performance, and as a result, they have been accused of measuring a different kind of ability than do other intelligence tests.

One scale that is widely used to screen for mental retardation is the Denver Developmental Screening Test (Frankenburg and Dodds, 1967). This is not exactly an intelligence test, but it consists of 105 items that assess a preschooler's general developmental progress. These items are divided into four areas: gross motor, language, fine-motor adaptive, and personal-social. Examples of gross motor items include rolls over, walks holding onto furniture, kicks ball, pedals a trike, and hops on one foot. Examples of language items include imitates speech sounds, combines two different words, uses prepositions, recognizes colors, and defines words. Examples of fine-motor and adaptive items include grasps a rattle, scribbles spontaneously, builds a block tower, and copies a square. Examples of personal-social items include plays peek-a-boo or pat-a-cake, uses a spoon, washes and dries hands, and buttons.

A number of tests have been developed to measure the intelligence of people with various kinds of handicaps. Obviously, if a person is blind or deaf or has severe motor problems, the Stanford-Binet or the Wechsler Tests will not accurately assess his or her mental abilities. Hayes has developed a test to measure the intelligence of visually impaired people. The test is made up basically of all of the purely verbal items from the 1937 Stanford-Binet. A test developed by Leiter is entirely nonverbal, requiring no verbal instructions from the examiner and no verbal responses from the person being tested. It is useful for assessing the mental capabilities of the hearing impaired, and is also frequently used for testing others with verbal handicaps or those whose native language is different from that of the examiner.

Another specialized test is the Peabody Picture Vocabulary Test (PPVT) (Dunn, 1959). This test measures only one ability—recognition vocabulary. The tester says a word and shows four pictures to the person being tested. The subject must indicate which of the four pictures best depicts the word. Items are arranged in order of difficulty to reflect mental ages of less than two years up to superior adult. Although this test only measures vocabulary, it is often used as a test of general intelligence. This practice is justified by the fact that on both the Stanford-Binet and the Wechsler Scales, vocabulary items correlate more highly with overall scores than do any other kinds of items. Also, scores on the PPVT generally correlate very well with broader measures of general intelligence. It has two advantages. First, administration of the test is very quick and very simple. Untrained people can be taught to use it in a short time, and administration usually takes about half as long as the Stanford-Binet. Second, because the only response necessary is pointing, the test can be used with individuals with severe speech defects or motor problems for whom conventional tests are useless. However, because of the limited range of abilities sampled, an IQ determined solely by the PPVT must be considered with caution, and some other test ought to be administered if at all possible.

All of the tests described above are individual intelligence tests; that is, they are administered to one person at a time, usually by a highly trained psychological tester. However, the only intelligence tests that most people are familiar with are group (paper and pencil) tests, tests that can be administered to a large number of people at once by a relatively untrained person. Most school systems obtain IQs on their children with such tests, and literally millions are given each year. Some of the more common tests of aptitude and achievement for school children include the California Test of Mental Maturity, the Kuhlmann-Anderson Measure of Academic Potential, and the Otis-Lennon Mental Ability Test. Also included in this category are college board tests such as the Scholastic Aptitude Tests and the Graduate Record Exams, although these have the specific goal of measuring academic aptitude and make no attempt to produce an IQ score. Paper-and-pencil tests correlate very well with individual intelligence tests for normal people who have had adequate schooling, but this excludes many people for whom mental retardation is suspected, and as a result, such tests are not widely used to diagnose retardation.

There is considerable concern that tests such as the Stanford-Binet and the Wechsler Scales are culturally biased because many of the questions are about objects and events that are found in white middle-class American culture. Children reared in other cultures or subcultures may not be familiar with this content and thus would do poorly on the test. This issue will be discussed in some detail in a later chapter. As a result of this controversy, a number of so-called culture-free tests of intelligence have been developed. These are tests in which there is no content that is specific to a particular culture. The best known of these is the Raven's Progressive Matrices. All of the items of this test are of the same form. A matrix is shown, with one item missing, and the subject must indicate what the missing item should be. Verbal instructions are minimized and none of the items uses any content from the real world. They all use abstract designs so that previous experience should not be important. Figure 2-2 shows an example of such an item. Another such test is the Cattell Culture Fair Intelligence Test. Both of these test the general ability to perceive relationships rather than specific knowledge. Another type of culture free test is the Porteus Mazes, which consists entirely of a series of mazes of varying degrees of difficulty. It supposedly measures planning and foresight. The Goodenough-Harris Drawing Test is popularly called the Draw-a-man Test because subjects are asked to draw the best man and woman that they can. The pictures are scored according to specific criteria, and a general measure of intellectual development can be obtained.

This list of intelligence tests is by no means complete. Many new measures of ability and aptitude are published each year, and the number of mental abilities tests currently on the market numbers in the hundreds. Many are quite specialized and are used primarily by industrial psychologists or personnel officers to measure specific aptitudes. The tests described in this chapter are the ones most frequently used in work with the mentally retarded.

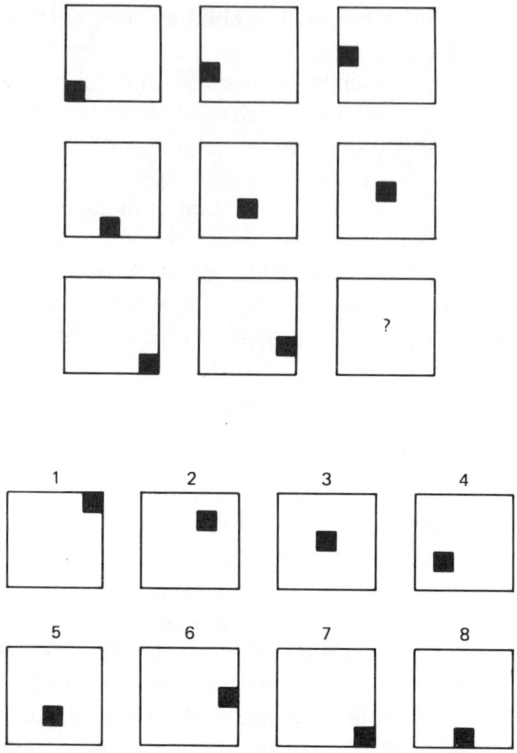

Figure 2-2 A sample problem from the Raven matrices.

Research on Intelligence Tests

The intelligence testing movement has generated an enormous body of research, far too vast even to be summarized here, but there are certain areas of research that require discussion because they have direct bearing on the fundamental nature of intelligence and thus have implications for the understanding of mental retardation.

Reliability, Validity, and Correlates of Intelligence Tests

There are two important criteria on which a test is evaluated: reliability and validity. Reliability refers to the stability of the scores. A test is reliable if the same individual receives about the same score if he or she takes the same test several times, takes alternate forms of the same test, or is tested by several different people. Obviously, if different testings produce widely different results, the scores are not very meaningful. The validity of a test refers to how well the test measures what it is supposed to measure. If a psychological test is designed to measure extroversion, then the test is valid to the extent that those people who are the most extroverted get the highest scores on the test. It is possible for a test to be reliable without being valid. For example, if a researcher decided to measure intelligence by measuring the diameter of a person's head, this test would presumably be reliable but not valid. Repeated testings would probably produce about the same scores, and several different people each measuring the same person would presumably arrive at the same result. However, skull size is not related to mental abilities within the normal range. Those people with large heads do not have any tendency to be any better in mental abilities or to do better academically than do people with small skulls. Thus, the test is not valid; it does not measure what it is supposed to measure. An example of a test with relatively low reliability is the Rorschach inkblot test in which people are asked to describe what they see in a series of inkblots. Quite frequently, the same person tested several times will produce different results, and different people may arrive at different interpretations of psychological dynamics using the same test with the same individual (McArthur, 1972).

The reliability of most intelligence tests is not usually seriously challenged. There is general agreement that repeated testings of the same individual will result in about the same IQ score as long as the interval between testing sessions is not too great. Specific reliability data are available in the manuals of each different test. It is also usually the case that different testers will arrive at about the same IQ scores for a given individual, although there is often some discrepancy (Schwarz and Flanigan, 1971). However, it should never be assumed that a given IQ score represents a precise measurement. There is always a certain amount of error in any test score, and a given IQ should probably be thought of as representing a range of about four IQ points in each direction. If someone achieves an IQ of 85 on a given test, his or her real IQ (as determined by a large number of testings under identical circumstances) might lie anywhere between 81 and 89. The specific range, called the standard error of measurement, differs slightly from test to test and for different age groups.

The validity of an intelligence test is far more difficult to measure, and most criticisms of intelligence tests center around their validity rather than their reliability. Even since the first crude attempts to measure mental abilities with tests of sensory acuity and reaction time, people have tried to demonstrate that intelligence tests do in fact measure intelligence. The early tests were considered failures precisely because they were not valid; they did not correlate with other measures of ability such as school performance or eminence. The Binet type tests were more successful because there was some evidence that they were measuring something similar to intelligence. Those children rated highest in ability by teachers and those children who achieved the best grades in school tended to do the best on this type of intelligence test.

It is logically impossible to demonstrate that an intelligence test is measuring intelligence unless one has an objective definition of intelligence, and, as we have seen, this is not the case. As a result, attempts to validate intelligence tests have had to resort to more indirect methods. The most common way to demonstrate that intelligence tests are measuring intelligence is to correlate them with school performance. There have been numerous such studies comparing intelligence test performance with various indicators of school success, and the results are remarkably consistent; intelligence test performance and school success as measured by achievement test performance, grades, or number of years of school completed, correlated between .50 and .60. For example, Dillon (1949) obtained IQ scores on 2600 seventh grades and then followed them through high school graduation. It was clear that IQ in seventh grade was a good predictor of how long a student would remain in school. Of those with an IQ of greater than 115 in seventh grade, 86 percent eventually graduated while of those with an IQ between 85 and 94, only 54 percent graduated.

However, the correlation, while high, is by no means perfect, which means that other factors besides mental ability are important in school success. Not surprisingly, there is a slightly higher relationship between IQ and achievement than there is between IQ and grades. This is presumably because teachers tend to take into account factors such as motivation and cooperation in assigning grades. Similarly, there seems to be more people who do well on intelligence tests and poorly in school than the reverse. There are more underachievers than overachievers (Herrnstein, 1973). This makes sense because it is difficult to imagine an individual who is doing much better than his or her intellectual potential will allow, but everyone is familiar with students who have high potential but who don't work very hard and as a result, do poorly in school. In fact, a major clinical use of intelligence tests is discriminating the underachiever from the student with little potential.

Other attempts to validate intelligence tests have tried to correlate IQ with success in life. To the extent that intelligence is a measure of adaptability, there ought to be a high correlation, but, in general, the relationship is not nearly as high as is the correlation between IQ and academic success. Some writers, such as Herrnstein (1973) argue that there is a fairly direct relationship; that is, people with high intelligence are far more likely to be successful as defined by income or being in a high status occupation than are people of low intelligence. To support this argument he cites a number of studies showing a positive correlation between intelligence and social status.

For example, Stewart (1947) investigated the occupations of more than 67,000 men who had taken the Army General Classification Test (an intelligence test used by military induction centers) during World War II. She discovered that the median intelligence level of people in some occupations was considerably higher than in others. For example, the median accountant had an IQ of 129, the median lawyer had an IQ of 124, and the median reporter had an IQ of 119, while the median painter had an IQ of 97, the median barber had an IQ of 93, and the median lumberjack had an IQ of 87. In general, those professions with higher average IQs tend to be the higher status occupations, and people in them tend to make more money. However, the relationship between intelligence and profession is oversimplified by such statistics. There is a wide range of IQs for nearly all of the professions listed, particularly the lower ones. What this means is that there are many people with well above average IQs in the lower income, lower status professions, and there are a few people with below average intelligence in the higher status professions.

Christopher Jencks and his associates (Jencks et al., 1972) have done an extensive study of the sources of various kinds of inequality in America; that is, inequality in income, inequality in status, inequality in education, inequality in intelligence, and so on, and they come to some interesting conclusions that somewhat contradict those of Herrnstein. For example, in regard to inequality in income, Jencks concludes that the most intelligent fifth of men in this country have incomes 35 to 40 percent higher than the least intelligent fifth, certainly a significant difference. "But in a society where the best paid fifth of all men earn 600 percent more than the worst paid fifth, disparities of this magnitude are not very significant," and even this relationship is confounded by other factors. There is no question that people with higher intelligence tend to get more education and there is a high relationship between amount of education and later income. Employers are much more likely to hire a more educated worker than a less educated worker even though there is little evidence that the more educated workers will be more productive. There is some evidence that more intelligent people make more money than less intelligent people in the same occupations, but again the relationship is not clear. In other words, Jencks concludes that IQ by itself plays a small role in how much money a person makes, although in conjunction with education, it is somewhat more significant. This conclusion suggests that IQ tests are measuring only a narrow range of possible abilities. These abilities are important in academic situations, but are far less critical once a person gets out of school. It is not very important for most of the population to be able to use esoteric words correctly or solve algebraic equations or understand complex analogies once they leave school, and most of the skills that are necessary for normal living are either learned by almost everyone or else are not correlated with intelligence. This conclusion has important implications for the study of mental retardation. There are numerous individuals, such as the case of Mary described in Chapter 1, who do badly in school and are labeled retarded for that reason, but once they leave school they are able to lead a relatively normal life.

The Stability of IQ

An implicit assumption that is usually made about IQ is that it is a relatively stable trait. If most people's IQs fluctuated considerably from year to year, it would not be a very useful measure. It is important to keep in mind that a stable IQ does not mean that individuals are doing equally well on the test from year to year; nearly all people will improve their performance on intelligence tests as they get older. A stable IQ means that individuals keep their relative place compared to their age mates as they grow older; that is, those who do best on the test when they are four also do better on the test when they are eight, even though all have improved. There has been a good deal of research investigating this assumption. The results have been interpreted in two ways; some people have concluded that research supports the concept of stable intelligence while others argue that research indicates that IQs are not very stable at all. Some of the best evidence bearing on this issue was collected by Bayley (1949) in a research project known as the Berkeley Growth Study. This study followed some 61 children from birth to 18 years old, administering intelligence tests to them at frequent intervals. Such a research design in which the same subjects are tested at several different ages is known as a longitudinal study. Figure 2-3 shows the correlation of IQ at various ages with IQ at age 18. It can be seen from this graph that a child's performance on an intelligence test before age 2 is not a good predictor of adult intelligence. Many nervous parents note carefully the age at which their child first sits up, takes the first step, and says the first word, presumably because children who develop faster in these abilities will be more intelligent later. This is not the case. There is essentially no relationship between the rate at which the child reaches various motor milestones and later intelligence. Children who turn out to be very intelligent do not walk at a younger age than do children of average or even below average intelligence. Intelligence tests do not begin to predict adult performance accurately until the child is about two years old. In fact, close scrutiny of tests used to measure the intelligence of young babies has not produced any individual items that correlate significantly with adult intelligence, although there is some evidence that girls who vocalize more as infants grow up to have higher IQs. Because of the lack of relationship between infant mental development and later mental capacities, it has been argued that the

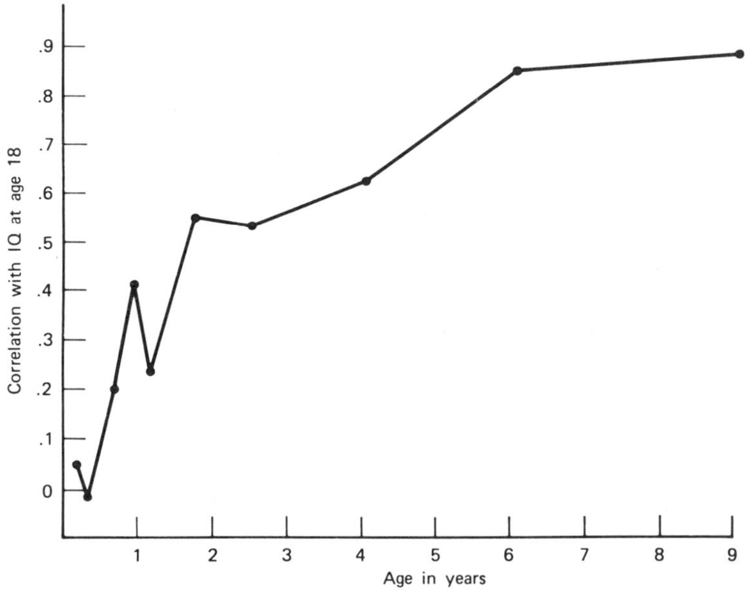

Figure 2-3 Correlation of IQ at various ages with IQ at 18. Adapted from Bayley, 1949.

process of intelligence does not begin to manifest itself until the child is 18 months to two years old. Perhaps not coincidently, this is the same age at which the child is beginning to acquire the rules of language and demonstrate primitive symbolic thought.

However, after the age of 2, IQ becomes increasingly more stable. The Berkeley Growth Study indicates that the correlation between IQ at age 8 and IQ at age 18 is an extremely high .84, suggesting that intelligence is a reasonably stable trait from school age on. However, other research suggests different conclusions. Honzik, Macfarlane, and Allen (1948) in a longitudinal study similar to the Berkeley Growth Study, found that the general shape of the graph of correlations was similar to that of Bayley described above, although somewhat lower. More importantly, however, they also examined how much individual children varied in their IQ as they developed. Because preschool IQs are unstable and do not predict adult performance very well, they only considered the stability of IQs from age 6 to 18. Table 2-1 shows the percentage of subjects whose IQ changed by various amounts during the school years. It can be seen from this table that 85 percent of the children showed IQ fluctuations of at least 10 points, and that more than a third fluctuated more than 20 points, a considerable change. A variety of different patterns were observed. Some children consis-

Table 2-1 Changes in IQ with Development

IQ Changes between 6 and 18 Years	Percent of Total ($n = 222$) (%)
50 or more IQ points	.5
30 or more IQ points	9
20 or more IQ points	35
15 or more IQ points	58
10 or more IQ points	85
9 or less IQ points	15

From M. P. Honzik, J. W. MacFarlane, & L. Allen, The stability of mental test performance between two and eighteen years, *Journal of Experimental Education,* 1948, **17,** 309–324. Copyright © 1948 by the Helen Dwight Reid Educational Foundation. Reprinted by permission of the foundation.

tently increased in IQ, others consistently decreased in IQ, while still others were highly inconsistent and variable. Many of these fluctuations could be attributed to environmental stresses such as illness, family discord, and the like, and thus, the instability may be exaggerated. The general trend of the change was in the direction of parental abilities, that is, as the children grew older, they became more like their parents in terms of mental ability.

The general conclusion of such longitudinal studies is that a person's IQ is likely to show some fluctuation either up or down as he or she grows older, but, for most people, the fluctuations will not be large. Whether one wishes to argue that IQ is a stable or unstable trait is, to some extent, a moot point.

This conclusion has some implications for mental retardation. Mental retardation is usually conceived of as a permanent condition. However, because mental abilities as measured by IQ tests can fluctuate, this means that a person who is considered mentally retarded at one point may not be considered retarded later on, particularly if the mental retardation was only mild. In other words, mental retardation might sometimes be a temporary condition.

The Heredity Environment Issue and Intelligence

One of the implicit characteristics of the popular concept of intelligence is that it is essentially fixed by heredity. During the early part of this century this idea was generally accepted, and the first intelligence tests in this country were assumed to be measuring native ability rather than acquired skills. Beginning in the 1930s, there was a gradual shift toward the belief that an individual's IQ level was largely a product of the environment rather than genes, and this is the more widely accepted viewpoint today. However, recent articles by Jensen (1969) and Herrnstein (1971, 1973) advocating a more important role for heredity in the determination of intelligence have resparked the controversy.

The question of the importance of heredity in the determination of intelligence is often misunderstood, although it has some very important implications for the understanding of some forms of mental retardation. It is important to remember that genes do not cause intelligence directly. A given individual's level of intelligence is always a product of a unique genetic potential interacting with a unique environment. It is possible for anyone, regardless of genes, to be mentally retarded if the environment is not auspicious, for example, if the individual were locked in a closet for much of his or her childhood. Similarly, it makes no sense to say that a certain percentage of someone's intelligence is determined by genes. An analogy can be drawn with the height of a plant. The height of a given plant is a result of the particular gene type of the seed, the quality of the soil, the amount of rain, and numerous other factors. If a given plant grows to be four feet tall, it makes no sense to say that it achieved this height because of the seed variety. It is equally nonsensical to say that 80 percent of the height was due to the genes.

However, it is reasonable to discuss the heritability of a given trait. Heritability is the percentage of differences between members of a population that can be attributed to differences in genes. Heritability only applies to a given population at a given point in time, and cannot be applied to individuals within that population. One extreme of heritability is that everyone is conceived with the identical potential for developing intelligence, and that all differences in mental abilities are due to the environment of the child. This would be a case of extremely low heritability. On the other hand, some traits, such as blood type, have a heritability of close to 100 percent; that is, virtually all of the differences in the trait can be attributed to differences in genotype.

Our plant analogy is again useful. Suppose a farmer plants a number of fields with the identical variety of seed, but some fields have good soil, and others have poor soil. The plants in the good fields grow considerably taller than the plants in the poor fields. However, the heritability of height in this population is near zero, since virtually all of the differences in height between plants are due to environmental conditions. Another farmer plants several different varieties of plants in fields that are virtually identical with respect to soil conditions, amount of rain, sunlight, and so on. The farmer observes that some varieties grow taller than others. Most of the differences in height are due to genetic differences, and, thus, height in this population has a high heritability. Notice that in neither case does it make sense to say that the height of a given plant is caused by the seed variety or the environmental conditions, even though the heritability is very high in one case and very low in another. Notice also that heritability may differ from one population to another with respect to the same trait.

The same thing is true of the heritability of intelligence. In a community in which all of the children are reared under virtually identical conditions, such as an Israeli kibbutz where all of the children are collectively raised, most differences in intellectual abilities would be attributed to differences in the heredity of the children, and thus the heritability of intelligence for this population would be high. Heritability would necessarily be somewhat lower in communities where there are a wide variety of child-rearing approaches and diverse environmental conditions, as in the United States.

Mental abilities are undoubtedly determined by a great many different kinds of genes, and, thus, a simple model of the inheritance of intelligence through a small number of dominant and recessive genes is inadequate. However, it is possible to estimate the heritability of intelligence test scores in a given population by examining the correlations in test scores between individuals of various kinships. Because of the theoretical importance of this type of research, a great deal of data has been collected, and the results are quite reliable. Table 2-2 shows the results of a number of such studies.

If heritability is high, the more genes two individuals have in common, the more similar in intellectual abilities they ought to be. In other words, siblings, who have half of their genes in common, ought to be more similar in mental

Table 2-2 Correlation Coefficients for Intelligence Test Scores between Varying Degrees of Relationship

Relationship	Median Correlation	Number of Studies
Unrelated persons reared apart	0	4
Unrelated persons reared together	.23	5
Parent-child	.50	12
Siblings	.49	35
Fraternal twins (Same sex)	.53	11
Identical twins reared apart	.75	4
Identical twins reared together	.87	14

Adapted from Erlenmeyer-Kimling & Jarvik, 1963.

abilities than are first cousins, who themselves ought to be more similar than second cousins. However, simply looking at the correlations in IQ scores between brothers and sisters is not useful in resolving the heredity environment controversy since they ordinarily share a very similar environment also. There are three types of comparisons in which heredity and environment are not confounded, and these are the most informative regarding heritability. The first of these is comparing fraternal twins to identical twins. Fraternal twins result from two separate ova being fertilized at the same time, and they have half their genes in common, just as siblings do. Identical twins result from one fertilized ovum splitting to produce two children, and they have all of their genes in common. However, there is little reason to assume that the environments of identical twins are more similar than the environments of fraternal twins. If the heritability of intelligence is low, the correlation of IQ between identical twins would not be much higher than for fraternal twins, but it can be seen from Table 2-2 that this is not the case. The correlation for identical twins is about .87 while it is about .53 for same-sexed fraternal twins, a large difference.

A second comparison is between identical twins reared apart versus identical twins reared in the same household. The phenomenon of identical twins being raised in separate homes would only result from unusual tragedies such as the death of the mother, and thus it is quite rare, but it is of such theoretical importance that several researchers have tracked down enough cases to gather reliable data. If the prime determinant of mental abilities was the environment, the correlation between identical twins reared apart ought to be relatively low because even though their genes are identical, their upbringing was different. However, it can be seen that the correlation coefficient is .75, lower than that for identical twins reared together, but still higher than any other degree of relationship.

The third important comparison is between adopted children, children reared in the same home but who are not biologically related. These are children with environments in common but no genes in common. This correlation is a relatively low .24, again suggesting that the heritability of intelligence is quite high.

Findings such as these are disconcerting to those who emphasize environmental determinants of differences in intelligence test scores because they indicate quite strongly that differences in environment do not seem to account for much of the differences in test scores. It is hard for an environmentalist to explain why identical twins who are reared in different environments, perhaps not even seeing each other, should be quite similar in their performance on intelligence tests while children reared in the same home who are unrelated should be so dissimilar. As a result of such data, Jensen (1969) and others have estimated the heritability of IQ in the United States to be about .81, meaning that 81 percent of the observed differences in intelligence between people can be attributed to differences in genetic factors.

This estimate has been widely challenged as being a gross misrepresentation of the truth. For example, Jencks et al. (1972) estimate the heritability of intelligence to be about half of Jensen's estimate. Even more important, however, the concept of heritability has been almost universally misinterpreted. It does not mean that an individual's level of intelligence is determined mostly by his genes. Moreover, it says nothing about the extent to which intelligence test scores can be altered by experience. There is evidence from a number of different sources that a child's experiences can have drastic effects on his later IQ. For example, the average intelligence of the American population has risen during the twentieth century. When the mental test that was administered to recruits during World War I was given to World War II soldiers, 85 percent of the latter scored above the World War I average, and there was certainly no significant changes in the U.S. gene pool during that time. Lee (1951) has shown that the IQ test scores of Negro children increased when they migrated from the South to Philadelphia, and the only possible explanation of this increase is the improved environmental circumstances of the North over the way that blacks were treated in the South at that time. The classic research demonstrating the importance of a stifling environment in lowering IQ was done by Skeels (1966). In the 1930s, he observed that a number of physically normal children who had been placed in a minimally stimulating orphanage were developing very slowly. These children received routine physical care but little attention from adults. However, when a number of them were removed from this environment and placed on a ward with mildly retarded girls who were able to give them almost constant attention, their rate of development improved dramatically. Thirteen such children were removed from the unstimulating orphanage, and almost all were eventually placed in foster homes. A comparison group of 12 children remained in the orphanage. In adulthood, the subjects who had been removed from the orphanage were all of essentially normal intelligence and living independently. They were engaged in occupations such as nursing instructor, real estate sales, and vocational counselor. Virtually none of the control group was living independently. Four of the twelve were institutionalized, and most had IQs in the mentally retarded range.

In conclusion, it is almost certainly the case that one's level of intelligence or IQ is affected by his genes. In other words, some peple are born with more potential for high intelligence than others. However, one's life experiences are important determinants of IQ also, and almost any child's level of functioning can be either raised or lowered considerably by differing environmental circumstances. A more detailed discussion of the kinds of environments that seem to be conducive to high (or low) intellectual functioning will be provided in a later chapter.

Single Trait Versus Multitrait Theories of Intelligence

One of the most important issues related to the study of intelligence is whether it is more profitable to conceive of it as a single trait, or whether intelligence is better conceptualized as a number of semiindependent abilities. The various Binet tests implicitly describe intelligence as a unitary ability. The Stanford-Binet test yields only a single IQ score, which is supposedly a measure of this single factor. No attempt is made to break this single score down into various subscores representing different abilities. Even though only a single ability is being measured, a vast multitude of different kinds of questions appear on the test, everything from drawing geometric figures to defining words, from repeating a span of digits to saying why various things are similar. It is possible to justify this approach because even though the various questions appear to be very different, they all correlate with each other; that is, subjects who do better at drawing geometric figures also do better at defining words and seem to have better memories for digits. Other IQ tests show a similar effect. Each of the 11 subtests of the WAIS correlates at least to a moderate degree with each of the others. Such seemingly different subtests as digit symbol and vocabulary have a correlation of .60 between them among young adults (Wechsler, 1955). On most intelligence tests, even though the items selected appear to be very different, those who perform well on some types of questions generally do well on all. Evidence such as this has led a number of people to propose a general intelligence factor that is an important determinant of all tests of intellectual abilities (e.g., Burt, 1972). This factor is often referred to as "g," a name given to the factor of general intelligence found by Spearman (1927).

The alternative point of view says that a single figure measuring general intelligence is not sufficient, that it is more important to describe individual strengths and weaknesses in various abilities included in general intelligence. The best-known example of this approach is David Wechsler, who develops tests that provide not only an overall IQ score, but also a verbal intelligence score, a performance intelligence score, and scores on 11 different subtests. The advantage of such an approach is obvious. An individual can achieve a given score on a test in many different ways. With rare exception, people do not do equally well on all subtests of the WAIS or WISC. Usually, a subject will do moderately better on some subtests and moderately worse on others, although there are usually not drastic differences between subtests. Thus, the idea behind the Wechsler tests is to provide a profile of these moderate differences in performance.

This issue has been most effectively dealt with by a statistical procedure known as factor analysis. Factor analysis attempts to determine underlying traits or factors through the use of correlations. The assumption is that if two or more subtests are determined by the same factor, they will correlate positively with each other. A discussion of factor analysis is beyond the scope of this book; it is sufficient to say that it is a useful technique for determining the underlying structure of a large body of data.

Unfortunately, for various reasons, different attempts to analyze the factor structure of intelligence have produced widely variant results. For example, the originator of factor analytic techniques, Charles Spearman, concluded from his research that there was a single predominant factor underlying mental abilities, which he labeled g, for general intellectual ability. One does not necessarily have to equate g with intelligence, but most people have.

The best known factor structure of intelligence is that of Thurstone (1946). His factor analysis produced no general factor, instead he found eight different underlying intellectual abilities: *space,* the ability to visualize objects spatially; *number,* facility with arithmetic and mathematics; *verbal comprehension,* the ability to deal with verbal concepts and reasoning; *word fluency,* the ability to produce appropriate words; *memory,* the ability to store and retrieve experiences and concepts; *induction,* finding principles; *deduction,* the use of principles in problem solving; and *flexibility and speed of thought.* He developed an intelligence test based on this model called the Primary Mental Abilities Test (PMA), which yielded a separate score for each ability.

The most outspoken exponent of the factor analytic, structural approach today is J. P. Guilford (1967) who has presented a model of the overall structure of intellect based on factor analysis. Guilford emphatically denies that there is any such thing as general intelligence. He argues that intellect is made up of 120 separate abilities, each one of which can be measured independently. The factors result from the interaction of five types of operations, four kinds of content, and six products of intellect. Figure 2-4 demonstrates this model. He and his associates are attempting to develop relatively pure tests of each of these factors (Guilford and Hoefpner, 1971).

Perhaps the ultimate in multiability theories of intelligence is the approach of a group of psychologists known as behaviorists (e.g., Thorne, 1970). Behaviorist theories have had an important impact on the understanding of mental retardation, and they will be discussed extensively in a later chapter. They tend to deny the whole concept of intelligence and even the concept of mental traits, arguing that these concepts are poorly defined and unobservable. Thus, at the very least, the concept of intelligence is irrelevant, and it is likely to be misleading because even though it does not exist, it is used

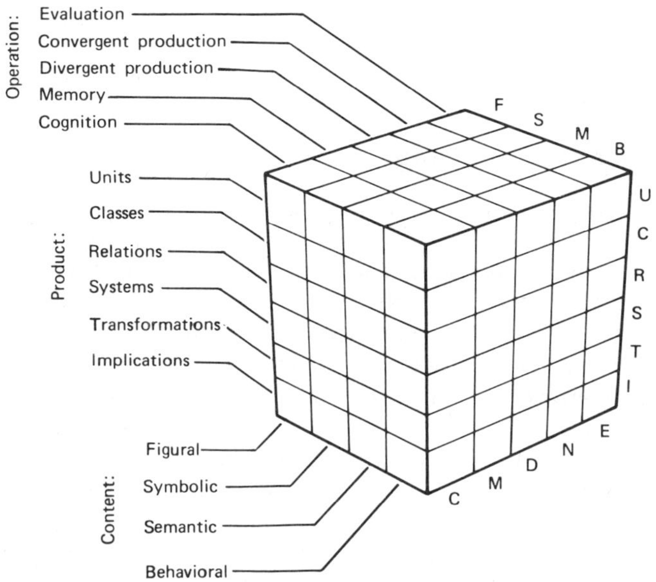

Figure 2-4 Guilford's model of the structure of intellect. From *The nature of human intelligence* by J. P. Guilford. Copyright © 1967 by McGraw-Hill Inc. Used with permission of McGraw-Hill Book Company.

as an explanation of behavior. Behaviorists consider mental abilities or intelligence to be little more than a large number of specific behaviors. Everyone, as a result of past experiences, has learned to make certain responses to certain stimuli, and our total potential at any time is nothing more than the total of these learned responses.

One's opinion on the general question of the unity of intelligence has some important implications for how one thinks about mental retardation. If we think of intelligence as being essentially a unitary ability, then our concept of mental retardation can simply be a deficit in this one ability. However, if we think of intelligence as being made up of a number of independent abilities, then a concept of mental retardation becomes considerably harder to define. The theory of general intelligence is out of favor today. Most people prefer to talk about mental *abilities* rather than a single, general mental *ability*. As a result, the concept of mental retardation has come under considerable fire. The rapid growth of the field of learning disabilities in education is one manifestation of this, as is the popularity of diagnostic tests such as the Wechsler Scales over IQ tests that produce a single score, such as the Stanford-Binet. It is far more important to understand the particular pattern of strengths and weaknesses of a child than it is to know his or her general level of functioning.

Criticisms of Intelligence Testing

Intelligence tests have had their critics right from the start, but in recent years the use of intelligence tests and the whole concept of intelligence have come under unusually vigorous attack. The principal argument against the tests is that they discriminate against those individuals who are outside the mainstream of American culture, particularly blacks and Mexican-Americans. One of the most consistent research findings with intelligence tests is that there is a considerable correlation between intelligence and socioeconomic status and between intelligence and race. On the average, those people who come from high-income families tend to have IQs some 20 points higher than those from lower-status families. Similarly, the average IQ of whites is slightly over 100, while the average IQ of blacks is about 85, a whole standard deviation lower than average. The usual interpretation of this finding is that tests are only measuring white middle-class knowledge and values and thus are invalid for minorities and the poor who, having been reared in a different subculture, cannot be expected to do well on questions measuring understanding of an alien society. It is certainly the case that the kinds of items selected for intelligence tests only measure a narrow range of abilities; vocabulary and abstract reasoning are overrepresented relative to mechanical abilities, practical experience, and the like. To illustrate this cultural bias, Williams (1971) has constructed a test based on the black subculture on which black children perform better than whites. The questions are almost all concerned with black slang, and the test is quite obviously not a valid measure of intelligence, but as was pointed out above, it is impossible to demonstrate that more traditional tests are actually measuring intelligence either.

As a result of such criticism, the use of intelligence tests has become more circumscribed. A recent Supreme Court decision (*Griggs* v. *Duke Power Co.*, 1972) specified that any test used to select job candidates must be demonstrated to be valid for that particular job. The case involved a power generating plant that used a general intelligence test to select employees for such jobs as shoveling coal. Because blacks do not tend to score well on such tests, they were kept in low-paying jobs. The court ruled that since the power company could not demonstrate that there was any relationship between performance on their test and the ability to shovel coal, they could not use the test. In a California case (*Diana* v. *Board of Education,* 1971), nine families of Mexican-American children who had been placed in special classes for the retarded on the basis of their poor performance on intelligence tests argued that the placement had been unfair because the test used in the placement decision had been based on English rather than on the child's native language. The court ruled that children whose primary language was other than English must be tested in their native tongue as well as in English, and that school districts must reintegrate most special class children of Mexican and Chinese descent back into regular classes. School systems all over the country are placing less emphasis on intelligence test scores in assigning children to classes, and an increasing number of schools are not using tests at all except in unusual cases.

Defenders of intelligence tests argue that the problem lies not with the validity of the tests, but with how the tests are interpreted. Many teachers and parents still have a tendency to think of intelligence as an innate capacity, fixed at birth and unaffected by the environment, although no one has taken this position in print for many years. This misinterpretation of the word has confused the issue. Obviously, intelligence tests are not valid if they are supposed to measure some kind of innate capacity. However, if one takes the more limited position that the tests are measuring potential for school success and accepts the fact that this potential could readily be affected by upbringing, then intelligence tests might sometimes be useful. There is no reason why different racial groups ought to perform exactly the same on tests of school performance, particularly if one group has not been exposed to conditions conductive to school success. If a badly malnourished child is weighed and found to be 20 pounds underweight for his or her age, no one accuses the scales of discrimination. Similarly, test advocates argue that IQ tests are only documenting the cultural disadvantage of minority children. They point out that intelligence tests predict school performance just as well for black children as they do for whites, and, in this sense, they are equally valid for the two groups (Cleary et al., 1975).

One question that is too seldom asked is why we need to know what a child's IQ is. Usually, it is not necessary to predict a child's school performance, and even if one did need this information, a child's past school performance is a far better predictor than is IQ. Schools sometimes justify the wholesale administration of IQ tests to children by saying that it helps to place children in the proper classes. However, grouping children by test scores has been declared illegal in at least one court case (*Hobson* v. *Hansen,* 1967), and there is little evidence that children who do well on intelligence tests learn differently or require a different type of teaching than do children who do poorly on them. If a certain child is having difficulty learning in school, it is usually more productive to attack the learning problem directly than it is to determine IQ first. Knowing a child's IQ is far more likely to have a negative effect than a positive effect on the teacher because if the child's record indicates a low IQ, the teacher is likely to consider the child a hopeless case and spend little time with him or her. In fact, Slack (1976) has suggested that no child has ever been helped by being given an IQ test.

Intelligence testing is experiencing a slow but well-deserved death. A great many Stanford-Binets and Wechslers are still being given, either because they are mandated by law or simply through inertia, but more and more psychologists and educators are questioning their value. More importantly, professionals are placing less emphasis on a simple IQ score in making decisions about a child. The older concept of intelligence tests measuring some sort of innate capacity has been rejected, and an intelligence test is now more likely to be used simply as a structured interview. The psychologist, by observing how the child attacks certain problems, can form a clinical impression of the child's behavior and make a guess about the nature of the child's problem. For example, if a child fails a number of low-level items but passes several questions on a much higher level, this can indicate some sort of emotional disturbance. Similarly, poor performance on certain subtests of the WISC or the WAIS can suggest neurological problems. The IQ itself is often considered to be a relatively unimportant output of the testing procedure. Hopefully, the days are long past when decisions about placement will be made solely on the basis of a test score. There are simply too many variables influencing performance for a score to mean much by itself. How a child does on a test is just one piece of evidence that must be considered along with other evidence in making diagnoses and prescribing remediation.

A good deal of confusion would be eliminated if the word intelligence were deleted from the English language. The word intelligence has too much surplus meaning and is too often misinterpreted to be useful. It refers, on one hand, to one's innate potential, in another case, it may refer to the level of functioning of a given child at one point in time, and at other times it can refer simply to the performance on a test. As a result, the use of the word intelligence will be minimized in the remaining chapters. However, it will often be necessary to refer to intelligence test scores and IQs, and it is important that you do not misinterpret what is meant by these terms.

Summary

The primary goal of this chapter is to remove some of the mystique that seems to surround intelligence tests. An intelligence test is nothing more than a collection of items that one person or a small team of people believe measure intelligence. These items are not based on any special insight that psychologists have about mental abilities. Their main value is that they have been standardized on large numbers of children so that norms are available.

No one has ever been able to adequately define intelligence, and, as a result, it is impossible to demonstrate that intelligence tests are in fact measuring intelligence. Because of the confusion surrounding the term, statements like "Susy does poorly in school because of her low IQ" should be avoided because they are misleading. Intelligence is not a thing or a process, and therefore it cannot cause behavior.

Many of the myths associated with the folk meaning of the word intelligence have been disproved by research. Intelligence is certainly not fixed, but can be readily influenced by a child's training or experience. In fact, some fluctuation in IQ either up or down during development is normal. Most people do not now think in terms of one unitary mental ability, but in terms of many mental abilities, with the possibility that a child can be strong in some areas of mental functioning and weak in others. While intelligence tests do a reasonably good job of predicting school performance, the relationship between IQ and success in later life is quite low. The general confusion and misunderstanding that is associated with the concept of intelligence has some important implications for defining, diagnosing, and understanding mental retardation, as Chapter 3 will show.

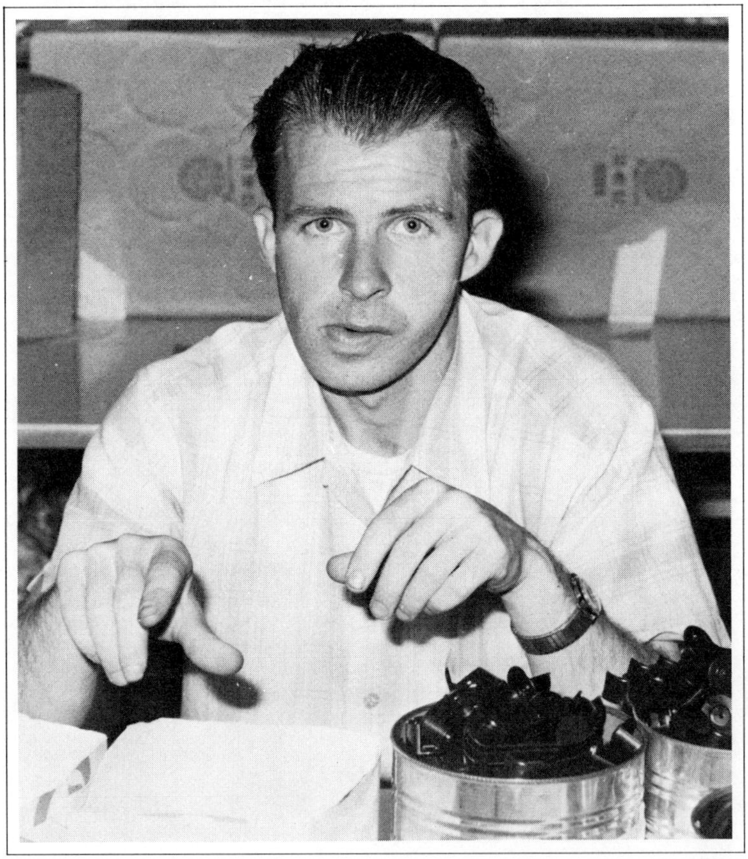

3

What Is Mental Retardation?

Much of the confusion and misinterpretation that is associated with the term intelligence has spread to the study of mental retardation. The result is that the label mentally retarded is frequently misunderstood, not only by the general public, but all too often by professionals as well. For example, it is widely assumed that once a person is diagnosed as mentally retarded, that person will always be retarded. This assumption stems directly from the old concept of fixed intelligence. Similarly, many people think of a retarded person as being unable to learn anything at all. This assumption is based on the notion of intelligence being a single, global ability. Even more important, there are occasional disagreements about who should be labeled mentally retarded and who should not. This is an important legal issue, because whenever special programs for the mentally retarded are established, the kinds of people who are entitled to these services should be clearly specified. In recent years, there have been several lawsuits (e.g., *Diana* v. *Board of Education,* 1971) in which it has been argued that a group of people have been mistakenly labeled retarded.

Defining Mental Retardation

Because of the legal status of the mental retardation label, it is important that retardation be defined clearly, reliably, and in such a way that all people who could benefit from special programming for the retarded be included, but excluding those people for whom the potential harm resulting from being so labeled would outweigh the benefits. Traditional attempts to define mental retardation can be placed roughly into three categories, definitions based on intelligence test scores, definitions based on a failure of social performance, and definitions based on the cause or essential nature of retardation, such as brain damage.

Definitions Based on Intelligence Test Scores

Intelligence tests were specifically designed to detect children who would not be able to benefit from a normal school curriculum—in other words, the mentally retarded—and their primary use has always been for this purpose. Some people have defined mental retardation solely in terms of performance on such standardized tests, that is, anyone with an IQ below a certain level, usually set at 70, is considered mentally retarded. This is the approach taken by test writers such as Wechsler and Terman (the author of the Stanford-Binet) who assign interpretive labels to various IQ ranges. In practice, many school systems define retardation largely in terms of IQ, using intelligence tests as the main criterion for determining eligibility for special classes. The primary advantage of this definition is that it is reliable and objective. People may disagree on the meaning of a certain IQ score, but there is not usually much disagreement between testers regarding an individual's IQ.

However, the previous chapter covered some major conceptual weaknesses in intelligence testing and concluded by warning against thinking of an individual's IQ as an absolute measure of potential. Attempts to define mental retardation solely in terms of IQ seem to be making this error. Another trouble with this approach is that there is not always a good relationship between performance on an intelligence test and the child's general level of adjustment. There are many cases where a child who has a low IQ still seems to making a satisfactory adjustment to the environment. Perhaps the most serious indictment of the use of intelligence tests to define mental retardation is that these tests discriminate against poverty children, particularly children from racial minorities and children whose native language is other than English.

Definitions Based on a Failure in Social Adjustment

Many writers prefer to define retardation not in terms of a score on a test, but in terms of how well the individual adjusts to the environment and culture. For example, consider the following two definitions:

> *Mental deficiency is a state of incomplete mental development of such a kind and degree that the individual is incapable of adapting himself to the normal environment of his fellows in such a way as to maintain existence independently of supervision, control or external support (Tredgold, 1937, p. 4).*

> *A mentally defective person is a person who is incapable of managing himself and his affairs, or being taught to do so, and who requires supervision, control, and care for his own welfare and the welfare of the community (Benda, 1954, p. 115).*

Both of these definitions imply that a retarded person is one who, on reaching adulthood, is incapable of leading an independent life. One difficulty with this approach is that an individual may be retarded in one environment but not in another. The obvious example is someone who has difficulty with academic skills such as reading or arithmetic. This person may be able to get along perfectly well in a simple rural culture and work as a farmhand but would be considered retarded in a modern urban culture where even the simplest jobs require filling out forms, making change, reading instructions, and other similar skills. For this reason, Kanner (1957) makes a distinction between relative and absolute feeblemindedness. The latter term refers to individuals who are so impaired in their mental functioning that they would be considered handicapped in any existing culture. Relative feeblemindedness refers to individuals who are handicapped in complex societies but would not be handicapped in simpler ones. As more and more jobs in our society require extensive educational backgrounds, in a sense, more and more people are becoming handicapped.

Another difficulty with defining retardation as a failure to adapt to the environment is that failure to adapt is very difficult to measure reliably. Different professionals may have very different ideas concerning what constitutes successful adaptation, and particularly where legal matters are concerned, it is important to have very explicit criteria of retardation so that several people evaluating an individual independently will arrive at a similar conclusion. A number of tests of adaptive behavior have been devised, but, in general, they are not as reliable as intelligence tests.

A third problem with defining mental retardation in terms of social failure is that deficits in adaptive behavior can result from other causes in addition to deficient mental abilities. There are many people with emotional problems that interfere with their ability to live independently, and since many cases of suspected mental retardation are complicated by emotional problems, it is often difficult to determine which is more important in preventing successful adjustment—the poor intellectual abilities or the emotional problems.

Definitions Based on the Essential Cause of Mental Retardation

A third approach to defining retardation involves definitions based on theoretical considerations about the cause or essential nature of retardation. The best example of this approach is the definition of mental retardation widely used in the Soviet Union:

> *Mentally retarded children. . . . have suffered from a severe brain disease while in the uterus or in early childhood, and this has disturbed the normal development of the brain and produced serious anomalies in mental development. . . . The mentally retarded child is sharply distinguished from the normal by the range of ideas he can comprehend and by the character of his perception of reality (Luria, 1963, pp. 5, 10).*

Thus, to Luria, brain damage is essential to retardation. Notice that the last sentence emphasizes the major qualitative leap between retardation and normalcy while most western theorists emphasize that retardation is on a continuum with normalcy.

The difficulty with definitions such as these is that they exclude large numbers of children and adults who probably ought to be considered retarded. There are many individuals who are functioning at an obviously retarded level, but there is no evidence of any defect in their nervous system. Theorists such as Luria argue that retarded behavior is prima facie evidence of some sort of nervous system defect, but this has yet to be proved. Such definitions of retardation are not satisfactory.

The Current Consensus: The AAMD Definition

By far the most widely accepted definition of mental retardation today is that adopted by the American Association on Mental Deficiency (AAMD):

> *Mental Retardation refers to significantly subaverage general intellectual functioning existing concurrently with deficits in adaptive behavior, and manifested during the developmental period. (Grossman, 1973, p. 11).*

This definition of retardation is so generally accepted that all students of retardation ought to be familiar with it. According to this definition, in order for a person to be classified as mentally retarded, three criteria must be met. First, there must be "significantly subaverage intellectual functioning." In practice, this means that the person must score at least two standard deviations below the norm for his or her age group on a standard intelligence test. This means that the person's IQ must be below 68 on the Stanford-Binet or below 70 on one of the Wechsler Scales. The specific test is not mentioned because there are cases where a specialized test such as the Hayes Binet (for the blind) must be used in order to determine an accurate IQ.

However, a low IQ by itself does not define retardation. The individual must also show a deficit in adaptive behavior. This criterion is somewhat more difficult to specify, but basically what it means is that the individual's adjustment to the demands of his or her natural and social environment must be impaired relative to his or her age mates. Because there are different social expectations at different ages, deficits in adaptive behavior will manifest themselves differently in younger children than they will in older children or adults. The *A.A.M.D. Manual of Terminology and Classification* provides some guidelines. For infants and preschoolers, adaptive behavior may be reflected in the following areas: sensory-motor skills, communication skills, self-help skills, and socialization. Delays in the development of these behaviors may represent potential deficiencies in adaptive behavior. For school-age children, adaptive behavior deficits may be manifested by difficulties in the application of basic academic skills to daily life activities, or in the application of appropriate reasoning and judgment in the mastery of the environment, as well as by deficits in social skills. In late adolescence and adulthood, vocational performance and social responsibility become important, and thus, adaptive behavior may be determined by the extent to which the individual is able to maintain himself or herself independently in the community.

Several scales have been developed to assess social adjustment. Probably the best known is the *Vineland Social Maturity Scale* (Doll, 1964). This is a checklist of items of adaptive behavior listed according to the age at which the average child is able to perform them. For example, the average child can be expected to perform the following social skills regularly between the second and third year: asks to go to the toilet, removes coat or dress, eats with a fork, gets a drink unassisted, cuts with scissors, and relates experiences. The following items are at the 6-year level: uses table knife for cutting, uses pencil for writing, bathes self assisted, goes to bed unassisted. The average 15 to 18 year old can be expected to communicate by letter, follow current events, have his/her own spending money, and buy all of his/her own clothes. The scale produces a social age that indicates the level at which the child is functioning. If the child is not able to perform many of the skills that most children of that age are able to perform, in other words, if the child's social age is well below his or her chronological age, this may indicate retardation.

Another such scale is the *Adaptive Behavior Scale,* published by the AAMD. This is specifically designed to assess and describe the adaptive behavior of mentally retarded people, and instead of having norms collected on a normal population as most assessment instruments do, the only norms are on retarded individuals, and instead of producing a single score, the end result is a profile of the individual's adaptive behavior on 10 scales of functional behavior and 14 scales of antisocial behavior. Its main value, however, is simply as a checklist of behaviors that can then be used as a guide for programming and as a way to measure progress over time.

The third criterion of the definition is that the deficit in adapative behavior and subaverage intellectual functioning must be manifest during the developmental period, which is from conception to age 18. This means that retardation is conceived as a developmental disorder. The individual who reaches adulthood after normal development can never be considered retarded. Those people whose intellectual powers have deteriorated because of senility or brain damage at adulthood are not retarded.

As we said before, if an individual is to be considered retarded, all three of these criteria must be met: the person must score at least two standard deviations below average on a standard intelligence test, adaptive behavior must be impaired, and the deficit must occur during the developmental period. There are many individuals who meet one or two of these criteria, but they are not retarded. For example, children from culturally deprived backgrounds frequently perform poorly on standardized intelligence tests, but they show little impairment in adaptive behavior. They have no trouble learning the skills necessary for survival in their world. They are not delayed in basic maturational milestones such as the age at which they begin to speak or the age at which they learn to dress themselves. They have no unusual difficulty in learning their way around the neighborhood or getting along with their peers. These children should not be considered retarded. Similarly, there are many people who are impaired in adaptive behavior in the sense that they cannot perform many of the social skills necessary for independent living such as holding a job or getting along with others. They may be institutionalized as psychotics or psychopaths or they may survive by depending on relatives, but if they perform in the normal range on intelligence tests, they are not retarded.

There is an important distinction between this definition of mental retardation and the popular use of the term. The AAMD definition makes no mention of either the cause of the retardation or its incurability. Mental retardation is defined solely in behavioral terms: people are considered mentally retarded if they act mentally retarded. However, retardation is often thought of as being a constitutional disorder—organic and permanent. Earlier definitions often made specific reference to this (e.g., Doll, 1941). If some mention of permanence is included in the definition, then it is possible for children or adults to be misdiagnosed, labeled mentally retarded because they showed retarded behavior, but later turning out not to be because they functioned independently. These people were called pseudoretarded. The current definition avoids this issue by making no mention of permanence; it is possible for a child to be genuinely mentally retarded at one point in time and not mentally retarded later on. This use of the term is still widely misunderstood. It is common for a teacher to make a statement like "When Johnny first came into my class, I thought he was mentally retarded because he didn't learn anything for the first three months, but now I know that he is not retarded because he is progressing better." In similar fashion, some psychological testers are still concerned with developing test methods to distinguish the truly retarded child from the child who only appears to be retarded [see Silverstein (1970) for a brief review]. Some psychiatrists feel that if a child's retarded behavior is a result of emotional disturbance, then the child should not be considered retarded. Such people feel that an important job of the clinician is to distinguish between the retarded and the pseudoretarded child, apparently on the assumption that the emotionally disturbed child is more amenable to treatment. The definition of retardation adopted by this book says that this is not a significant issue. Emotional disturbance or cultural deprivation or other adverse circumstances can produce mental retardation just as real as can brain damage.

Levels of Mental Retardation

Because the label mentally retarded includes so many different kinds of people, the AAMD has developed a system of diagnostic classification of the retarded based on the individual's level of functioning, principally the IQ. Individuals with IQs between two and three standard deviations below normal are labeled *mildly retarded,* those with IQs between three and four standard deviations below normal are called *moderately retarded,* those with IQs between four and five standard deviations below average are labeled *severely retarded,* and those who score greater than five standard deviations below normal are called *profoundly retarded.* Table 3-1 translates this system into IQ scores for the Wechsler and Binet tests.

The last column of Table 3-1 shows the adult mental ages of each of the four levels. This gives a good indication of the expected level of functioning of an individual at various levels. For example, a mildly retarded adult is usually capable of doing most of the things that a child from 8 to 11 years

Table 3-1 Levels of Mental Retardation

Level	Binet IQ (s.d. = 16) [a]	Wechsler IQ (s.d. = 15)	Mental Age at Adulthood
Mild	68–52	69–55	8.3–10.9 yr
Moderate	51–36	54–40	5.7–8.2 yr
Severe	35–20	39–25	3.2–5.6 yr
Profound	≤19	≤24	≤3.1 yr

[a] s.d. = standard deviation.

old is able to do, such as reading and calculating to the third- to fifth-grade level, taking care of personal needs such as dressing and grooming with negligible assistance, holding down a simple job, manifesting essentially normal coordination, and showing adequate social interaction. A moderately retarded adult can be expected to function at the level of the average 5 to 8 year old. This person needs occasional assistance with personal care and grooming, can read only at a minimal level if at all, and probably cannot live independently, but could hold a job if special provision were made for the handicap as in a sheltered workshop. A severely retarded adult would be functioning at the level of the average preschooler. While this person could look after basic bodily needs such as dressing, feeding, and toileting, and could probably communicate with simple language, he or she would certainly require considerable supervision throughout his or her life. This person would not be able to get around town independently, may have some coordination problems, and may not be able to hold a job even in a sheltered workshop. A profoundly retarded person has a mental age of less than 3 years at adulthood. Thus, many profoundly retarded people cannot even be expected to take care of basic bodily needs. Most are not fully toilet trained, many need assistance with dressing, some do not even feed themselves. This category also includes many bed cases who never even learn to walk. Language skills would be minimal.

The AAMD classification in use from 1961 to 1973 also included the category *borderline retarded,* which was defined as an IQ from one to two standard deviations below average, in other words, a Wechsler IQ of 70 to 85. Thus, under this system, retardation is defined as functioning more than one standard deviation below normal and included a great many more people. The justification for including the borderline category was that modern society is becoming so complex that even the simplest jobs require a minimal level of academic skills, and as a result, many people with IQs below 85 would require some asisstance or guidance in such matters as locating and obtaining a job, renting an apartment, personal money management such as opening a bank account, buying insurance, paying taxes, and so forth. While this is probably true to some extent, these people are no longer considered retarded according to the more recent classification system. The reason for this change is that in the past decade a good deal of concern has developed about the stigmatizing and degrading effects of being labeled retarded. If a person is classified as retarded by being placed in a special class in school or by being institutionalized, friends, relatives, and potential employers may react to that person differently and expect different behavior. In addition, the individual's self-esteem may be severely damaged. A second reason for dropping the category of borderline retardation is that research (Cobb, 1972) has consistently indicated that the vast majority of people in this IQ range as able to lead independent and productive lives. As a result, the AAMD suggests that this condition be called borderline intelligence rather than borderline retarded.

The AAMD classification of mental retardation is the most widely accepted one today, but there are other classification systems. An obsolete scheme involved the categories of moron, imbecile, and idiot. A moron was an individual with an IQ of 50 to 75, an imbecile was a person with an IQ of 25 to 50, and an idiot was someone with an IQ of less than 25. These labels are no longer used because the terms have come to have degrading connotations. Educators classify retarded children into the categories of educable mentally retarded (EMR), trainable mentally retarded (TMR), and severely mentally retarded (SMR). The label EMR corresponds roughly to mild retardation, and TMR corresponds roughly to moderate mental retardation. The origin of the labels is obvious. Educable refers to the fact that these people can be taught basic academic skills such as reading, writing, and arithmetic. Trainable children cannot ordinarily learn academic skills beyond a very basic level such as writing their name or reading MEN and WOMEN on bathroom doors, but they can be trained in basic self-care skills and simple vocational abilities. The severely mentally retarded and the profoundly retarded are also sometimes referred to as custodial or subtrainable retarded people because frequently they cannot even be taught basic self-care skills. They have traditionally been excluded from the public schools (although education-for-all legislation is changing this situation rapidly).

Diagnosing Mental Retardation

Because mental retardation is defined in behavioral terms, proper diagnosis can technically be made only by a psychologist. In practice, this is not always the case, however, and there are a number of different ways in which children are diagnosed as retarded. Who makes the initial diagnosis and the age of the initial diagnosis depend on how severe the retardation is. If the retardation is profound or if it is accompanied by obvious physical abnormalities or associated with a specific syndrome such as Down's syndrome (mongolism), then the child may be diagnosed as retarded at birth. However, diagnosis at birth is the exception. Because so little in the way of adaptive behavior is expected from a newborn, a child who will later be diagnosed as severely retarded may be considered normal for many months after birth. Severe retardation is often diagnosed by delayed motor development and general apathy, but such gross motor skills as rolling over, sitting, and walking are often only slightly delayed in moderately retarded children and frequently not delayed at all in mildly retarded children. Occasionally, moderate retardation is not diagnosed until the child is two to four years old when the parents notice that their child is not developing as rapidly as other children are. An important diagnostic clue is delayed language. Children who are more than mildly retarded almost always manifest some delay in the acquisition of language. (However, there are also many perfectly normal children whose language is delayed, so delayed language by itself is not clear proof of retardation.) Thus, the customary diagnostic procedure for moderate, severe, or profound retardation is that the parents will notice some peculiarity in their child and bring this to the attention of a physician, who will then normally refer the child to a specialist for further clarification. A psychologist will usually measure the child's mental development, and if there is any suspicion of neurological damage, various tests such as skull X rays and electroencephalograms may be made.

However, many mildly retarded children are not classified as such until they reach school age. The early development of many mildly retarded children does not differ significantly from normal; these children acquire basic skills such as walking, language development, and social skills at about the same rate or only slightly delayed from normal children, and as a result, the parents do not suspect anything until the child enters school. Thus, the first suspicion of mild retardation is usually made not by the parents but by the teacher. If a child is having unusual difficulties in school, the most frequent procedure is for the teacher, with the consent of the principal and the parents, to refer the child to the school psychologist for assessment. The school psychologist will normally administer a standard intelligence test and then determine whether the child is retarded or not. The psychologist may also recommend placement in a special class. Unfortunately, psychologists frequently rely solely on an intelligence test in determining retardation, ignoring the child's adaptive behavior (Adams, 1973).

Thus moderate, severe, and profound retardation are usually seen by the public as primarily medical problems. The kind of diagnosis done is usually medical; that is, the physician will determine that the child has Down's syndrome or that the child suffered a brain injury at birth. Mild retardation, on the other hand, is more often seen as an educational problem. It is supected by a teacher and diagnosed by a psychologist, and frequently a physician is not consulted at all. Most mildly retarded children present no unusual medical disorders which can account for their poor school performance. However, most individuals with IQs below 50 are characterized by some specific biological abnormality. In neither case do the people doing the initial diagnosis adhere strictly to the AAMD definition. Physicians frequently make a diagnosis based strictly on medical criteria (because the child has brain damage he or she is retarded) while schools tend to rely heavily on academic performance and test scores, ignoring adaptive behavior outside the school. Mercer (1973) has shown that these two approaches result in different kinds of people being diagnosed as retarded. She asked all of the medical agencies and all of the schools in a community to supply the names of all mentally retarded people in their files, and she discovered that there was little overlap between the two lists. There were a large number of people that the schools considered retarded that medical agencies did not, and there were a few people that physicians considered retarded that schools did not.

The random fashion in which the diagnosis of mental retardation and other developmental disabilities is made is slowly being changed by the establishment of various types of screening clinics designed to provide a wide range of diagnostic procedures to children born at risk, that is, children born to low-income families who do not ordinarily receive adequate medical attention. These screening clinics generally administer a short developmental test and assess the child's vision and hearing as well as providing a complete physical examination. The purpose of these clinics is to detect any abnormalities of development as young as possible because it is usually the case that the younger any disorder is discovered, the greater the probability that it can be effectively treated.

Intelligence Testing with the Mentally Retarded

One of the paradoxes of the intelligence testing movement is that the primary use of intelligence tests is to diagnose mental retardation, and thus, almost all of the children tested are abnormal in some way. Despite this, the various tests have almost always been developed on and standardized on a population of normal children. Any child for whom brain damage, emotional disturbance, mental retardation, or other abnormality is suspected is routinely dropped from the standardization sample. For this reason, it is important to verify that widely used intelligence tests such as the WISC and the Stanford-Binet are as reliable and valid with the mentally retarded and with other handicapped groups as they are with normal children.

Fortunately, there has been a good deal of research addressed to this question (see Silverstein, 1970 or Sattler, 1974 for general reviews). This research concluded that, in general, the Stanford-Binet and the various Wechsler tests are about as useful with the retarded as they are with normal children. For example, a number of people have determined that test-retest reliability of the Stanford-Binet and the WISC are adequately high (Scarr, 1953; Throne, Schulman, and Kaspar, 1962). However, Silverstein (1970) pointed out that the correlation between the Stanford-Binet and the WISC is only about .74. This is high, but not high enough to suggest that the two tests are measuring exactly the same abilities. An additional problem is that

Wechsler IQs tend to be slightly higher than Binet IQs for retarded people, although this would be expected because the standard deviation for the Wechsler tests is slightly lower.

An interesting theoretical question is the extent to which the relative degree of difficulty of various items and subtests is similar for retarded and nonretarded people. If there are certain kinds of questions on which retarded people seem to do particularly badly or particularly well, this could suggest that the general structure of mental abilities is different for retarded people, and it could also have implications for special education. One of the easiest ways to answer this question is to look at the relative degree of difficulty of various subtests of the WISC. Silverstein (1970) reviewed 10 studies in which this was done, and he discovered some important generalizations. Retarded subjects almost always tend to do best on the nonverbal subtests, object assembly and picture completion in particular. Most retarded subjects do the poorest on the subtests of vocabulary, arithmetic, and information, all verbal subtests. There is also a general trend for retarded subjects to have a slightly higher performance IQ than a verbal IQ. In other words, retarded people seem to have unusual difficulty with verbal abstraction abilities and relatively less difficulty with tests of nonverbal comprehension.

Achenbach (1970) performed a similar study with the Stanford-Binet. He matched 54 retarded subjects with nonretarded subjects of similar mental age (the nonretarded subjects were of necessity considerably younger), and then he compared performances between the two groups on individual items. There were no significant differences between the two groups on the vast majority of the items, although this was not surprising since the two groups were matched on overall test score. However, there were a number of items that clearly favored the nonretarded subjects, and these tended to be those measuring abstract verbal abilities such as explaining the difference between two things or explaining verbal absurdities. There were also items that favored the retarded subjects, and these tended to be nonverbal and relatively free from abstract thinking such as drawing, copying, or naming the days of the week.

These studies indicate that mentally retarded children have a particular deficit in verbal abstract abilities, even when they are compared to nonretarded children of a much younger age. However, they do not appear to be as impaired on items assessing nonverbal and nonabstract abilities. This observation has led Jensen (1970) to suggest that there are two levels of intellectual abilities. Level 1 refers to simple association skills such as is required in rote learning, and Level 2 refers to more abstract kinds of abilities. Retarded children are only significantly impaired in Level 2 abilities. This theory is discussed in detail in a later chapter.

The Growth and Decline of IQ in the Retarded

As normal children develop there is no consistent tendency for their IQ to either increase or decrease. However, there is general agreement that the IQ of most retarded children drops as they get older, at least during the developmental years. The best research in this area is that of Fisher and Zeaman (1970). They analyzed the IQ scores of all of the residents of a large state institution for the retarded who had been tested more than once. Using this data, they were able to determine the extent of decline in IQ with age for various levels of retardation. Figure 3-1 shows their results. Notice that between the ages of 5 and 16, the average IQ of these subjects dropped some 15 points. There was also a tendency for those subjects with lower IQs to show more of an IQ decline during development.

This decline can be largely explained as a statistical artifact of the way that IQ is computed. If one plots mental age (i.e., the overall score on the test) as a function of age, it rises rather consistently for normal subjects until some-

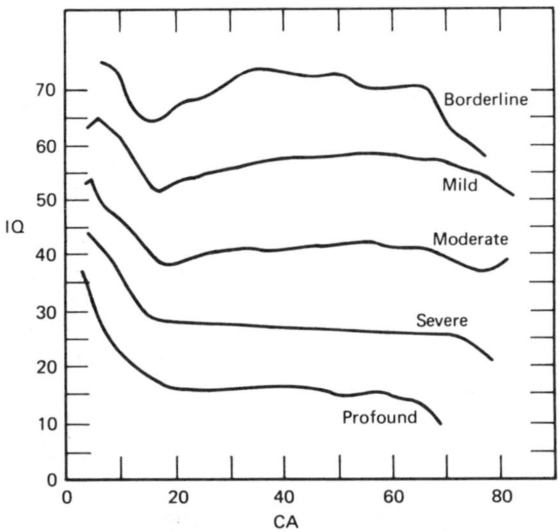

Figure 3-1 Age changes in IQ for the five levels of retardation computed semilongitudinally. From M. A. Fisher & D. Zeaman. Growth and decline of retardate intelligence. In N. R. Ellis (Ed.), *International review of research in mental retardation.* Vol. 4. New York: Academic Press, 1970. Copyright © 1970 by Academic Press. Reprinted with the permission of the publisher and the author.

where around the age of 16, when it begins to level off, and it increases only very slightly after that time. However, Fisher and Zeaman found that retarded people begin to plateau at a younger age than do nonretarded people. Thus, not only do the mental abilities of retarded people as measured by intelligence tests grow more slowly than do those of nonretarded people, but these abilities stop growing sooner, and this accounts for the drop in IQ of retarded people during their developmental years.

However, during adulthood there is some tendency for the IQs of retarded people to rise again. This can be attributed to the fact that there is still some improvement in mental abilities during the twenties and thirties, and perhaps later. The Fisher and Zeaman study found this, as have numerous other studies that have followed retarded people into adulthood (e.g., Charles, 1953). This means that some people who are considered retarded while they are growing up will "outgrow" their mental retardation as they get older.

The Prevalence of Mental Retardation

For both theoretical and practical reasons, it is important to have an idea of how many retarded people there are in the general population. This figure, known as prevalence, is usually expressed as the number of retarded people per thousand people in the general population. For example, if research indicates that the prevalence of mental retardation is 20 per thousand, this means that 2 percent of the people are retarded, and in a community of 30,000 people, we would expect to find about 600 mentally retarded individuals.

However, determining prevalence is not always easy. First, there is the general problem of locating all of the retarded people in a given population. The usual method here is to survey clinics and agencies for lists of cases, but this method can expect to underestimate the retarded population since there will always be some cases of obvious retardation who have escaped the notice of the establishment for one reason or another. The one exception to this is schools, since school systems presumably have a relatively complete list of children of school age and have made some attempt to distinguish the retarded. However, there is a second problem. Depending on how mental retardation is defined, prevalence figures will be significantly different. It is obviously not feasible to give everyone in the community an intelligence test and a test of adaptive behavior, so other criteria have to be used, and since different agencies use different criteria for diagnosis, then discrepancies arise between studies. Even if IQ scores were available for everyone, an arbitrary cutoff point would have to be decided on, and different kinds of agencies tend to use different cutoff points. The most recent AAMD guidelines place the cutoff point at IQ 70, but many school systems have an IQ cutoff at 75 or even 80 for mental retardation. The old AAMD classification system in effect until 1973 placed the retardation cutoff point at IQ 85. Obviously, if the category of borderline retardation is included, there will be a great many more retarded people in the country than if it is not included.

In theory, it should be very easy to predict the prevalence of mental retardation from the normal curve. Recall that the distribution of IQ is based on the assumption that intelligence is normally distributed as shown in Figure 2-1. Thus, given a specific IQ, it should be possible to specify the percentage of scores below it. For example, 16 percent of a set of scores ought to lie below one standard deviation below the mean. In other words, 16 percent of the population ought to have an IQ below 85. Two percent of a set of scores ought to be more than two standard deviations below the average, and this means that 2 percent of the population ought to have IQs below 70. Similarly, about one person in a thousand ought to have an IQ below 50 and so on. Unfortunately, this is not a very useful way to estimate the prevalence of mental retardation for two reasons. First, in order for a person to be considered retarded not only must that person have a low IQ but he or she must also be impaired in adaptive behavior. The majority of people with IQs between 85 and 70 are probably not impaired in adaptive behavior, and a smaller but still substantial percentage of those with IQs below 70 show little adaptive deficit. In other words, not everyone with a low IQ is retarded. Second, the normal curve is a reasonable description of the distribution of intelligence within the normal range, but the farther a given IQ is from the average, the less well the normal curve predicts its incidence. There are a great many more individuals in the moderate, severe, and profound ranges of mental retardation than one would predict from the normal curve. Table 3-2 shows the expected prevalence of various types of retardation as well as the actual estimated prevalence from one study. According to the

Table 3-2 Mentally Retarded Population of the United States

IQ Range	Number Calculated from Normal Curve [a]	Estimated Prevalence	Excess
0–20	50	87,500	84,450
20–50	155,529	350,000	194,471
50–70	5,224,255	5,276,755	52,500

H. F. Dingman & G. Tarjan, Mental retardation and the normal distribution curve, *American Journal of Mental Deficiency,* 1960, **64,** 991–994.

[a] Based on a U.S. population of 175 million.

theoretical distribution, profound retardation ought to be virtually nonexistent (exactly as common as the prevalence of IQs 180 to 200), but obviously it isn't. Similar discrepancies are observed for the severely and moderately retarded. There is a simple explanation for this divergence from theory. The factors that are responsible for producing differences in IQ, whether they be genes or upbringing, tend to produce a normal distribution. It is a natural law that when a variable is determined by a large number of independent, random factors, the result is that the distribution of this variable will resemble the normal distribution. For example, height is normally distributed. However, intelligence can occasionally be drastically lowered by the presence of a single major organic defect such as a metabolic error or brain damage due to accident. The introduction of this new factor results in more cases of extremely low intelligence than would be predicted. Zigler (1967) has proposed that the distribution of IQs is more accurately described as two separate normal distributions, one including the vast majority of the population with a mean of 100 and the other including those with some sort of organic brain damage with an average of about 35. These two distributions would be superimposed upon one another as in Figure 3-2*a*, resulting in a slightly skewed overall distribution as shown in Figure 3-2*b*, which seems to be a close approximation of reality.

There have been a number of studies investigating the prevalence of mental retardation in the general population. The results have not been entirely consistent between studies, but there are certain generalizations that can be made. The most frequent method of determining prevalence is to survey all of the various agencies in the community for names of people they consider retarded. A typical example of such a study was done in Onondaga County, New York (Goodman et al., 1956). This survey queried all public and private agencies that would have records of cases of retardation. The request was for the names of all those with confirmed or suspected retardation who were under 18 years old. They found 3787 cases of retardation in this manner, which yielded a prevalence rate of 35.2 per thousand. However, this survey has been criticized (Kirk and Weiner, 1959) for having a criterion of retardation that was grossly overinclusive and hence, overestimated the prevalence. Many cases of suspected retardation presumably turn out not to be retarded. Kirk and Weiner cite a prevalence study done in Hawaii in 1956 that yielded a prevalence figure of 23.6 cases per thousand among school-age children, considerably lower than the Onondaga study. The Hawaii study defined retardation much more strictly. If group IQ scores were available, students with IQs below 65 were considered retarded. If such scores were not available, older children were considered retarded only in both reading and arithmetic skills were three years below grade level. First and second graders were classified retarded only if they

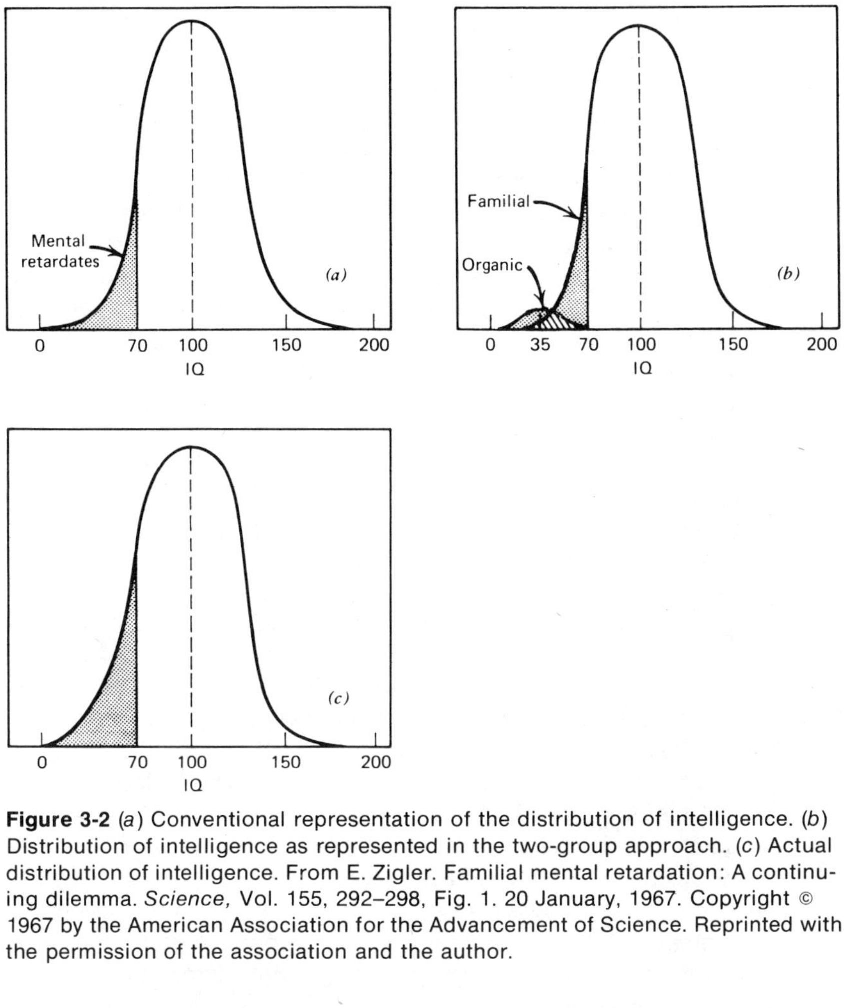

Figure 3-2 (*a*) Conventional representation of the distribution of intelligence. (*b*) Distribution of intelligence as represented in the two-group approach. (*c*) Actual distribution of intelligence. From E. Zigler. Familial mental retardation: A continuing dilemma. *Science,* Vol. 155, 292–298, Fig. 1. 20 January, 1967. Copyright © 1967 by the American Association for the Advancement of Science. Reprinted with the permission of the association and the author.

could not read a preprimer and do sums below 10. Kindergarteners were considered retarded only if they were unable to succeed in readiness activities in language and number. Because of the strict criteria, this study might well have underestimated the prevalence.

A recent prevalence study by Jane Mercer (1973) deserves special note. In her research, an adaptive behavior scale developed by Mercer and her co-workers was administered to all residents of 2661 households in Riverside, California. These households were selected to have the same proportion of whites, Mexican-Americans, and blacks as in the overall population of the community, as well as representing all geographic and socioeconomic levels of the city in proper proportion. The scale was administered to a total of 6907 people, 1026 preschoolers (seven months to 5 years), 1875 school age children (6 to 15 years old), and 4006 adults (16 to 49 years old). For preschoolers, the adaptive behavior scale measured predominantly developmental skills such as locomotion, language skills, self-help, and response to social situations. The school-age items of the scale contained a number of school-related items (whether the children had repeated a grade, whether they enjoy reading, whether they can count to twenty, whether they use a dictionary, etc.) as well as general measures of socialization (whether the children are active members of an athletic team or club, whether they go to the movies, whether they get along with their siblings, etc.). The adult questions involved occupational competence and general socialization (whether they visit neighbors, whether they read a newspaper regularly, etc.).

In addition, the Stanford-Binet intelligence test was administered to 660 individuals randomly selected from the nearly 7000 who had been given the adaptive behavior scale. Thus, this is one of the few prevalence studies that actually measures both adaptive behavior and intelligence independently, as is required by the current definition of mental retardation. If a person is considered retarded when he or she achieves an IQ below 84 on the Stanford-Binet and is in the lower 16 percent on the adaptive behavior scale, then the prevalence of retardation in Riverside is estimated to be 34.7 per thousand, a figure that is quite comparable to other prevalence studies. However, this study also indicates that IQ alone cannot be used as a measure of retardation because there were a great many people who had low IQs but no apparent impairment in adaptive behavior. Mercer labeled these people the quasi-retarded. Similarly, there were a number of people who had problems with adaptive behavior but whose IQ was not in the retarded range. These people were called the behaviorally maladjusted. If only those individuals who scored in the lowest 9 percent on both scales are considered retarded, then the prevalence rate is reduced to 18.9 per thousand. Mercer concluded that most other prevalence studies were overestimating the overall prevalence of retardation.

Farber (1968) has summarized a number of the best prevalence studies. Table 3-3 shows the results of 10 of these projects. Most of the discrepancies can be explained by considering the differences in criteria of retardation employed; that is, those studies that adopted a rather strict and restrictive criterion of mental retardation report somewhat smaller prevalence figures than do studies with more liberal criteria such as the Onondaga study. Perhaps the best general summary statement of this research is that 2.5 to 3 percent of the general population is mentally retarded.

If mental retardation is defined as the lowest 2.5 percent of the population, there would be over 5 million mentally retarded people in the United

Table 3-3 Prevalence Studies of Mentally Retarded Children in the United States, with Year, Location of Study, Age Range, and Prevalence Estimate per 1000 Population

Year	Location	Report	Age Range	Estimate of Prevalence (per 1000)
1953	New Jersey	Howard [a]	school age	15.2
1953	Onondaga, N.Y.	Goodman [b]	under 18	35.2
1954	Philadelphia	Ferguson [c]	preschool	32.2
			school age	33.9
			adulthood	19.2
			all ages	23.2
1954	Georgia	Wishik [d]	0–20	37.0
1956	Hawaii	Weiner [e]	Grades K–12	23.6
1956	Delaware	Jastak [f]	All ages (through adult)	
			–at 25% cut-off pts.	83.3
			–at 9% cut-off pts.	20.3
			–at 2% cut-off pts.	3.8
1957	Maine	Levinson [g]	5–20	29.9
1958	Illinois	Farber [h]	6–15	18.8
1957–8	Wyoming	— [i]	6–21	50.2
1963	Middle-sized City, California	Mercer [j]	All ages (through adult)	36.1

From *Mental retardation: its social context and social consequences* by Bernard Farber. Copyright © 1968 by B. Farber. Reprinted by permission of Houghton Mifflin Company.

[a] John W. Howard, ed., *Found, A Report of the Committee to Study the Education of Handicapped Children* (Trenton: New Jersey Department of Education, 1954.)

[b] Melvin B. Goodman, Ernest M. Gruenberg, Joseph Downing, and Eugene Rogot, "A Prevalence Study of Mental Retardation in a Metropolitan Area," *American Journal of Public Health,* 46 (June, 1956), pp. 702–707.

[c] Robert G. Ferguson, "A Study of the Problem of Mental Retardation in a Large Urban Community," *American Journal of Orthopsychiatry,* 27 (1957), pp. 490–501.

[d] Samuel M. Wishik, "Handicapped Children in Georgia, A Study of Prevalence, Needs, and Resources," *American Journal of Public Health,* 46 (February, 1956), pp. 195–203.

[e] Samuel A. Kirk and Bluma B. Weiner, "The Onondaga Census—Fact or Artifact," *Exceptional Children,* 25 (January, 1959), pp. 226–228, 230–231.

[f] Joseph F. Jastak, Halsey M. McPhee, and Martin Whiteman, *Mental Retardation, Its Nature and Incidence* (Newark, Delaware: University of Delaware Press, 1963).

[g] Elizabeth J. Levinson, *Retarded Children in Maine, A Survey and Analysis* (Orono, Maine: University of Maine Press, 1962).

[h] Bernard Farber, *Prevalence of Exceptional Children in Illinois in 1958* (Springfield: Illinois Superintendent of Public Instruction, 1959), Circular—Census 1A.

[i] *Wyoming Mental Ability Survey, 1957–1958* (Cheyenne: State Department of Education, May 10, 1959).

[j] Computed from data in Jane R. Mercer, Edgar W. Butler, and Harvey F. Dingman, "The Relationship between Social Developmental Performance and Mental Ability," *American Journal of Mental Deficiency,* 69 (September, 1964), pp. 195–205.

States based on the 1970 census. In other words, the number of mentally retarded people exceeds the total population of such states as Georgia or Wisconsin. Others have made even higher estimates. The President's Panel on Mental Retardation (1962) estimated that in 1970 there would be 6.5 million mentally retarded people in the country. The prevalence of this condition is exceeded by only four other major health problems: mental illness, cardiac diseases, arthritis, and cancer.

Of the total retarded population, the vast majority are mildly retarded. It is estimated that only about 15 percent of all retarded people have IQs below 50. For example, the President's Panel on Mental Retardation (1962) estimated that 86.7 percent of the retarded population was mildly retarded, 10 percent was moderately retarded, and only 3.3 percent of the total retarded population was severely or profoundly retarded. Several studies of trainable level retardates have confirmed these general estimates. For example, Abramowicz and Richardson (1975) reviewed 27 prevalence studies of children with IQs below 50. Almost all of these studies reported a prevalence rate of between three and five per thousand, and they concluded that the "true" estimate was about four per thousand, a figure quite consistent with the estimate made by the President's Panel on Mental Retardation. This means that there are some 800,000 people in the United States whose intellectual functioning is so impaired that they will probably never lead independent lives.

Differences in Prevalence in Different Segments of the Population

Mental retardation is not found equally often in all segments of the population but is far more likely to occur in some groups than it is among others. These differences in prevalence provide some important insights into the nature of mental retardation.

Sex Differences

All of the prevalence studies summarized by Farber found more retarded males than females. For example, the Onondaga study (Goodman et al., 1956), which used a very liberal definition of retardation, reported that 64 percent of their cases were males. In other studies, the exact proportion of males to females varied somewhat, but the overall conclusion is unquestioned; there are more retarded males than females in a ratio of about three to two. In other words, about 60 percent of retarded people are males, and only about 40 percent females.

There are several reasons why this might be true. First, for reasons that are presently unknown, male fetuses and neonates are more susceptible to various kinds of trauma. Male babies are more likely to be born prematurely, they are more likely to suffer various kinds of brain damage, and male fetuses are more likely to be aborted or miscarried. Even after birth, males are more susceptible to the various dangers of the physical environment than are females, and this is only partially because of their more active life-styles.

However, differences in biology probably only account for part of the predominance of male over female retarded people. Psychosocial factors are also very important. Parents treat boys and girls quite differently, and these differences in treatment might well contribute to differences in mental functioning. For example, parents are frequently more tolerant of aggressive and acting out behavior among boys than among girls, and this means that boys are less likely to apply themselves to schoolwork and other intellectual pursuits. Some families encourage their sons to be independent while they encourage their daughters to be dependent, and this means that boys have a greater opportunity for social failure.

A third contributing factor is that boys who are doing poorly are more likely to be diagnosed as retarded than are girls. Boys who are not going well in school tend to become behavior problems to a much greater extent than do girls. They tend to call attention to themselves and make themselves obvious, while a girl who is having academic difficulties is more likely to sit quietly in the back of the class and not cause any problems. Many teachers tend to prefer quiet children to disruptive children, even if they are not as bright. As a result, boys are much more likely to be referred to the school psychologist for testing or to the principal for disciplining than are girls. Thus, they are more likely to be diagnosed as retarded. This does not mean that there are more retarded boys than girls, it simply means that a poorly functioning boy is more likely to come to the attention of a psychologist or other authorities than are girls because they tend to express their frustrations in more overt ways. Evidence for this argument comes from the Mercer study described above. Mercer (1973) determined prevalence in several different ways. In one study, she used the traditional approach of surveying all of the agencies in the community that could possibly have a list of mentally retarded individuals: schools, police, medical facilities, rehabilitation agencies, private service groups, and so on. Virtually all types of agencies reported more retarded males than females. However, in the field survey described above, when an adaptive behavior scale and an intelligence test were administered to a representative sample of the community, the sex difference disappeared, and she found almost exactly equal numbers of males and females. However, the ratio of behaviorally maladjusted (those who failed the adaptive behavior scale but not the intelligence test) males to females was almost two to one.

Prevalence Differences at Different Ages

Most prevalence studies find clear differences in the prevalence of mental retardation at different ages. For example, in the Mercer study where she queried various agencies for lists of the mentally retarded, after eliminating duplicates (those individuals nominated by more than one agency) she had a list of 812 names. Of these 812 people nominated as mentally retarded, only 7 percent were under 5, 72 percent were 5 to 19, and 21 percent were over 19. These percentages can be compared to 13 percent of the general population who were under 5, 39 percent between 5 and 19, and 48 percent of the population who were 20 or older. In other words, there were about half as many mentally retarded preschoolers and half as many mentally retarded adults, but twice as many mentally retarded school children as would be predicted if retardation were evenly distributed across ages. Most other prevalence studies have found a similar phenomenon, an almost negligibly small prevalence of retardation among preschoolers, a gradually increasing number of mentally retarded among school age children, reaching a peak at about 14, then a sharp decrease in prevalence among the population older than 16.

If we accept the traditional clinical approach to mental retardation, that is, that mental retardation is an essentially permanent condition originating from birth or shortly after, then this finding is disconcerting; we would expect to find the prevalence of retardation to be about the same among all age groups, making minor allowances for the few who become retarded during the school years as a result of accidents or the differential death rates of retarded people. However, this is clearly not the case.

Explanations of this phenomenon can be placed in two general categories. One interpretation is that there are numerous cases of retardation among preschoolers and adults that remain undiagnosed because there is no mechanism in society for systematic screening of intellectual abilities among these age groups. When retarded children go to school, the retardation is diagnosed by the teacher and school psychologist. However, after they leave school, agencies dealing with the mentally retarded lose contact with them, and, as a result, they are no longer counted in prevalence studies. In other words, the proportion of the population who is retarded does not differ very much from one age group to another, and the differences in prevalence found at different ages are a result of inaccurate reporting procedures. This conclusion is supported by the Mercer study, which found that when intelligence tests and adaptive behavior scales are actually administered to a large number of randomly selected people, the prevalence of retardation is relatively constant across age groups.

A second interpretation is that a person can be retarded in some situations but not in others. One of the defining characteristics of mental retardation is an impairment in adaptive behavior, and this impairment must be culturally defined. Since schools are situations where great demands of an intellectual nature are made, one might expect that there are more retarded people in school situations than in other situations. In other words, many people who are considered retarded in school are no longer retarded once they leave an academic situation. No one is naive enough to argue that schooling has cured the retardation, but because intellectual demands are no longer imposed on these people, they are no longer retarded.

This interpretation is supported in a classic study by Charles (1953) who followed up 151 cases of people who had been labeled mentally retarded during their school years. At the time of the study, the average age of the subjects in the group was 42 years old. The majority were leading independent, productive lives. About 80 percent were married, only slightly less than the national average. Over half owned or were buying their own home. Thirty-three percent of the males and 42 percent of the females had been entirely self-supporting since school, and at the time of the study, 83 percent were employable and usually had employment. The range of occupations was wide: some were in management positions, others in clerical or sales positions, others were skilled laborers, although not surprisingly, many were in unskilled labor categories. Only nine were institutionalized. One interesting finding was that 16 percent had died, a figure considerably higher than would be expected by chance. This study demonstrated quite conclusively that many people labeled retarded by the schools go on to lead independent, useful lives.

Socioeconomic and Racial Differences in Prevalence

Special classes and other treatment programs for the mentally retarded have become very much a political issue because retardation is found far more frequently among the poor than among the more well-off families in this country. For example, Mercer (1973), in her survey of agencies dealing with the retarded, found that while only 40 percent of the population of her community lived in low-income housing districts, 59 percent of the retarded individuals reported by these agencies lived in low-income housing areas. However, this discrepancy is largely limited to the mildly retarded. Mild retardation is almost exclusively found among low-income groups. Moderate, severe, and profound retardation are found in all income groups with only a slight overrepresentation in low-income families. This observation has some extremely important implications for the definition of, treatment of, and prevention of mental retardation. It has been widely suggested that there are two qualitatively different forms of mental retardation: one group labeled cultural-familial, which is found almost exclusively in the low-income groups and which is characterized by only mild retardation and the lack of other physical problems, and the other group labeled organically retarded, which is characterized by much lower IQs and by obvious organic disorders. Cultural-familial retardation is far more common than is organic retardation. This is such an important area of retardation that all of Chapter 7 is devoted to the relationship between social status and mental functioning.

A related finding is that retardation is much more prevalent among racial minorities such as blacks and Mexican-Americans than it is among whites of Northern European descent, a group that Mercer calls Anglos. For example, in her prevalence study, 82 percent of the community population was Anglo, 10 percent were Mexican-Americans, and 7 percent were black. However, of the 812 retardates on the records of various agencies, 32 percent were Mexican-American, three times as many as in the general population, and 12 percent were black, nearly twice what should be expected. A large part of this discrepancy can be explained by the fact that racial minorities tend to be in the lower income groups. However, this issue is also discussed in detail in Chapter 7.

Changes in Prevalence Over Time

A general trend in prevalence studies is that more recent studies tend to show a higher prevalence of mental retardation than do studies done many years ago. Research done around the turn of the century reports a prevalence several orders of magnitude lower than do more recent studies summarized above. Farber (1968) summarized the results of seven such projects done between 1906 and 1916. The range of prevalences reported in these seven studies is 3.82 to 7.35 per thousand with a mean of 4.68. Compare this figure with the prevalence of 35.2 per thousand reported by Goodman. Certainly, part of the reason for this discrepancy is that earlier studies were less thorough and more cases were missed, but the primary reason for the difference lies in changing definitions of mental retardation. Prior to the era of widespread testing and universal public education, an individual had to be rather severely deficient in order to cause alarm, and presumably many people who would now be considered mildly retarded could survive perfectly well in a simpler society. As society becomes more complex, a larger percentage of the population becomes unable to cope with independent living and thus, is likely to be labeled mentally retarded. This trend will probably be reversed in the future, and it is possible that the term mentally retarded will be reserved only for the more severely mentally handicapped people. The elimination of the category of borderline retardation is an example of this trend.

Modern medical research has also had effects on the prevalence of mental retardation, but the effects have been in both directions. There now exist medical cures and prevention for many syndromes of retardation such as cretinism, galactosemia, and phenylketonuria. In addition, improved obstetric techniques have drastically reduced the incidence of brain damage at birth. However, one negative effect of modern medicine is that many children who were born prematurely or had congenital deformities who in earlier times would have died can now be saved but are mentally retarded.

Summary of Prevalence Research

The research on prevalence clearly illustrates many of the problems with the current conception of mental retardation. The prevalence figure that a given survey arrives at is directly dependent on the method used to obtain the data, and different surveys produce quite different results. There are certain cases, perhaps 8 to 10 in a thousand, whom virtually everyone would agree are mentally retarded. This group would include all of the moderately, severely, and profoundly retarded as well as some cases of mild retardation. There are a great many more individuals, perhaps 20 to 25 in a thousand, who would be considered retarded some of the time by some people, but not mentally retarded under different circumstances. This distinction is similar to Kanner's relative and absolute feeblemindedness discussed above. The best example of a child who is relatively retarded is the child who has enough difficulty with academic subjects to be labeled mentally retarded by the school system and assigned to a special class, but when the child goes home at the end of the day or leaves school permanently, he or she is able to function relatively effectively. Such a child is considered mentally retarded by teachers and other school personnel, but is not considered retarded by family, friends, or neighbors. The President's Committee on Mental Retardation (1970) refers to such people as "six-hour retarded children" suggesting that they are retarded for only a part of each day.

Mercer's (1973) landmark study provides support for this distinction. She surveyed a number of people in the same community in which she had done her other surveys, and she asked them if they knew of any retarded people in the neighborhood. A total of 243 individuals were nominated; these nominees had a mean IQ of only 55, substantially lower than the IQ of 64, which was the mean of those named as retarded by the schools and other agencies. Also, the racial and socioeconomic differences that were so predominant in those named by the latter were nonexistent in the group of retarded nominated by lay people. Thus, the person considered retarded by a nonprofessional must have an IQ somewhat lower than that required for a professional to consider him or her retarded, and almost all of the people considered retarded by professionals but not by lay people are from culturally deprived or minority backgrounds.

In the first chapter, it was mentioned that one of the difficulties with labeling is that there is usually a grey area, a group of people who do not fit neatly into one category or the other. One of the characteristic problems of determining the prevalence of mental retardation is that this grey area is so large. Probably the majority of the people who have been labeled retarded fall into this area of relative retardation. This means that it is impossible to determine with any precision exactly how many retarded people there are in the country. Certainly, there is good reason to be skeptical of the 3 percent figure that is so widely cited by groups interested in emphasizing the importance of the problem of mental retardation, but any other prevalence estimate is likely to be equally suspect. In a very real sense there is no such thing as a true prevalence of mental retardation.

Criticisms of the Concept of Mental Retardation

As the above chapter implies, the area of the definition of mental retardation is in a good deal of ferment, and an increasing number of people are beginning to challenge the traditional ways that mental retardation has been conceptualized and delineated.

Many of the criticisms are directed toward what is widely referred to as the medical model, or what Mercer (1973) refers to as the clinical perspective. In this frame of reference, mental retardation is seen as comparable to a disease in medicine. There is an underlying condition, mental retardation, which causes symptoms, such as academic problems and inadequate adaptive behavior. This condition exists in the individual independently of whether it is diagnosed or not. It is possible for there to be a case of undiagnosed retardation just as there could be a case of undiagnosed rheumatic fever. Similarly, it is possible for retardation to be misdiagnosed, that is, a person is labeled as retarded because he or she shows some of the symptoms of retardation, but in fact is not retarded. If we adopt the assumptions of the medical model, then the crucial step in the treatment process is the diagnosis. Once a proper diagnosis is made, then the correct treatment can be initiated based on the diagnosis of underlying cause.

This medical model is misleading in a number of ways when it is applied to mental retardation. Mental retardation is not a disease. Mental retardation and low intelligence should not be used to explain behavior because no one knows what low intelligence is and the only way that low intelligence and mental retardation can be inferred is by observing the behaviors that they are supposed to cause. Many behaviorists (e.g., Neisworth and Smith, 1973) have suggested that it is more productive to talk about children with retarded behavior rather than retarded children. This may appear to be a trivial distinction but it avoids some of the logical traps described in Chapter 2 in which the label is seen as the cause of the behavior. Such an outlook suggests that the most productive treatment approach is to treat the symptoms directly and ignore any underlying cause. For example, if a child is having trouble reading in school, it will be far more productive to give the child intensive training in reading than it will to determine whether the child is retarded or not by administering an IQ test. This approach is directly contrary to the medical model, which suggests that treating the symptoms while ignoring the underlying cause is futile.

Mercer (1973) criticizes the current view of mental retardation from a somewhat different point of view. She suggests that mental retardation is a social role rather than an inherent characteristic of individuals. A social role is a category into which people are placed, and people placed in this category are expected to act in certain ways. From this point of view, a person is defined as being mentally retarded if other people consider him or her to be mentally retarded. The above chapter cited a good deal of evidence to support this view. The majority of people who are labeled retarded in this country fall into the category of relative rather than absolute retardation; their retardation is not inherent within them but results from the interaction of the individual with the environment. The same individual in a different environment would no longer be retarded. This is very different from a medical disorder. A person with cancer continues to have cancer wherever he or she goes, but it is possible for a child to be retarded at school but not at home.

Mercer provides a good demonstration of this point. In her community, there was a parochial school system in addition to the public schools. The public schools gave all of their pupils group intelligence tests and employed several school psychologists whose primary function was to diagnose retardation. The parochial schools had no testing, no special classes, and reported that they did not service the mentally retarded. There were a number of obviously slow children in the parochial schools, but they attended the same classes as everyone else and had no chance of being labeled retarded because there was no mechanism for it. If children attended the parochial school system, they could not be mentally retarded. However, if one of these slow children should happen to transfer to the public school system, the child might very well "become" mentally retarded by being diagnosed as such.

An even more extreme version of the same argument is that labeling a child as retarded provides a convenient mechanism for a teacher or in some cases even a parent to get rid of an unwanted child. If a teacher has a child who is a disciplinary problem, the teacher can refer the child to the school psychologist where the child may be diagnosed as retarded and sent to a special class. Special classes for the retarded have often been accused of being a dumping ground for undesirable children, and the mechanism for placing children there is to label them as retarded. Evidence for this comes from the fact that there is usually a considerable amount of overlap in abilities between children in a special class for EMR children and the lower functioning children in a regular class. (Garrison and Hammill, 1971).

Braginsky and Braginsky (1974) have used a similar argument to suggest that some of the children in institutions for the retarded are placed there because their parents or society do not want them around. Their research on children placed in such institutions indicates that many are functioning as well or better than many children on the outside, and the main reason why they are there is that there is no other appropriate home for them outside the institution. Virtually all came from poor homes, and they had either been actively rejected by their parents or else they had to be removed from their home because their family was such a bad influence on them. They suggest that in many cases, the decision to institutionalize the child was made prior to the diagnosis of retardation, and the diagnosis was made solely to make the placement legally possible. They conclude that "mental retardation, like mental illness, is not a psychological concept, but rather a sociopolitical one. It is another of the many myths perpetrated by a society that refuses to recognize its needed social reforms. The camouflage of the politics of diagnosis and incarceration have led to an enormous expenditure of time, effort, and money in a useless search for psychological and biological factors when the real problem exists in society" (Braginsky and Braginsky, 1974, p. 30).

The points made by Mercer and by the Braginskys are important because they stimulate thinking, and they point out some of the weaknesses in the more traditional ways of thinking about mental retardation, but their position should not be taken too literally. They tend to imply that there are no differences at all between most people who are labeled retarded and the general population, and this is clearly not true. While some people who are labeled retarded are more capable than some people who are not labeled, the diagnosis of retardation is not made on an entirely capricious basis. There will always be people who lack the mental abilities to successfully adjust to society, and thus, mental retardation is more than a sociopolitical concept.

Perhaps the most serious criticism of the concept of mental retardation is simply that it is not very useful. The knowledge that a person is retarded says very little about what kind of programming, therapy, or other services may be required. There are virtually no teaching methods that work better for retarded children than they do for nonretarded children, and there is little educational justification for placing all of the children who have been labeled retarded in a special classroom segregated from all the "normal" children. There is general agreement today that far too much effort was devoted by diagnosticians in the past to determining what the proper label was for a child's problem, and not enough effort devoted to determining what types of teaching and therapy would best be able to improve the functioning of a particular child.

Criticisms such as those described above have begun to have a major impact on public policy. The label mentally retarded is certainly used a good deal more cautiously now than was the case a few years ago. One example of this trend is the elimination of the category of borderline retardation. Most psychological testers and educators are now less concerned with labeling and categorizing children and are more oriented toward determining the strengths and weaknesses of each individual case. Treatment is now more likely to be oriented toward individual problems rather than toward specific diagnostic categories. Most government funding is now earmarked for "children with developmental disabilities" or for "children with special needs" rather than for specific diagnostic categories. If this trend continues, it will have important implications for the study of mental retardation. It is possible that future prevalence studies will report much smaller prevalence figures for example. In fact, in a few years, the diagnostic category mentally retarded may not even exist any more.

Summary

Traditional attempts to define mental retardation have fallen into three categories: those based on low IQ, those based on general social incompetence, and those based on some sort of constitutional defect such as brain damage. The most widely accepted definition of mental retardation today is that adopted by the American Association on Mental Deficiency, and it represents a combination of the first two approaches. A person labeled mentally retarded must score at least two standard deviations below average for his or her age group on a standard intelligence test and must show significant impairments in adaptive behavior. Also, these deficiencies must develop during childhood or adolescence. This definition of retardation makes no mention of cause. Mental retardation can be just as easily caused by an unstimulating environment or an emotional problem as it can by a biological defect. It is also important to note that mental retardation is not defined as a permanent condition; it is possible for people to be mentally retarded when they are 10 years old and not retarded when they are 15.

Most studies of the prevalence of mental retardation conclude that about 3 percent of the population of the United States is retarded. However, it is meaningless to try to precisely specify the prevalence because minor differences in how retardation is defined can result in major differences in prevalence estimates. Some researchers feel that the 3 percent figure is far too high since the majority of these 3 percent represent the relatively retarded, those people who are handicapped in situations where demands of an academic nature are made but who are able to function adequately otherwise.

There are considerable differences in the prevalence of mental retardation among different segments of the population. Among these differences are the following. (1) Mental retardation is found more often among males than among females in a ratio of about three to two. (2) Mental retardation is found far more often among children of school age than it is among either preschoolers or adults. (3) Mental retardation is found far more often among low income families and among racial minorities.

Findings such as these have prompted many people to criticize the traditional clinical view of mental retardation, the view that mental retardation is a permanent condition inherent within the individual and analogous to a disease in medicine. It might be more productive to consider it the result of an interaction of a given set of abilities with a given set of environmental expectations. Thus, as society becomes more complex, more people become mentally retarded. Many people who are considered mentally retarded by the schools are able to adjust to adult life with a few problems once they leave school, and thus they no longer have an impairment in adaptive behavior.

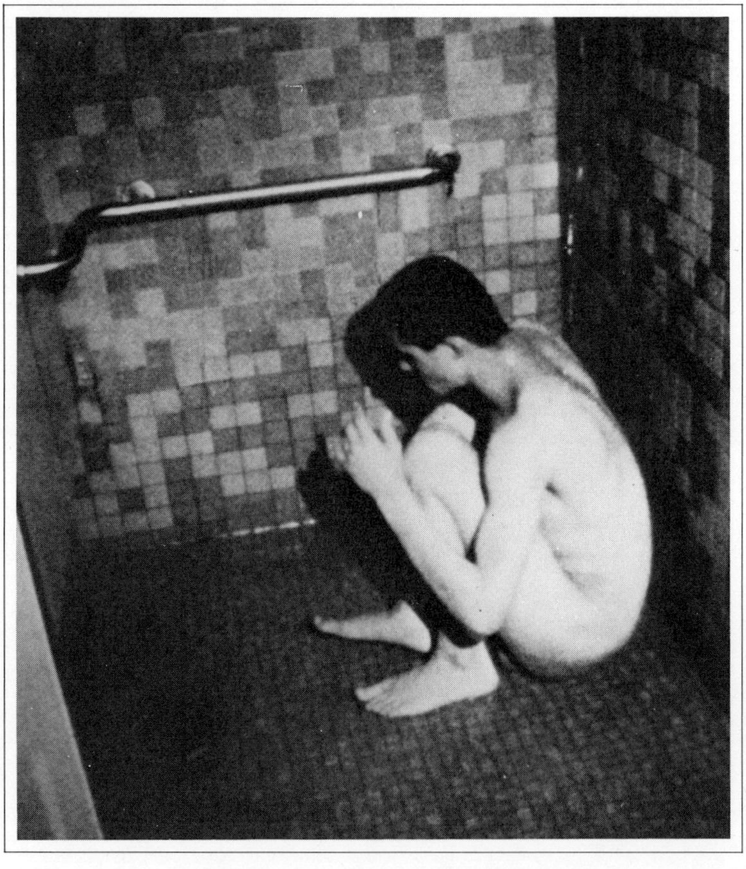

4

A Brief History of Mental Retardation

Mental retardation in its various forms has presumably existed as long as man, and there is even evidence of the equivalent of mental retardation in animals. However, the period prior to about 1800 can safely be considered pre-history as far as the study of mental retardation is concerned. Before this time, there was no scientific study of retardation to speak of, and there was little attempt to provide the retarded with special treatment or training. Early writings make little distinction between the retarded and other types of handicapped people such as the insane, criminals, deaf mutes, or epileptics. There are sporadic references to fools, idiots, and "those without reason" in ancient and medieval writings, but little is said about them. They were occasionally retained by noblemen for entertainment; many court jesters would apparently now be diagnosed as retarded. In other places handicapped people were thought to be closer to God and were treated with special reverence. For example, the astronomer Tycho Brahe retained a fool as a close companion and frequently sought his advice, much as the ancient Greeks sought counsel from the Oracle of Delphi, who was apparently an epileptic. Other people, particularly early Protestants, felt that retarded people were possessed by the Devil, and many people who would now be considered retarded became victims of witch hunts and other forms of persecution. For the most part, however, the retarded were merely tolerated. They were given basic care by their families, and they helped with the work wherever they could, but no special provisions were made for them.

Early Pioneers

In the late eighteenth and early nineteenth centuries, there developed a widespread concern in Western Europe and America for previously neglected peoples such as slaves, prisoners, and the insane, and a number of people took an interest in the mentally retarded. This early history of the treatment of retardation is largely a story of individuals, who by their own work, stimulated others to treat all sorts of handicapped people more humanely.

Jean Itard

The first of these noteworthy individuals was a Frenchman named Jean Itard. As a young man he achieved some distinction as a physician, and be became medical director at the Institution for Deafmutes in Paris. In 1798, a child of 11 or 12 years old was found in the woods near Aveyron. This child was mute and manifested no evidence of training or exposure to other people. He was hailed by some as an example of man in his natural state, untainted by culture, because he subsisted on nuts, roots, and berries, and wore no clothes. He could withstand extreme cold and heat and apparently relied much more on his sense of smell than do civilized men. The boy was diagnosed as hopelessly defective by various physicians, but Itard took an interest in the case and requested an opportunity to train the boy. Itard had been influenced by the English philosopher John Locke, who believed that everything a person becomes is determined by that person's environment, and that man's capabilities were almost infinite if he were raised properly. Thinking in this way, Itard believed that the boy could acquire all of the abilities of a civilized man with proper training.

Itard employed a wide variety of techniques in his attempt to socialize and educate the boy, whom he called Victor. For example, he tried to train the boy's senses one at a time by blindfolding him and teaching him to discriminate between the sounds of a bell and a drum. He trained his memory by placing a chestnut under one of three cups and permitted him to select one. He taught Victor basic social skills such as dressing, eating with utensils, and toilet training. Itard was not as successful in teaching him to speak, and at the end of the program, Victor could speak two words, *lait* (milk) and *O Dieu* (God). After five years of training, Itard had made considerable progress; he had transferred Victor from an incontinent, insensitive, emotional animal to a partially civilized human who could recognize objects and understand many words. However, Itard considered his experiment a failure because Victor was still unable to take care of himself, and he was eventually institutionalized. However, Itard was able to demonstrate that even a child who was diagnosed as an idiot could be taught many social skills if he were exposed to a systematic training program, and in this way, he made a major contribution to the attitudes of society toward retarded people.

Edouard Seguin

After Itard's failure with Victor at the turn of the century, little was done with mentally retarded children for about three decades. In 1835, one of Itard's students, Edouard Seguin, undertook the education of an idiotic boy. After a year and a half of training, his pupil "was able to make better use of his senses, could remember and compare, speak, write, and count." Seguin's success earned him a great deal of distinction, and he began to treat more retarded children and systematize his method. In 1846, he published a text on the training and treatment of the retarded that won him worldwide recognition, including a personal letter from the Pope for his humanitarian work. Two years later, revolution broke out in Paris, and Seguin emigrated to the United States where he continued his work, first as the head of a training school in Pennsylvania and later as a consultant in New York. In 1876, Seguin was elected the first president of the Association of Medical Officers of American Institutions for Idiotic and Feebleminded Persons, which was the forerunner of the present American Association on Mental Deficiency. Seguin's importance lies primarily in the fact that he was among the first to demonstrate that, with proper training, many mentally retarded people could be taught to do a great deal more than anyone else had thought possible. His system of education was called the Physiological Method. Much of the theory underlying it is now obsolete, but many of his specific educational techniques are still being used today. He believed in exercising the muscles through daily activities directed toward the child's own needs and capabilities, and he developed a number of activities toward training the muscles and the senses.

Samuel Howe

The name usually associated with the origin of the mental retardation movement in the United States is Samuel Howe. He graduated from Harvard Medical School in 1824 and then spent six years in Greece working with refugees. On his return, he became interested in deaf and blind children, and he began to take blind children into his home. Shortly afterward, he was offered a house and garden in Boston for his work, which became the Perkins

Institution for the Blind. Howe was the director of the institution until his death. He developed new teaching methods for the blind and deaf, but was also an avid campaigner for the rights of all kinds of oppressed and handicapped people, including the mentally retarded. In 1846, he was appointed the head of a commission to "inquire into the condition of idiots of the commonwealth, to ascertain their number, and whether anything could be done for their relief" (Kanner, 1964, p. 41). The commission's report made an impassioned plea for better treatment and training of the retarded, and the Massachusetts government provided Howe with funds to establish an experimental school for idiots. The school was a success and was incorporated on a permanent basis in 1855 under the name of the Massachusetts School for Idiotic and Feebleminded Youth. It is still in existence today as the Fernald State School.

The Institution Movement in America

Pioneers like Itard, Seguin, and Howe were able to demonstrate that with humane treatment and proper education it was possible to train the mentally retarded far beyond the level that most people thought was possible, and these three, along with other lesser known individuals, initiated a widespread social movement during the nineteenth century for a better treatment of the mentally retarded. In the United States, this movement took the form of establishing state training schools for the retarded where they could be given special treatment. The first such institution was Howe's in Massachusetts, but New York State followed three years later with an experimental school in Albany called the State Asylum for Idiots. Similar schools were established in Pennsylvania, Ohio, and Connecticut in the next decade, and by 1898, there were 24 such public institutions for the retarded in 19 states (Kanner, 1964). These institutions started with the noblest of intentions, to educate and "cure" retarded children, and these early training schools developed relatively advanced training and educational programs to teach music, carpentry, physical education, and other social skills as well as the traditional academic subjects. However, the institution movement quickly became sidetracked from its initial lofty aim. There were two reasons for this. First, the institutions grew quickly in size. Howe's initial experimental school had 10 students, but by 1917, the school had grown to more than 1500 residents. It was easy to provide high quality training for a small number of retarded children, but individual attention, so vital to the development of any youngster, retarded or not, becomes a rarity in a large state institution. A second reason for the change in the role of the institution was the fact that it quickly became apparent that good intentions and proper training would not by themselves "cure" retardation, and it became clear that most of the residents of these institutions would remain there indefinitely. Thus, the purpose of the institution shifted from that of a special educational center to a permanent care facility to provide for the needs of those who were unable to look out for themselves in society. As a result, the kind of child accepted by the institution began to change. At first, the training schools would only accept the most promising cases, but as their function changed, they began to accept more and more "hopeless" individuals, which only accelerated the change in institutional roles.

Eugenics and Social Darwinism

At the same time that Howe and Seguin were fighting for more humane treatment for the retarded, developments were occurring in the sciences that were to have profound effects, both positive and negative, on the attitudes of society toward the mentally retarded. In 1859, Charles Darwin published his revolutionary book *The Origin of Species* in which he proposed his theory of evolution by natural selection. Darwin suggested that the species of man had evolved from lower forms, and that the cause of this process of evolution and improvement was natural selection; that is, those species that are adaptive and able to cope with the stresses of life will increase while those species that are weak and poorly prepared to cope with life's adversity will die out, as did the dinosaurs. From Darwin's theory it was a logical step to assume that man was still evolving according to the laws of natural selection. Some individuals, some families, and some races are better able to cope with life because of superior endowments, both mental and physical, and these people will increase faster than those less well equipped. For example, if a certain family was very susceptible to a disease such as tuberculosis, more members of that family would die off without producing offspring, while members of a second family that was more resistant to tuberculosis would multiply. Extending this theory to political and social science, many people argued that it would be poor policy to interfere with this process of natural selection because by permitting those less favored by heredity to survive and bear children, the overall quality of the species would degenerate. Darwin himself took this position in a later book.

> *With savages, the weak in body or mind are soon eliminated; and those that survive commonly exhibit a vigorous state of health. We civilized men on the other hand do our utmost to check the process of elimination; we build asylums for the imbecile, the maimed, and the sick; we institute poor laws; and our medical men exert their utmost skill to save the life of every one to the last moment. There is reason to believe that vaccination has preserved thousands who from a weak constitution would formerly have succumbed to small-pox. Thus the weak members*

> *of civilized societies propagate their kind. No one who has attended to the breeding of domestic animals will doubt that this must be highly injurious to the race of man. It is surprising how soon a want of care, or care wrongly directed, leads to the degeneration of a domestic race; but excepting in the case of man himself, hardly any one is so ignorant as to allow his worst animals to breed* (Darwin, 1874, p. 149).

Thus, many people felt that any attempt to improve the lot of the poor, the weak, the insane, or the mentally retarded would be destructive to the species and counter-evolutionary. The assumption was that these people were inferior members of the race and ought to be allowed to die out.

In such an intellectual climate, the mentally retarded were bound to suffer, and feeblemindedness became the particular target of many "social Darwinists." In the late nineteenth and early twentieth centuries, people began to do research demonstrating that retardation ran in families and that it was closely related to a variety of social ills such as crime, alcoholism, prostitution, and other immorality. The best known of this research was a book called *The Kallikak Family* by H. H. Goddard (1912). He traced the ancestry of an inmate of an institution for the feebleminded for whom he invented the pseudonym Deborah Kallikak. Her great-great-great grandfather Martin Kallikak fought in the Revolutionary War. During the war, Martin fathered an illegitimate son, Martin Jr., by a retarded girl that he met in a tavern. "From him (Martin Jr.) have come 480 descendants; 143 of these we have conclusive proof were or are feebleminded while only 46 have been found normal. The rest are unknown or doubtful. Among those 480 descendants, thirty-six have been illegitimate; there have been thirty-three sexually immoral persons, mostly prostitutes; there have been twenty-four confirmed alcoholics; three epileptics; eighty-two died in infancy; three were criminals; eight kept houses of illfame" (Goddard, 1912). After the war Martin Kallikak Sr. married a girl of good family and from this union has come another line of very different character. There were 496 direct descendants, all of whom were respectable citizens; they became doctors, lawyers, educators, tradesmen, one even founded a university.

When intelligence tests became available, Goddard and others administered them to criminals, delinquents, and prostitutes, and he concluded that the majority of these people were also retarded. Such research could only have adverse affects on the way retarded people were treated. In the middle of the nineteenth century, a retarded person was seen as an unfortunate individual who deserved help. Gradually, however, this attitude changed to a view of a retarded person as a degenerate form of man whose very existence lowered the quality of the human race and who was seen as a rather direct threat to the future of the species.

A closely allied movement that flowered in the early twentieth century was eugenics, or selective breeding for desirable traits. Inspired by Galton, Goddard, and others, eugenicists proposed that the species could be improved for future generations if those with low intelligence were not encouraged to reproduce while those with the greatest mental abilities had many children. Naturally, the mentally retarded became one of their prime targets. Numerous solutions were proposed, but only two achieved widespread popularity. One was to segregate retarded people from the rest of society, at least during their reproductive years, in order to assure that they would not reproduce. Thus, institutions developed a new purpose, isolating the retarded from the rest of humanity. The second solution was sterilization. In 1907, Indiana became the first state to pass a law authorizing the sterilization of retarded people, and other states soon followed. By 1926, 23 states had sterilization laws, and a year later, the U.S. Supreme Court upheld their legality. By 1958, when the practice of sterilization had largely died out (although the laws remained), over 31,000 mentally retarded people had been sterilized (Davies, 1959). This represented only a small proportion of the total number of retarded people in the nation, but the figure is a good reflection of the negative attitudes that were widely held during that time.

The Beginning of the Scientific Study of Mental Retardation

Of course, developments in the sciences also had numerous positive effects on the treatments of the retarded. An important development in the latter part of the nineteenth century was the recognition that mental retardation was distinguished from mental illness. At the same time, there was an increased awareness that retardation itself was not a unitary condition; instead, there were many causes of retardation and many different levels. One source of confusion in researching the history of any kind of mental disorder is the inconsistency and inadequacy of terminology prior to the twentieth century. For example, early institutions in Europe were designed only for cretins (one kind of mental deficiency caused by an underactive thyroid gland). However, it is apparent that these institutions provided service for all different kinds of retarded people and that these educators were only vaguely aware that all retarded people were not cretins. The syndrome known as mongolism or Down's syndrome was discovered by Langdon Down in 1866. However, consistent with the ethnic and racial thinking prevalent at the time, he saw mongolism as an example of degeneration, a regression from a higher race (Caucasian) to a lower race (the Mongol, or Oriental). The first serious attempt to classify the retarded according to etiology was a book by William Ireland, *On Idiocy and Imbecility,* published in 1877. He classified retardation into 12 subdivisions according to etiology.

Much of the terminology is now obsolete, but he showed a clear recognition that there were numerous different types of retardation.

The scientific study of mental retardation took a giant step forward with the development of intelligence tests. Prior to Binet's first test in 1905, there was no simple or standard way to diagnose retardation. Several writers mention that idiocy is immediately apparent to the untrained eye, a fact that is only partially true and certainly misleading. The first person to use intelligence tests in America was Goddard, the author of the study of the Kallikak family. Goddard was immediately struck by their usefulness. He proposed a classification system based on levels of retardation that was prevalent for many years. Idiots were those with mental age below 2, imbeciles were those with a mental age between 3 and 7, and morons had a mental age between 7 and 12. The category of moron was a new one, and many people were alarmed that so many individuals living in their community would be classified as retarded. If it is assumed that everyone with a mental age below 12 is retarded, the research on intelligence tests given to draftees during World War I indicates that nearly half the adult population falls into this category. This finding provided ammunition for eugenicists who argued that this was clear evidence that the intellectual ability of the average American was at a low level and declining (Sarason and Doris, 1969).

Largely because of the influence of the eugenics scare and the general social indictment of the retarded, the early decades of the twentieth century were not distinguished by notable progress in the treatment of the retarded. The one exception to this trend was the development of public school special classes for the retarded in some of the larger cities. The first special class for retarded children was opened in Providence, Rhode Island, in 1896, and in the next few years, a number of other cities followed suit. In 1905, New Jersey became the first state to provide a training program for the teachers of the mentally retarded. However, the number of special classes grew slowly, and until the 1950s, most communities provided little or nothing in the way of special education for the retarded. During this time, retardation was seen as largely an institutional problem rather than a responsibility of the local communities. Retarded children who were not institutionalized were either placed in regular classes where they received little or no special attention or else they did not attend school at all.

Changing Attitudes toward the Retarded

During the 1930s, there were some developments in politics and in psychological research that were to bring about a gradual but rather profound change in the attitudes of society toward its handicapped citizens in the years following. In the 1930s, the country was too concerned with the Great Depression to worry about providing better services for the disabled, but the Depression and accompanying New Deal changed the attitudes of many people toward the role of the government in the welfare of the citizens. Because so many people were facing dire poverty, apparently through no fault of their own, people began to feel that the government had a major responsibility to provide assistance for its less fortunate citizens. The result was increased welfare and social security programs, and later, this feeling was to carry over to the mentally retarded.

Another important development during this period was the questioning of many previously unchallenged assumptions about intelligence. Research at the University of Iowa indicated that one's intelligence was not as fixed as was generally believed. Numerous cases were documented of people whose IQ rose substantially as a result of being exposed to better environmental circumstances. Such findings weakened the assumption that mental retardation was a hopeless condition. The most stifling environment of all was found to be an institutional environment where the residents received little attention or stimulation. As a result, the image of the institution began to change from a very positive one, a place where hopelessly retarded people could be cared for, where they would receive special training, and where they could be segregated from the rest of society for their own good and the good of society, to a much more negative image, a place where people were locked up against their will and where their intelligence was further lowered as a result of the stifling conditions.

It was not until after World War II that these changes in attitude began to have any positive effects. A major milestone in the history of the mentally retarded in America was the formation of the National Association for Retarded Children (NARC) in 1950. This was an organization made up of parents of retarded children and other interested citizens, which was instrumental in organizing nurseries, day care centers, special classes, activity centers, recreation programs, and sheltered workshops. Now for the first time, the retarded had an effective lobby to influence legislation and to look out for the best interests of retarded children. The organization grew rapidly, and by 1960, it had a membership of 50,000. It presently has a membership of about 250,000 and has changed its name to the National Association for Retarded Citizens. Its very formation signified a breakthrough since it indicated that an increasing number of parents, rather than being ashamed of their retarded child, were willing to work for better services for them. Throughout the 1950s and 1960s, partially under the impetus of the NARC, services for the mentally retarded grew rapidly. Special classes in the public schools multiplied, not only for higher-level retarded children, but even for trainable and severely retarded children, a group that had been almost com-

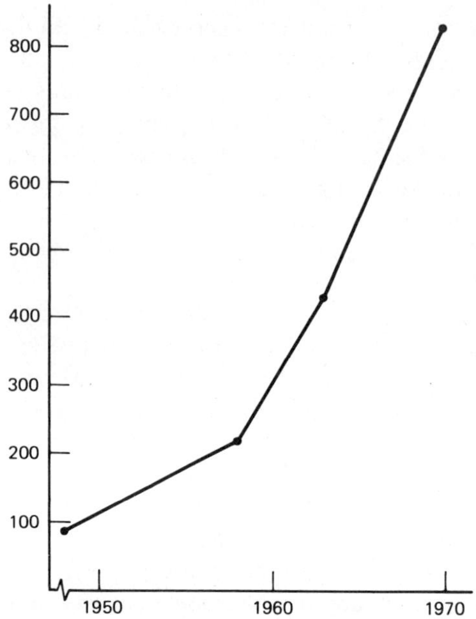

Figure 4-1 Number of mentally retarded children enrolled in special programs in the U.S., 1948–1970. (Enrollments in thousands.) From the *Statistical Abstract of the United States, 1975.*

pletely neglected previously. Most states passed laws requiring school districts to provide quality special education for everyone who could benefit from it, and funds were allocated to facilitate this. Special education has evolved from being the neglected stepchild of education to become almost a glamor field, with school districts competing to establish the most progressive programs and with many of the brightest college students aiming for careers in special education. Figure 4-1 shows the growth in total enrollment in classes for the mentally retarded over the postwar period.

Federal Involvement in Mental Retardation

The President's Panel on Mental Retardation

Up through the early 1960s, the federal government had virtually no involvement in programming for the retarded. Programs were funded almost entirely by the states, by individual communities, or by private sources.

However, President Kennedy had a particular interest in retardation, and shortly after he took office in 1961, he established a special committee called the President's Panel on Mental Retardation with a mandate to prepare a national plan to combat mental retardation. The panel's report, submitted a year later, made a number of innovative recommendations and became a sort of master plan for government programming for the retarded. Among the proposals made by the panel were the following:

1. Developing mental retardation research centers at universities and institutions.
2. Developing a continuing government program for the collection of population statistics on the incidence, prevalence, and personal and social characteristics of the mentally retarded.
3. Establishment of an Institute of Learning to do research in learning processes, particularly in the retarded, accompanied by increased government spending to support basic research.
4. Encouraging more students to go into areas of medicine, research, and teaching that deal with the mentally retarded by increasing the number of fellowships and scholarships.
5. Improving genetic counseling for parents.
6. Improving prenatal and postnatal care for infants in high-risk areas.
7. The establishment of a domestic Peace Corps to attack the problem of cultural deprivation.
8. Developing programs for early screening of infants for possible developmental delay and the availability of expert diagnosis and evaluation for everyone suspected of mental retardation.
9. Establishment of community referral services to coordinate service and provide life consultation for retarded citizens.
10. Planning community-based recreational facilities and activity centers for retarded children and adults.
11. Making special education available to everyone who needs it.
12. Providing preschool enrichment programs for retarded and deprived children.
13. Expanding federal programs for vocational rehabilitation to include more retarded individuals.
14. Increasing efforts to encourage employers to hire retarded people.

15. Limiting institutional care to those whose needs can best be met by this type of service.
16. Establishing a legal protection service for the retarded to protect their legal rights.
17. The development of public awareness programs to educate the public about mental retardation.

This report was an extremely important document because it highlighted the changing public attitude toward the retarded. The emphasis of the recommendations was on local communities providing services rather than relying on state-run institutions to deal with problems. For the first time, the federal government was recognizing that mental retardation was a major public problem and that it had a responsibility to develop a coordinated program to attack it.

Inspired by President Kennedy and the President's Panel report, the remainder of the decade saw a number of landmark laws passed to provide federal assistance to the mentally retarded on broad fronts. Two major pieces of legislation were passed in 1963: the Mental Retardation Facilities and Community Mental Health Centers Construction Act, which authorized federal funds for the construction of facilities for the diagnosis, treatment, training, and custodial care of the mentally retarded as well as providing for the construction of a number of comprehensive mental retardation research centers, and a second bill, which authorized money for grants to the states to begin comprehensive mental retardation planning on a coordinated interagency basis. The Elementary and Secondary Education Act of 1965 was one of the most important pieces of legislation to come out of President Johnson's Great Society program because, for the first time, massive federal money for the support of education was authorized. An amendment to this bill provided support for a wide variety of experimental educational programs for handicapped children, including the mentally retarded. In 1970, Congress passed the Developmental Disabilities Services and Facilities Construction Act, which expanded the money available for construction of facilities for the retarded.

Other federal programs were modified to fill the needs of retarded individuals. For example, Social Security payments to retarded people were greatly expanded to permit a retarded person to continue to receive dependency benefits after becoming 18, the age when such payments usually cease. The Office of Vocational Rehabilitation has been involved in providing job training for handicapped citizens for many years, but it was only in the 1960s that this office began to realize its responsibility toward the mentally retarded; and an increasing number of retarded persons have been rehabilitated each year. In 1971 for example, more than 35,000 mentally retarded people received vocational training under this program, about 12 percent of the total (*MR Source Book,* DHEW, 1972).

A trend that accelerated rapidly during the 1960s was the deemphasis of institutions as the primary facility for retarded individuals. During this decade, the number of state institutions almost doubled, from 108 in 1960 to 190 in 1970, but this disguises the fact that the new institutions were much smaller in size and were considerably less dehumanizing. As an indication of the improvement in care, the average amount of money spent per institution resident per day in 1960 was only $4.20, but by 1970, this figure had increased by 150 percent to $11.64. In 1968, a milestone was reached when for the first time since the institution movement began more than 100 years ago, the total number of retarded people in institutions decreased from the preceding year.

The 1970s: The Courts Step In

The decade of the 1970s has been characterized not so much by progressive new federal legislation, but by a number of very influential court decisions that have reaffirmed that retarded people are entitled to the same legal rights as are other citizens. In 1971 (*Wyatt* v. *Stickney*), a federal judge in Alabama ruled that people placed in a state institution against their will (as is the case with virtually all institutionalized mentally retarded people) are entitled to a full range of treatment services including medical, psychological, and educational attention. The judge ordered the state to hire additional staff and to otherwise provide additional professional services. Immediately, parent groups in other states initiated similar suits, charging the institutions with everything from inadequate medical attention to involuntary servitude. While other courts have somewhat watered down the Alabama decision (e.g., *Burnham* v. *Georgia,* 1972), virtually all of the states have now started programs to improve programming in their institutions and eventually to phase the large state institution out completely.

A Pennsylvania legal decision had an even wider impact. In *Pennsylvania Association of Retarded Children* v. *Commonwealth of Pennsylvania* (1972), a parent group filed a suit on behalf of 13 mentally retarded children who had been excluded from all forms of publicly supported education. At that time, Pennsylvania, like virtually every other state in the union, had a law specifying that any child deemed "ineducable and untrainable" was excused from public schooling, and, in practice, the word excused meant excluded. It was estimated that more than 14,000 children were being denied public school education under this law. The court ruled that all children, even the most severely retarded, were entitled to a free public education, and they ordered the state to identify, locate, and place all previously excluded children starting with the next school year. The court also ruled that each child must be placed in a program appropriate to the child's needs. This decision had far-reaching implications. Immediately, other states began to pass similar education-for-all legislation in an effort to avoid having such a program forced on them by the courts. In November 1975, Congress passed the Education of All Handicapped Children Act (PL 94-142), which made education-for-all the official policy of the federal government. Under this law, Washington would encourage the states to provide education and training to even the most severely handicapped by picking up a percentage of the cost. The amount of federal money available to the states and localities for education of the handicapped is scheduled to expand to more than three billion dollars by 1982. Thus, it is likely that, by the early 1980s, the United States will have truly universal public education.

The Pennsylvania decision also ruled that no child could be placed in a special class (or be removed from a special class to a regular class) without the informed consent of the child's parent. This decision is further evidence that the courts are beginning to recognize that retarded people have the same civil rights as anyone else, and that any decision which effects the child's welfare must be governed by the rules of due process. In many states, a child cannot even be given an intelligence test without the consent of the parents. The primary purpose of this policy is to provide parents of minority children with an opportunity to protest their child being labeled retarded.

Normalization

If there is a single word that best describes the current direction of services for the retarded and other handicapped people, that word would be *normalization.* Normalization refers to a philosophy of treatment and services that attempts to make the lives of retarded people as much like the lives of everyone else as possible. This represents a significant change in policy from just a few years ago, when services for the retarded were more likely to stress the differences between retarded people and nonretarded people, and as a result, they were likely to be segregated from the normal population in facilities where their life-style was extremely abnormal. One example of this normalization idea is the deinstitutionalization movement, the attempt to get as many retarded people as possible out of the large, oppressive state institutions and back into their home communities. An institution is the least normal living environment of all. People live in large, impersonal wards where they have no privacy and no control over their lives, and recent experience has demonstrated that many of those institutionalized retarded people can live far better in a small group home or a foster home where their life-style resembles that of everyone else to a much greater degree. A second example of normalization is the mainstreaming movement in public education in which many retarded and other handicapped children who in earlier decades would have been placed in special classes segregated from the mainstream of education are now provided with special services in a regular classroom with all the other students their own age. Both of these movements represent a change in outlook from emphasizing the differences between retarded people and everyone else toward stressing that retarded people are really not very different from many people considered normal.

Summary

Prior to the early 1800s there were virtually no programs for the mentally retarded or other handicapped people, but in the early nineteenth century a number of pioneers developed a special interest in securing better treatment for the retarded. For example, a Frenchman named Jean Itard attempted to educate an apparent "wild child" who had been found in the woods. One of Itard's students, Edouard Seguin, also attempted to train several retarded children and wrote what is probably the first text on the education of the mentally retarded. In the United States, Samuel Howe established the first training school for the mentally retarded in the 1850s.

For the next hundred years or so the center of services for the mentally retarded was the state residential institution. Early institutions were established with the noble goal of providing good services and training to the mentally retarded, but they became sidetracked from this lofty aim as they became more crowded and as they accepted more severely handicapped people.

During much of this time a major theme in social thought was "Social Darwinism," the application of Darwin's theory of the survival of the fittest to human society. Thus the mentally retarded were considered to be a threat to the future of the species. This belief was supported by research that indicated that mental retardation ran in families and that it was often associated with delinquency and immorality.

These negative attitudes toward the mentally retarded began to change slowly as scientists discovered more about the nature of mental retardation. Research indicated that intelligence was determined as much by upbringing and environment as it was by heredity and that one of the most stifling environments of all was an institution. Also, during the Depression there came about a fundamental change in the attitudes of the nation's citizens away from the ideas of rugged individualism and toward the idea that the government ought to help its less fortunate citizens. As a result, after World War II services for the mentally retarded grew rapidly. For example, the number of mentally retarded children enrolled in special classes increased nearly tenfold between 1948 and 1970. In 1962 a panel appointed by President Kennedy made a report on the status of the mentally retarded in the United States, and the recommendations of this committee formed the basis of government policy for a number of years. Largely as a result of the President's Panel report, the federal government began to fund programs for the mentally retarded on a massive scale. A fundamental shift in this programming was that the prime locus of service was not to be the state institutions, but the retarded individual's own community.

The 1970s have been marked not so much by landmark legislation as by court decisions that have affirmed the basic rights of retarded citizens. These include the right to full educational services for even the profoundly retarded and the right of treatment for those people institutionalized involuntarily. The single word that best describes the direction of programming in the 1970s is normalization, the attempt to make the lives of the handicapped as normal as possible.

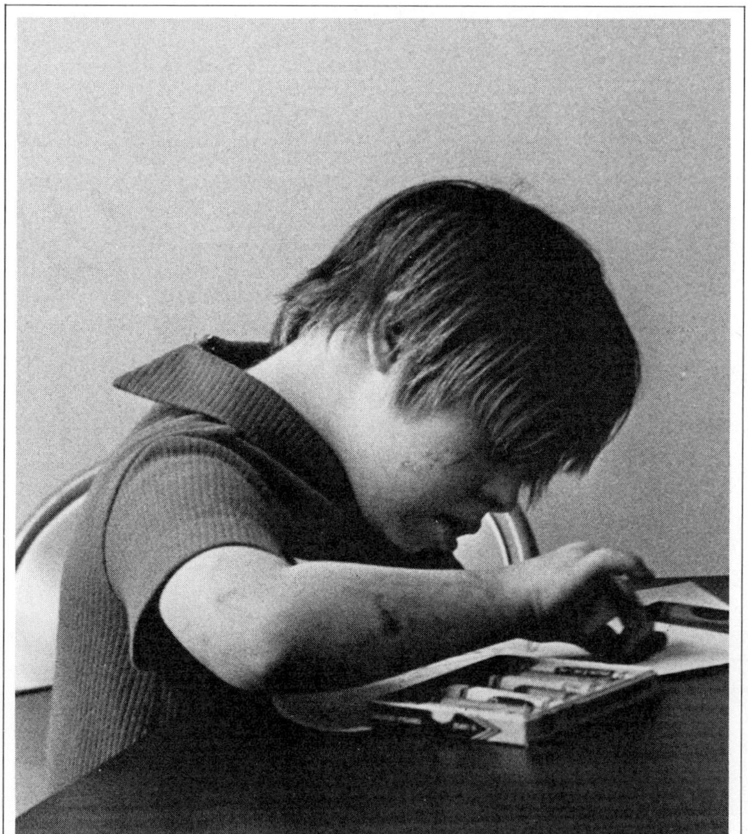

5

Biological Causes of Mental Retardation

It is possible to make a distinction between two broad categories of mentally retarded people. One category consists of all those people for whom there is substantial evidence that their diminished mental abilities are due to a specific organic cause such as a disorder in brain metabolism or specific nervous system damage. These people are often referred to as the organically retarded. Medical and biological science has made vast strides in the past few decades in determining many of these causes, and new syndromes of organic retardation are being discovered even today. The second category is considerably larger and includes those people for whom there is no apparent organic cause for their lowered intellectual capacities. These individuals have been labeled the culturally retarded (the term preferred by those who believe that this type of retardation has its origins primarily in the individual's psychosocial environment), the familially retarded (the term preferred by those who advocate a hereditary cause), and the functionally retarded. This book uses the latter term because of its more neutral connotation. Most individuals who are functionally retarded manifest only mild mental retardation, and most come from low-income families, while the organically retarded tend to be more severely impaired, and they are distributed with much less lower-class bias.

This chapter discusses some of the more common and better known syndromes and causes of organic mental retardation. These will be described using the classification system

Table 5-1 Major Categories of Organic Retardation

1. Infections and intoxications
2. Trauma or physical agents
3. Disorders of metabolism or nutrition
4. Gross brain disease (postnatal)
5. Unknown prenatal influences
6. Chromosomal abnormality
7. Gestational disorders
8. Retardation following psychiatric disorders
9. Retardation due to environmental influences

adopted by the AAMD (Grossman, 1973). This system divides the mentally retarded into nine broad categories based on the etiology (cause) of the retardation, with a tenth category, "Other." Table 5-1 lists these categories. The present chapter will discuss the first seven of these.

Infections and Intoxications

Prenatal Infections

An infection is a condition or disorder caused by microorganisms such as a virus or bacteria. Occasionally such a microorganism can attack the nervous system, resulting in mental retardation. The time when this is most likely to happen is prenatally, when the nervous system is just beginning to develop. Frequently an infection will cause either very mild symptoms or no symptoms at all as it infects the mother, but when it spreads to the child developing in her uterus, it causes serious and permanent malformations and abnormalities.

Rubella. The best known and the most serious of the various prenatal infections that can result in mental retardation is rubella, known colloquially as German measles. In adults and children, the rubella virus usually causes a mild sickness characterized by swollen glands and a skin rash. However, if a woman becomes infected with the rubella virus during the embryonic stage of pregnancy, the virus can also affect the developing child, producing a variety of serious defects. The last epidemic of rubella was in 1964–1965, and it is estimated that more than 30,000 infants were affected in some way (Holmes et al., 1972). The primary symptoms of congenital rubella are hearing loss, visual defects, mental retardation, and heart defects. In one study of 376 children whose mothers had had rubella during the first three months of pregnancy, the following symptoms were noted. One hundred and eight (29 percent) had cataracts, and 158 (42 percent) had other eye disorders. Nerve hearing loss was noted in 252 (67 percent) and 182 (48 percent) had heart disease. One hundred seventy of the 376 (45 percent) were mentally retarded. About half of these were only mildly retarded, but many others were severely retarded, and a number of the mentally retarded also had cerebral palsy (Cooper et al., 1969). There is a clear relationship between the time of infection and the severity of the symptoms. One study found that 47 percent of infants born to mothers infected during the first month were abnormal, but only 22 percent of those infected during the second month and 7 percent of those infected during the third month were abnormal (Michaels & Mellin, 1960). The overall incidence of defects is somewhat below that reported in other studies, but it clearly indicates the relationship between the time of infection and abnormality. Within the past few years, a vaccination against rubella has been developed, and thus, there is hope that this disease can be eliminated as a cause of retardation.

Syphilis. Another virus that can produce serious congenital defects is syphilis. Fortunately, syphilis can be readily detected and easily cured with penicillin if treated promptly, and as a result, the incidence of infants born with congenital syphilis has declined dramatically from earlier times. Syphilis was virtually eliminated in the United States in the 1950s, but, in the past decade, there has been a resurgence, and it is quite common again among adults. Because the disease can be so readily cured, its increasing incidence can only be accounted for by ignorance and the fact that many people are ashamed to seek medical help for a venereal disease. The incidence of congenital syphilis has increased slightly in the past few years, but it is still not a major medical problem, partially because a blood test for syphilis is required for a marriage license in most states.

A developing child is usually only infected if its mother has contracted the disease within two years and has not been properly treated. Many children with congenital syphilis die at birth, but for the survivors, the chances for a complete recovery are good if prompt treatment is initiated. The untreated disease has a long course, with different symptoms at different stages of development. In infancy, the syphilitic child may have skin lesions, a chronic runny nose with nasal hemorrhaging, and enlarged liver and spleen. As children, mental retardation becomes apparent, and it is frequently accompanied by other abnormal behavior and seizures. In addition, a characteristic saddle nose begins to develop. Adults with congenital syphilis have a characteristic skull shape, enlarged in the front, with saddle nose deformity, mental retardation, and seizures. Another frequent symptom is atrophy of the visual system, resulting in blindness (Holmes et al., 1972).

Other Infections. There are a number of other lesser known viruses that usually produce no symptoms in adults but can cause various birth defects if they infect a developing embryo. For example, cytomegalovirus is believed to infect about one in 3300 newborns. The effects of this infection are extremely variable. Some infants show no symptoms at all, but most show signs of neurological impairment and many are mentally retarded. Occasionally, the virus will produce cranial abnormalities such as hydrocephaly, an enlarged skull due to fluid pressure, or microcephaly, an unusually small skull (McCracken et al., 1969).

Toxoplasmosis is a disease caused by a protozoa. Like cytomegalic infection, the effects are quite variable. In one study of 300 infected children, slightly more than half showed signs of neurological disorders, with 26 percent also showing cranial abnormalities. Eye disorders were even more frequent (Couvreur and Desmonts, 1962).

Infections After Birth

Although most organic retardation originates prior to or during the birth process, it is possible for a child to be born with an intact nervous system but become mentally retarded some time after birth as a result of an injury or infection of the brain. The most common source of postnatal neurological damage is infection. There are a number of viruses that can produce permanent brain damage. Meningitis refers to an inflammation of the meninges, the membrane that protects the brain and spinal cord. It can be caused by a number of different types of microorganisms. The usual clinical picture is a child who was developing normally until contracting an acute illness. The illness is accompanied by high fever and later by signs of brain infection such as convulsions, headache, delirium, paralysis, and even coma. After a period of time, the child recovers, but the evidence of brain defect persists, and the child is either retarded or has a motor disability or a sensory impairment such as nerve deafness. The degree of impairment from meningitis varies widely; some children show no permanent effects, others are severely retarded.

Encephalitis refers to infection of the brain itself, and it also is often responsible for postnatally acquired mental retardation. Like meningitis, there are a number of different viruses that can produce it, and the symptoms are quite varied.

Intoxications

Another category of causes of mental retardation is intoxications, better known as poisons. This category refers to disorders in which a foreign substance of some sort enters the system of the child, either prenatally or after birth, and causes permanent damage of some sort.

Maternal Antibodies. There is an unusual set of circumstances in which a mother actually produces antibodies that attack the blood cells of the developing fetus and cause brain damage, mental retardation, and frequently death. About 85 percent of the population contains a substance in their blood called the Rh factor. These people are called Rh positive, and those without this factor are called Rh negative. Rh factor is transmitted genetically by a single gene, with Rh positive being dominant. Thus, if an Rh-negative woman marries an Rh-positive man, the offspring will probably be Rh positive. Ordinarily, this causes no problems, because the mother's blood and the blood of the developing fetus are separated, but occasionally, a few blood cells from the fetus get into the circulatory system of the mother. When the mother is Rh negative and the child is Rh positive, this causes the mother to produce an antibody to attack the foreign substance. This antibody can cross the placenta and enter the circulatory system of the fetus and cause the child's blood to clot and not distribute oxygen normally. The production of this antibody does not usually cause problems in the first pregnancy, but subsequent preganancies in which the fetus is Rh positive are in grave danger. In many cases, the problem is so severe that the infant is aborted or stillborn, but in less severe cases, the child is born with a condition known as erythroblastosis fetalis, which is characterized by the destruction of red blood cells. If the child survives, there may be severe neurological damage resulting in mental retardation, spasticity, and nerve hearing loss. There are a number of diagnostic symptoms. At birth, the child may be lethargic and hypotonic (insufficient muscle tone). Soon afterwards, a type of jaundice called kernicterus develops. The child may be feverish, and signs of nervous system damage may appear, such as unusual posture and hypertonicity (excessive muscle tension).

Until recently, this condition was an important cause of mental retardation. The traditional medical treatment is a complete blood transfusion in which all of the infant's blood is replaced with blood from donors. This procedure is generally effective in clearing up the condition, but there is evidence that lowered intelligence may still result in some cases (Gerver and Day, 1950). More recently, a preventive drug has been developed which, if administered to an Rh-negative mother within a few days of the birth of her Rh-positive child, prevents the formation of the antibodies. As a result of these developments, Rh incompatibility is a far less important cause of retardation than it used to be.

Drugs. Various drugs that the mother takes during pregnancy can have adverse effects on the developing child, and in some cases, drugs can cause delayed development. Drugs are an important concern because most women take several drugs during pregnancy, and a great many new drugs are introduced each year. The most dramatic example of the adverse effects of a drug on the developing child is the effect of the sedative thalidomide, which when taken by a woman during pregnancy, results in gross deformities of the child such as the absence of limbs. In theory, any drug that has been approved for use in this country has been demonstrated to be safe by careful research, but it will probably be just a matter of time before there is another tragedy similar to the one surrounding thalidomide.

The type of drug that concerns most public health officials is the nonprescription, nonmedical drugs such as alcohol, nicotine, and heroin. While there is no demonstrated relationship between the occasional consumption of alcohol and an increase in birth defects, Jones et al. (1973) have identified a syndrome of congenital disorders that is common among the children of alcoholic mothers. One of the characteristics of this syndrome is microcephaly and lowered mental abilities.

While at the present time, smoking has not been directly implicated as a cause of mental retardation, mothers who smoke during pregnancy are significantly more likely to give birth to a premature or small-for-date child (Pasamanick and Knobloch, 1966), and there is a clear relationship between prematurity and deficits in mental abilities.

Similarly, heroin and related drugs such as morphine or methadone can interfere with the normal development of the infant, and infants born to heroin-addicted mothers often display characteristics of drug withdrawal shortly after birth.

One category of drugs that is increasing in popularity very rapidly are the mild tranquilizers such as Librium, and at least one study (Milkovish and Van den Berg, 1974) has found some evidence of an increase in birth defects among children of mothers who took such drugs while they were pregnant. However, the increase in birth defects was only slight.

Other Prenatal Toxic Conditions. There are several other prenatal conditions that have been linked to birth defects, brain damage, and diminished mental abilities in the child. For example, one of the more common complications of pregnancy is a condition called toxemia. This disorder is characterized by swelling, edema, and high blood pressure. The cause is not known in most cases. While most offspring of mothers who had toxemia develop normally, the prevalence of mental retardation in these children is increased. Birch et al. (1970) studied the pregnancy and birth histories of more than 100 mentally retarded children in Scotland and found that more than 10 percent of the pregnancies of the mentally retarded children had been complicated by moderate to severe toxemia, compared with less than 3 percent of the control (nonretarded) pregnancies.

Various kinds of radiation can have drastic effects on a developing embryo or fetus. Small doses of ordinary X rays are apparently harmless, but if a pregnant woman is exposed to larger amounts of radiation for therapeutic purposes such as the destruction of a tumor, there is a high probability that the child will have serious birth defects or will not survive. For example, Murphy (1929) followed up 625 pregnant women who had been exposed to therapeutic doses of radiation and found gross birth defects in a third of the infants. There were a wide variety of defects, but the majority had involvement of the central nervous system, and the most frequent effect was microcephaly. Plummer (1952) found a greatly increased number of birth defects among the offspring of women who had been pregnant while exposed to the atomic blast over Hiroshima during World War II. Physicians are now very careful in using radiation therapy with pregnant women, but new uses of radiation are being developed regularly, and this could become a more important cause of birth defects in the future.

Almost any kind of health problem that the pregnant mother has can have a negative impact on the unborn child. Pregnant women who have heart disease, high blood pressure, or dibetes are more likely to have premature babies or other birth complications. Even maternal emotions can apparently have an effect on the development of the fetus. Davids, Devault, and Talmadge (1961) reported that mothers who received higher scores on an anxiety questionnaire had a higher incidence of pregnancy complications. Perhaps the higher level of stress hormones such as adrenaline can somehow affect the fetus.

Lead Poisoning. While most organic mental retardation can be traced to conditions prior to or during the birth process, one important toxic condition that generally develops some time after birth is lead poisoning. Lead poisoning has only recently gained attention as a possible important cause of mental retardation. The prime source of lead poisoning is paint that was manufactured before the 1940s. Many children, particularly low-income children, develop the habit of eating unnatural food substances, a condition called pica (Chisolm and Kaplan, 1968), and if they eat paint chips containing lead, they can suffer permanent brain damage. The symptoms of acute lead poisoning are similar to those of other neurological traumas, for example, convulsions, optic atrophy, perceptual difficulties, and sometimes lowered intelligence. While the effects of severe lead poisoning are well known, little is known about the effects of chronic ingestion of small quantities of lead over an extended period, and this is a serious problem among low-income children. Recently a number of cities have started screening programs for lead poisoning in poverty children, and several such programs report that more than 5 percent of inner city children have dangerously high levels of lead in their blood (Guinee, 1972).

Trauma and Other Physical Agents

Disorders Associated with the Birth Process

A second major category of causes of mental retardation is trauma and physical injuries. Unlike most other organic causes of mental retardation, which have their origins in conditions prior to birth, physical injury is unlikely to occur during the prenatal period because the developing fetus or embryo is fairly well protected by the mother. The time when physical injury is most likely to occur is the perinatal period, the time of the actual birth. The birth process is fairly complex, and there are many things that can go wrong.

Perinatal Anoxia. The most crucial aspect of the birth process is the transfer of respiration from the mother to the child. All during gestation, the child receives its oxygen from the mother's blood, but as soon as the child becomes detached from the mother's circulatory system, this source of oxygen is no longer available, and the child must breathe on its own for the first time. Cells need a constant supply of oxygen to function, and if the child is without oxygen for more than a few minutes, cells begin to die. Brain cells are among the first to succumb, and they are unique in that they cannot be replaced. The condition of lack of oxygen is known as anoxia. There are several ways that anoxia can develop. If the birth is long and complicated, the placenta may become detached from the wall of the uterus before the child is born, resulting in a time when the child is not getting oxygen from the mother, but is not yet able to breathe on his own. If the umbilical cord develops a kink or becomes wrapped around the child's neck, this can produce anoxia. Anoxia can also develop if the child does not begin to breathe immediately after birth. This is particularly likely to occur if the mother has been heavily sedated during labor. Apparently, the drug enters the circulatory system of the child and slows down the metabolic rate. Perhaps the best follow up study of anoxic infants is that of Graham et al. (1962). They found that preschoolers who had been anoxic at birth were significantly lower than a comparison group on a number of measures of mental functioning including the Stanford-Binet, a vocabulary test, and a concepts test. There was also a higher incidence of indications of neurological damage.

Mechanical Injury. During the birth process, the newborn is subject to a number of physical stresses. In the normal birth, the infant's head is down and this opens up the birth canal. The bones of the skull are still flexible, and frequently, the head of a newborn is misshapen. Ordinarily, this is not a cause for alarm, but occasionally, if the stresses of birth are too great, internal hemorrhaging may occur, resulting in brain damage. This is particularly likely if the labor is very short or if the infant, instead of being born head first, is presented buttocks first, a breech delivery.

In the case of multiple births, all of these perinatal hazards are increased. Because there are two or more fetuses developing at the same time, any effects of maternal malnutrition are multiplied. Twins are more likely to be born prematurely, and there are more likely to be other birth complications when two children are born at the same time. Several studies have documented that fact that on the average, twins have slightly lower IQs than do single births (Vandenberg, 1968).

Postnatal Trauma and Child Abuse

After infection, the most frequent cause of postnatally acquired retardation is physical injury of some sort, resulting either from an accident or from deliberate aggression. Obviously, these injuries take a wide variety of forms, and there is no precise pattern of symptoms. The importance of postnatal physical injury as a cause of retardation is uncertain because parents will occasionally attribute retardation in their child to a fall when in fact this is not the cause.

One variant of physical injury that has only recently received attention is the battered child syndrome, injuries that result from deliberate punishment by the parents or other caretaker. Estimates of the frequency of child abuse are difficult to obtain because parents generally deny that they inflicted the wound, and physicians are often reluctant to accuse parents unless child abuse is undeniable. Parents inflict a wide variety of injuries to their children, everything from burning to beating to bone breaking. As with many other causes of retardation, child abuse is more frequently found in the lower socioeconomic groups, although many cases have been discovered even among well-to-do families. The seriousness of the problem is illustrated by a survey by Kempe et al. (1962) who surveyed a number of hospitals and district attorneys and found 749 reported cases of child abuse in a one-year period. Among these cases were 78 fatalities and 114 children suffering from permanent brain damage. In a follow up of 50 children hospitalized for child abuse, Elmer and Gregg (1967) found that 8 had died and an additional 5 were in institutions for the mentally retarded. They found a high rate of speech disturbances, emotional disorders, and lowered intellectual functioning among the remainder.

Disorders of Metabolism or Nutrition

A third category of causes of mental retardation is conditions that result either from the child not getting proper nutrition or from the child not being able to properly metabolize what is eaten due to an inherited disorder. This latter group will be discussed first.

Inherited Metabolic Disorders

Phenylketonuria (PKU). Occasionally an individual is born with an inherited inability to properly metabolize one or more of the essential amino acids, which are the building blocks of proteins. Almost all of these conditions are extremely rare, but one that is very important is called phenylketonuria, usually shortened to PKU.

PKU is transmitted by a single recessive gene, and it is a classic example of Mendelian inheritance. There are apparently two possible genes that can occupy a certain position on one of the chromosomes, one of which results in a normal individual and can be designated the *N* gene, the other can result in an individual with PKU and will be designated the *p* gene. Every individual receives two of these genes, one from each parent. The combination of genes that an individual has is referred to as his genotype, and thus there are three genotypes that are possible for this particular locus. An individual can have two *N* genes, designated an *NN* genotype, he can have two *p* genes, a *pp* genotype, or he can have one of each, an *Np* genotype. Individuals with an *NN* genotype are always normal for this trait, individuals with a *pp* genotype always have PKU, and individuals with one gene of each type, an *Np* genotype, are also normal. Because when one gene of each type is present, the trait of the *N* gene is present, the *N* gene is called dominant and the *p* gene is called recessive. It is common practice to designate dominant genes with an upper-case letter and recessive genes with a lower-case letter.

The vast majority of the population, probably about 98 percent, are of the *NN* genotype, and this means they do not have PKU and that none of their children can have the disorder. However, about 2 percent of the population have the genotype *Np*. These people also do not have PKU and probably do not even know that they carry the *p* gene. However, these individuals are known as carriers, and if two carriers happen to marry, then they are capable of producing children with the disorder. Each parent will contribute one of his two genes to each child, and each gene has an equal probability of being donated. Each parent will, on the average, donate an *N* gene half the time and a *p* gene half the time. Thus it can be proven mathematically that a child resulting from the mating of two carriers (*Np* genotype) has a 25 percent chance of having the *pp* genotype and thus having PKU. A child from such a marriage has a 50 percent chance of having an *Np* genotype, thus being normal but a carrier. A child also has a 25 percent chance of having an *NN* genotype, thus not even being a carrier. Notice that while the probability is one in four that any given child will have PKU if both parents are carriers, this does not mean that exactly one fourth of their children will have this trait. It is possible for such a couple to have five or six children with none having PKU, and it is possible that they will have three or four children with PKU in a row.

PKU results from the body's inability to properly metabolize one of the basic amino acids, phenylalanine. The *N* gene is apparently responsible for the manufacture of the enzyme phenylalanine hydroxylase, which converts phenylalanine to another amino acid, tyrosine. Individuals lacking the *N* gene cannot produce the enzyme, and thus this vital metabolic reaction does not occur. As a result, phenylalanine is converted to phenylpyruvic acid, which is secreted in relatively large quantities in the urine.

The disease was discovered in 1934 by Dr. Asbjorn Følling, a Norwegian physician. A concerned mother had referred her two severely retarded children to him, and in the course of his examination, he noticed a musty odor to their urine. Chemical analysis indicated that the smell was due to phenylpyruvic acid, a substance not usually found in normal urine. Følling surveyed several hundred severely retarded institutionalized children and found a number of others with high phenylpyruvic acid. He labeled the new disease imbecilitas phenylpyruvica, but this name fortunately did not achieve wide acceptance. Others began to do research on the disorder, and the nature of the disease and its mechanism of transmission were gradually discovered.

The most important symptom of PKU is low intelligence. The majority of those afflicted are profoundly retarded, and nearly all of the remainder have IQs of less than 50 at adulthood (Knox, 1960). At birth, the child's nervous system is intact and development may proceed normally for a few months, but brain damage occurs gradually, probably because of poisoning by excess phenylalanine. This brain damage results in a progressive deterioration of abilities over the course of development. Occasionally, a child will say a few words, but loses the ability to speak as he or she grows older. Delayed development is almost always evident by the end of the first year. Most cases of PKU also have some brain wave abnormality, and about 20 percent have epileptic seizures (Woolf, 1970).

Several studies have reported a higher incidence of behavioral disturbance among those afflicted with PKU than is found among others of similar IQ. For example, Johnson (1969) asked the ward personnel of an institution to rate inmates on a variety of scales. Those with PKU were significantly more likely to be rated high on such characteristics as hyperactivity, self-destructiveness, destroying ward property, attacking others, and requiring restraint.

Another symptom of the disorder is insufficient pigmentation of the skin, eyes, and hair, which means that most children with PKU are light-skinned blue eyed blonds. However, this condition is not usually severe enough to be useful in diagnosing the disease.

PKU is one of the few syndromes of retardation for which there is a cure of sorts. In the early 1950s, several independent researchers hypothesized that the brain damage was due to excessively high accumulations of phenylalanine in the blood. Therefore, several children with PKU were put on a diet low in phenylalanine, and there was marked improvement in their condition. For example, one research team reported the following cases: "The patient, a two year old girl, was severely retarded, unable to stand, walk, or talk. She showed no interest in her surroundings, was uninterested in food, and spent her time groaning, crying, and head banging." After several weeks on the low phenylalanine diet, "the child learned to crawl and stand, she no longer banged her head or cried continuously." When she was put back on a regular diet, there was an immediate regression (Bickel, Girrard, and Hickmans, 1953).

For the past decade, it has been common medical practice to test all newborn infants for PKU. This can be done either by testing the urine for excess phenylpyruvic acid, or more commonly now, with a blood test, the Guthrie test. Children who are identified as having PKU can then be put on a low phenylalanine diet. This is a difficult task, since virtually all foods containing protein have phenylalanine, so the diet must be largely synthetic, and as a result, it is quite expensive. Several such diets are now available commercially. Mothers often report difficulty keeping their children on the diet, since the various synthetic foods don't taste very good. The physician must check the child's blood periodically to insure that the child is getting enough phenylalanine to keep him or her alive, but not enough to cause brain damage. Normally, the child with PKU is raised almost exclusively on the synthetic diet, supplemented by a few protein-free foods, until reaching school age, when most children can be put on a regular diet with no apparent ill effects.

There have been numerous studies on the effects of the special diet. All of them report considerable improvement in the behavior and intelligence of children reared on the diet when compared to untreated children, but there is some disagreement regarding the magnitude of the effect. Some studies (e.g., O'Grady, Berry, and Sutherland, 1971) report no significant difference in intelligence between PKU children reared on the diet and normal siblings, but most research indicates that the average IQ of treated PKU children is still in the borderline range (editorial, *British Journal of Medicine,* 1968).

The screening of newborns for PKU, which is now required by law in most states, has also contributed new knowledge about the disorder. For example, incidence figures have risen considerably, and PKU, while still relatively rare, is now recognized as being more widespread than was previously believed. Hudson (1967) reports that the incidence of PKU among newborns in England has appeared to increase from one in 25,000 to one in 10,000. Some cases have been found where individuals with PKU have normal intelligence even though they have had no treatment (Dyken and Culley, 1969). This has led some people to suggest that there may be several different varieties of the disorder. Like many disorders produced by hereditary factors, incidence differs widely among different ethnic groups. Mass screening in Ireland has found one newborn in 4842 to have PKU, suggesting that gene frequency is higher among Celtic stock (Cahalane, 1968). In a Massachusetts study, the incidence was one in 10,000 (Effron, 1967), and in an Ontario study, the incidence was one in 14,321 (Hanley et al., 1969). However, the disease is virtually unknown among the Japanese and certain Jewish sects.

Galactosemia. A disorder known as galactosemia is similar to PKU in some ways. It is transmitted by a single recessive gene that results in an inability to properly metabolize galactose, a carbohydrate that results from the digestion of milk. There are a number of early signs. Infants with galactosemia are frequently born with slightly lowered birth weights, and the first complaint is frequently failure to thrive; galactosemic infants do not gain weight and have frequent vomiting and diarrhea. The poison that accumulates usually leads to liver damage, which results in jaundice and frequent death in untreated cases. About half the cases develop cataracts early in life. The symptoms are quite variable, and mental retardation, while frequent, is by no means a universal characteristic. Like other inherited metabolic disorders, galactosemia is treated with a change in diet. When milk is entirely eliminated from the diet, many of the symptoms clear up almost immediately. Children are placed on a virtually milk-free diet, and many galactosemic adults report that milk causes stomach distress. However, the diet is not generally totally effective in preventing lowered intelligence, and research indicates that the average IQ of children with treated galactosemia is about 90. In one study, the mean IQ of 44 treated patients was 91, and 8 had IQs below 70. Eighty percent of these children had repeated at least one grade in school (Nadler, Inouye, and Hsia, 1969). It seems that carriers of galactosemia also have an inability to digest large quantities of galactose, and study of their digestive enzymes indicates that they have only about half of the normal amount of the enzyme which galactosemic children are completely lacking (Brandt, 1969). Thus, carriers can be quite readily identified.

As is the case with many such disorders, recent research has discovered that there are a number of variants of the basic syndrome. Also, screening has produced a number of cases of clear galactosemia with no clinical signs. They have no digestive problems, no liver damage, and have normal mental abilities. This complicates the problem of estimating the prevalence. Clinical surveys report a frequency of one in 70,000. However, estimates based on gene frequency suggest that the incidence ought to be about one in 25,000 to 30,000 (Butler, 1969).

Disorders of Lipid Metabolism. There are a group of related disorders called the lipidoses, which result from an excessive accumulation of lipids or fats in nervous tissue and elsewhere in the body. Most are very rare. There is no known cure for any of them, and death almost always occurs at a young age. The best known of these is Tay-Sach's disease or infantile amaurotic familial idiocy. This disorder is much more frequently found in individuals of Eastern European Jewish stock than in other ethnic groups. The incidence of the disease has been reported to be as high as one in 10,000 in New York, which has a large Jewish population, but is much rarer elsewhere (Crome and Stern, 1967). As with other inborn errors of metabolism, the child appears to be functioning normally at birth, but excess lipids begin to accumulate. This results in apathy, mental deterioration, blindness, hypersensitivity to sound, convulsions, and spasticity. A classic diagnostic sign is a cherry red spot on the retina of the eye. Death invariably occurs within a few years. There are other lipidoses that begin at a later age and have a more gradual onset, but these are extremely rare. Depending on the age of onset, the syndrome is known as Bielschowsky-Jansky's disease, Spielmeyer-Vogt disease, or Kuf's disease.

Hurler's Syndrome. A disorder called Hurler's syndrome results from an error in muco-polysaccharide metabolism. The disorder is also called gargoylism because many of the facial and body features are somewhat misshapen. There is wide variation in the symptoms. Some of the more frequently observed manifestations are short stature, hump back, enlarged liver and spleen, a large, slightly misshapened head, thick, heavy eyebrows, corneal clouding, snub nose with chronic nasal discharge, thick lips and large tongue, thick lowset ears, hearing loss, short, clawlike fingers, short, thick neck, and progressive retardation. Few cases will show all of these symptoms.

The child with Hurler's syndrome appears normal at birth and may develop normally for a few years. Once the symptoms become evident, the child shows gradual deterioration of abilities, resulting eventually in profound retardation. Death usually occurs before adulthood. The disease can be diagnosed by a characteristic substance in the urine. There is no cure at the present time.

There are two different modes of inheritance of Hurler's syndrome. The more usual cause is a simple recessive gene pair, but there is also a sex-linked gene locus that produces essentially identical symptoms, but is generally less severe. The sex-linked variant occurs exclusively in males.

Endocrine Disorders

Hypothyroidism (Cretinism). Another class of congenital metabolic disorders that can cause diminished mental abilities are the endocrine disorders, conditions caused by a defect in the level of one of the body's hormones. The most important endocrine disorder is hypothyroidism or cretinism. Prior to the twentieth century, cretinism was quite common in many parts of the world, and, in fact, the word for cretinism in French and German was synonymous with mental retardation until the last century (Crome and Stern, 1967). The term cretinism refers to the condition of low levels of thyroid hormone, and thus is more commonly called hypothyroidism (the prefix hypo- means below or lowered). The thyroid gland is located in the neck and its function is to secrete thyroxin or thyroid hormone. This hormone is responsible for maintaining a proper metabolic rate, and if too little of it is secreted, body metabolism slows down and a number of symptoms appear such as lethargy, slow heart beat, hair loss, obesity, and mental dullness. A condition commonly associated with hypothyroidism is goiter, a large growth in the neck resulting from a swelling of the thyroid gland. The traditional cause of goiter and some hypothyroidism is an iodine deficiency in the diet. For the past 50 years or so, iodine has been added to salt, and, as a result, goiter and hypothyroidism due to iodine deficiency have been virtually eliminated from developed countries, although it is still widespread in many undeveloped regions of the world.

Occasionally, however, the hypothyroidism is present at birth. This is a more serious condition usually called cretinism. Congenital cretinism has a number of different causes. In some cases, the thyroid gland does not form at all. In other cases, radiation during pregnancy can effect thyroid development. If the mother has an iodine deficiency, this can lead to hypothyroidism in the developing child. Various drugs taken during pregnancy can produce the syndrome. In many cases, there is a genetic cause. A number of different inherited metabolic defects have been identified that lead to congenital hypothyroidism.

In all cases, the symptoms are similar. At birth, the child may be heavier than usual, with a flat nasal bridge, puffy eyes, and a thick tongue. Most parents quickly notice that their child is very quiet and lethargic, and this is frequently the first sign that something is wrong. Growth is markedly slowed, and many cases are dwarfed. Cretins have a hoarse voice and a short, thick neck, with broad hands and short, stubby fingers. The skin is dry, flaky, cold, and greyish, and hair is sparse and brittle. Both mental and motor development are retarded, and the retardation is often severe. For many years now, the condition has been treated with thyroid medication, the hormone being obtained from animals. Most of the symptoms clear up immediately after treatment is initiated. However, in some cases irreversible nervous system damage has occurred prior to birth, and, as a result, the retardation, although it is not as severe as it otherwise would have been, it is still present. In one study of 22 patients with congenital cretinism in which thyroid medication was begun in the first six months, only 10 had IQs less than 90. However, if treatment is not begun in the first year, 49 of 50 cases with congenital cretinism had IQs below 90 (Smith, Blizzard, and Wilkins, 1957). If the condition develops some time after birth, it is far less serious. Treatment is almost always successful, and mental development is frequently not retarded even without treatment.

Malnutrition

Malnutrition is another cause of mental retardation that, like child abuse and lead poisoning, has recently received a good deal of attention because it is found predominantly among low-income groups and because it is at least in theory entirely preventable. However, to simply state that malnutrition causes mental retardation is an oversimplification of a complex matter, and there is some disagreement about the nature of and the extent of the relationship.

For ethical reasons it is very difficult to do good research on the relationship between diet and mental abilities in humans. It has frequently been observed that in families where nutrition is presumed to be inadequate, there is a higher incidence of mental retardation, and the overall level of mental functioning in such families appears to be lower; but malnutrition is found almost entirely among the poor, and in virtually all cases where malnutrition is suspected, there are a number of other major problems such as inadequate medical care, crowded and unsanitary living conditions, a lack of intellectual stimulation, and the general stresses that usually accompany poverty, and as a result it is extremely difficult to determine the effects of diet on mental abilities independently of these other factors. This problem is further complicated by the fact that it is virtually impossible to collect reliable data on what people eat, and the diet of the child in a low-income family may differ considerably from day to day, being entirely adequate some of the time but extremely deficient at other times.

Estimates of the extent of malnutrition in the United States vary widely. The figure that is most commonly cited is a government estimate that about 10 million Americans suffer from hunger and malnutrition (Birch and Gussow, 1970). However, this certainly does not mean that all, or even most of these 10 million people have suffered diminished mental abilities as a result. While there is little question that prolonged, severe malnutrition that results in such diseases as kwashiorkor can cause brain damage and mental retardation, such severe malnutrition is quite rare in this country. Most of these 10 million people suffer from mild to moderate subnutrition in which there is frequent hunger and a poorly balanced diet, but life itself is not usually threatened, and the relationship between such subnutrition and diminished mental abilities is less clear. The extent and the permanency of the intellectual deficits, if any, depend on a variety of factors such as the age of the individual, the extent and type of malnutrition, and the presence of other detrimental conditions, and thus it is impossible to state with any certainty the extent to which malnutrition is a cause of mental retardation in the United States.

The problem of malnutrition as a causative factor in mental retardation can be divided into two parts, the nutritional condition of the mother during pregnancy and the diet of the child after birth.

Prenatal Nutrition. The nutritional state of the mother during pregnancy is an important determinant of the overall physical and mental development of the child. This has been clearly demonstrated in research with animals. For example, Chow and his associates (Chow et al., 1971) found that when the diet of rats was reduced by 50 percent during pregnancy and lactation, the offspring showed marked growth retardation accompanied by decreased learning capacity and hyper-emotionality.

The research with human subjects is less clear, but a number of research projects support the same conclusion. For example, Burke et al. (1943) evaluated the diets of more than 200 U.S. women and found that children born to mothers on poor diets were more likely to be premature or stillborn, and they functioned less maturely shortly after birth than did the children of well-nourished mothers. In a classic study, Harrell, Woodyard, and Gates (1955) found a large number of pregnant women living in extreme poverty in rural Virginia and who were presumably not eating a proper diet for pregnancy. Some of the women were given vitamin supplements throughout their pregnancy while others were given a placebo, a pill with no nutritional value. When the resulting children were three to four years old, their intelligence was measured with the Stanford-Binet. The children of the mothers who had been given the vitamin supplements were significantly higher in IQ than were the control subjects who had been given the placebo. However, the difference between the two groups, while statistically significant, was less than four IQ points.

A number of researchers do not accept the general conclusion that prenatal malnutrition results in an increase in birth complications or lowered mental abilities in childhood. For example, McGanity et al. (1955) studied the diets of more than 2000 U.S. women whose nutrition ranged from good to poor and concluded that nutrition during pregnancy was not an important influence on the course of pregnancy or the health of the newborn. Thomson (1968) and others argue that early in pregnancy a mother will store a good deal more protein and other nutrients than will be needed under normal circumstances, and if the nutritional demands of the fetus are large, the fetus takes priority, and thus malnutrition will have few effects unless the food shortage is severe and long lasting.

There is evidence that the mother's diet during her own childhood may be an important factor in the eventual well being of her children. If a girl does not get sufficient food while she is growing up, there may be pelvic deformities and other abnormalities that affect the developing fetus. Gruelich, Thoms, and Twaddle (1939) found that the pelvic shape most adequate for childbearing was found in 73 percent of economically well-off student nurses, but in only 37 percent of poor clinic patients. The most obvious result of poor nutrition during childhood is short stature, and there is a clear relationship between short mothers and birth complications, stillbirths, and prematurity (Baird, 1949). A similar finding has been reported with rats. Cowley and Griesel (1966) fed female rats a low protein diet from weaning. These rats were mated at adulthood, and their offspring showed deficits in learning mazes.

Postnatal Malnutrition. There are several good studies documenting the fact that postnatal malnutrition can result in long-term intellectual deficits and brain deficiencies, at least when the malnutrition is severe and prolonged and occurs within a few years of birth when the brain is developing rapidly. For example, Stoch and Smythe (1963) followed up a group of South African children who had been hospitalized for malnutrition and compared them to other children of similar economic background who had presumably received an adequate diet. At the end of a seven-year period, the malnourished group averaged 22.6 IQ points lower than the comparison group. Cravioto, DeLicardie, and Birch (1966) used height as a measure of nutritional status in an extremely poor Guatemalan village. It is universally recognized that one of the first symptoms of poor nutrition is stunted growth, and, as a result, it is reasonable to assume that among the very poor, height is a good measure of prior nutritional status. They found a clear difference between the tallest fourth of the children and the shortest fourth of the children on a test of sensory integration, a measure of mental development with little cultural bias. Chase and Martin (1970) followed up 19 children who had been treated in a Denver hospital for malnutrition. These children had a mean DQ (Developmental Quotient, a ratio comparable to IQ) of only 82, far below what would be expected even for culturally disadvantaged children, and 17 points below a comparison group.

It is clear from research with animals that the age of the organism is crucial in determining the effects of malnutrition. In general, the younger the child, the more severe and more irreversible will be the effects. In people old enough that their nervous system is no longer developing, malnutrition must be severe for there to be much effect on the nervous system, and these people are more likely to recover completely if adequate nutrition is restored. If malnutrition occurs during the period of rapid development of the nervous system, particularly during the first six months when brain cells are still forming, the effects are likely to be far more severe and, for the most part, irreversible (Winick, 1970).

However, even though malnutrition is not severe enough to cause permanent neurological damage, it is clearly the case that if children do not have enough to eat, they are more likely to be apathetic and less likely to be interested in learning. Children who are concerned about where their next meal is coming from are not going to be very interested in learning to read, and if they don't have very much energy because of low calorie and protein intake, they are not going to be very curious about their surroundings or make the effort to get involved in school activities. Thus, this is a result of subnutrition that operates indirectly to reduce mental abilities, and, even though there is no organic damage, the result is the same.

Postnatal Gross Brain Disease

The category of postnatal gross brain diseases includes a number of disorders that do not begin to manifest themselves until after birth. Most are extremely rare, and only two syndromes will be discussed here: tuberous sclerosis and von Recklinghausen's disease (neurofibromatosis). Both fall into the general category of neurocutaneous dysplasias, which refer to hereditary conditions that result in developmental disorders of the skin and nervous system.

Tuberous Sclerosis. Tuberous sclerosis is characterized by the formation of numerous hardened (sclerotic) nodules on the surface of the cerebral cortex. These sclerotic areas result in mental retardation and epileptic seizures. The nodules are generally not present at birth but gradually form during development, and, as a result, the retardation is often progressive; that is, the person becomes more impaired as he or she gets older. Many adults are profoundly retarded. In addition to the retardation and epilepsy, a third characteristic symptom is a skin rash on the face that vaguely resembles acne except that it is usually confined to a region around the nose. Like the nodules in the brain, the rash is not present at birth, but gradually forms when the child is four to six years old. Other symptoms include nodes on other organs such as the heart or the kidneys and various other sorts of skin disorders.

Tuberous sclerosis is somewhat unusual in that it is transmitted by a dominant gene. This means that only one of the abnormal genes need be present in order for the syndrome to manifest itself. There are very few serious disorders that are transmitted in this way because a disorder that is produced by a dominant gene cannot skip a generation, and there are no carriers. Everyone who carries the gene also has the disorder. However, the tuberous sclerosis gene has variable expressivity. This means that it can manifest itself in several different ways. While about two thirds of those with the disorder are mentally retarded, some people who carry the gene show only mild symptoms and no retardation. Some cases are presumably never even diagnosed.

von Recklinghausen's Disease (Neurofibromatosis). A related disorder is called neurofibromatosis or von Recklinghausen's disease. The characteristic symptoms are skin tumors and spots on the skin the color of coffee with milk in it. The tumors may vary from barely noticeable lumps to hideous growths. Like tuberous sclerosis, neurofibromatosis is transmitted by a dominant gene with variable expressivity. It is found in about one of 3000 births, but only about one fourth of the cases are mentally retarded, and many of these are only mildly impaired (Holmes et al., 1972).

Unknown Prenatal Influences

This category includes a number of congenital malformations of the brain or skull that are frequently associated with mental retardation. In most cases the cause is unknown, although some have an apparent genetic basis.

Hydrocephaly

Hydrocephaly is one of a group of disorders known as the cranial anomalies. This group of syndromes is so called because the characteristic feature is a distortion of the shape of the skull. There are several kinds of cranial disorders, and almost all of them produce mental retardation, but most are quite rare. However, there are two that are relatively more common than many of the syndromes discussed above: hydrocephaly and microcephaly.

Hydrocephaly, colloquially called water on the brain, is a condition in which cerebrospinal fluid accumulates in the head, creating pressure on the brain and skull. This fluid is normally drained from the central nervous system and absorbed in various ducts, but in hydrocephaly, a blockage occurs somewhere in the drainage system or else the drainage ducts are not properly formed. As a result, the fluid cannot drain properly and the resulting pressure causes the skull to enlarge. A large and rapidly growing head, particularly in the front, is the usual diagnostic sign. Occasionally, the head can reach grotesque proportions, with the skull circumference being well over double the normal head size. In this extreme condition, the bones of the skull are very thin and widely separated and the head readily develops pressure sores. The pressure on the brain can cause considerable damage, with the result that many cases are profoundly retarded, and other signs of brain damage such as spasticity are frequent. Occasionally, the pressure pushes the eyes out of their usual orientation resulting in a condition known as the setting sun syndrome because only the tops of the pupils are visible above the lower lids. Not surprisingly, many cases die in infancy. The incidence of hydrocephaly in one study was 0.6 per thousand live births (Nelson and Forfar, 1969).

There are a number of different causes of the disorder and a number of variants of the condition. It is rarely familial. Sometimes the drainage system is malformed, in other cases, the condition results from infection, either pre- or postnatally. Other cases are due to physical trauma. However, in a good many cases, the cause is unknown. It is usually present at birth, but there are many cases of hydrocephaly developing after birth, usually as a result of infection. After the bones of the skull have closed, the skull does not enlarge. Interestingly, the condition is more frequent among children of older mothers, but there is no evidence that it is due to a chromosome disorder. It is more frequent among lower economic status families than among higher income groups. The prognosis is very mixed. Many cases are spontaneously arrested and the individual may show no signs of mental deficit although the head may still be abnormally large. Other cases have normal intelligence but with motor impairment. The degree of retardation can be anywhere from borderline to profound. Many cases are treated with surgery in which a mechanical shunt is inserted in the head to bypass the blockage. This operation must generally be done soon after birth and is not always successful in alleviating the condition because considerable brain damage may have occurred prior to birth.

Spina Bifida

There are a number of other congenital malformations of the nervous system that frequently accompany hydrocephaly. Spina bifida is a condition in which the spinal column is not properly formed and there is an opening in the bony case protecting the nerves. In some cases, the neural tissue is unimpaired, and there are no symptoms other than a dimple on the back. In other cases, however, considerable tissue protrudes through the opening, and there is a sac on the back. This sac is called a meningocele if it contains no nerve tissue and a myelomeningocele (or meningomyelocele) if there is nerve tissue in the sac. Particularly in the latter case, there may be paralysis below the point of the bifida. These conditions are usually repaired with surgery soon after birth. Spina bifida is relatively common, with an incidence rate of 3.2 per thousand births (Nelson and Forfar, 1969). It does not produce retardation by itself, but it is usually accompanied by other malformations, in particular hydrocephaly, and, as a result, it is a condition frequently found in retarded populations.

If a similar condition exists on the head, it is called a cranial bifida or encephalocele. In this case, there is an opening in the back of the skull with tissue protruding. In extreme cases, there is a large sac on the back of the head containing considerable brain tissue. Retardation and other signs of brain damage such as spasticity and blindness almost always accompany cranial bifidas. It is not as common as spina bifida (0.7 per thousand births), and nearly half the cases do not survive despite surgery (Holmes et al., 1972).

Microcephaly

Microcephaly is a general term meaning small skull. It is usually defined as a head circumference of more than two standard deviations below average for age and sex. As such, microcephaly frequently accompanies other syndromes of retardation such as Down's syndrome, PKU, and retardation caused by prenatal infections or radiation. A small skull usually, but by no means always, suggests retardation. In one study of 202 microcephalic children, 27 (13 percent) had normal intelligence. However, of these 27, many had signs of minimal brain dysfunction (Martin, 1970).

However, there is a syndrome of pure or primary microcephaly in which the cause is either unknown or produced by a recessive gene. In this case, the retardation is usually severe, and spasticity is common. There is a characteristic appearance to these people. The skull is very small, but the face is of normal size, resulting in a small forehead and peculiar shape to the skull.

Chromosome Abnormalities

One of the most important categories of organic syndromes associated with mental retardation is the category of chromosome aberrations. All normal human beings have 46 chromosomes in each cell in their body (with the exception of sex cells). These 46 chromosomes can be divided into 23 pairs, and under certain conditions these chromosomes can be examined under a microscope. Figure 5-1 shows the 46 chromosomes of a normal male sorted into pairs and categorized into one classification system. The letters refer to groups of chromosome pairs that cannot always be distinguished from each other under the microscope because they are so similar.

Each chromosome contains many thousands of genes, and thus, with one exception, it makes no sense to say that a given chromosome is responsible for given characteristics. The one exception is the last chromosome pair. These are called the sex chromosomes because they determine the sex of the individual. There are two types of sex chromosomes, a relatively large one, which is referred to as the X chromosome, and a very small one, called the Y chromosome. Normal males have one of each, an X and a Y, and normal females have two X chromosomes.

Occasionally an individual is born with something other than the normal

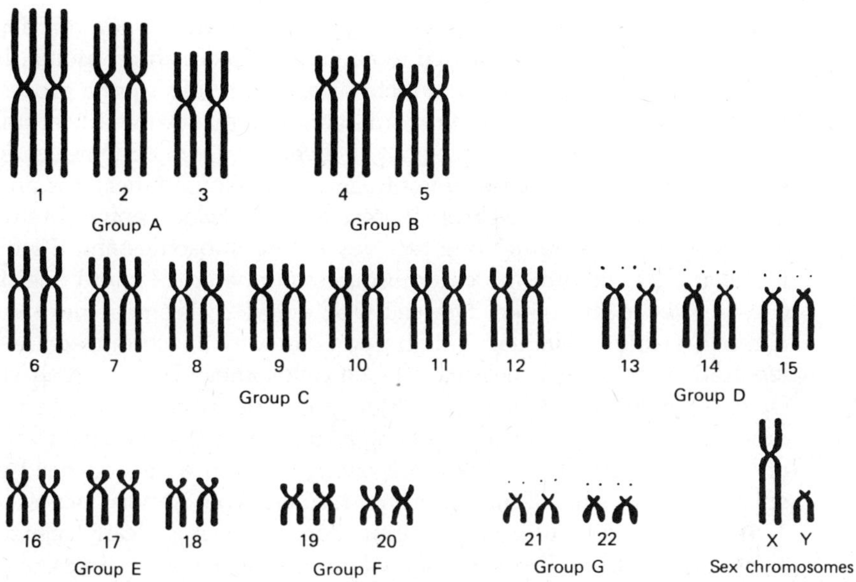

Figure 5-1 Normal human chromosomes. From U.S. Department of Health, Education and Welfare. Antenatal diagnosis of Down's syndrome. Bethesda, Md.: National Institute of Child Health and Human Development, 1974.

complement of 46 chromosomes, usually 47, but occasionally 48 or more, and in the case of one syndrome, only 45. The presence of this extra chromosome material results in various abnormalities that range in severity from barely noticeable to lethal. One of the more common symptoms associated with the presence of an extra chromosome is lowered intelligence.

Down's Syndrome (*Mongolism*)

Chromosome aberrations are of two basic types, those in which the extra chromosome is an autosome (any chromosome other than an X or Y chromosome) or those in which the extra or missing chromosome is a sex chromosome. The former will be discussed first. By far the most important aberration is Down's syndrome or mongolism, which results from the presence of an extra chromosome number 21. Because there are three of chromosome 21 rather than the usual two, another name for this disorder is trisomy 21. The labels mongolism and mongoloid are more widely used than is Down's syndrome, but they are not considered to be as acceptable any more because of their racial connotations (There is no relationship at all between Down's syndrome and the Oriental, or Mongol race.).

There are actually three different types of Down's syndrome depending on how the individual happened to acquire the extra chromosome. In about 90 percent of the cases, the extra chromosome results from a process called nondisjunction. Normally, in the formation of gametes, the 46 chromosomes of the parent cell are divided equally between the two daughter cells so that each has 23 chromosomes, one of each type. Nondisjunction is an error in this process in which the chromosomes are not divided equally between the two daughter cells, rather one receives 24 chromosomes and the other 22. In trisomy 21, both of the chromosomes numbered 21 go to one daughter cell, neither to the other. The cell with only 22 chromosomes never produces a viable individual, but the gamete with 24 chromosomes can be fertilized, producing a cell with 47 chromosomes. The resulting child has Down's syndrome. Thus, in nondisjunction, both parents have normal chromosomes, and there is no such thing as a carrier. The probability of parents of a child with Down's syndrome giving birth to a second child similarly afflicted is very small if the syndrome resulted from nondisjunction.

An interesting feature of nondisjunction is that it is clearly related to the age of the mother. Table 5-2 shows the probability of mothers of different ages giving birth to a child with Down's syndrome. Mothers in their early twenties have about a one in 1500 chance of having an afflicted baby while for mothers in their late forties, the probability increases to about one in 65. The age of the father appears to be irrelevant, which suggests that the nondisjunction must occur in the formation of the ovum rather than the sperm. The exact reason why this is the case is unknown.

A second error that can produce the identical syndrome is called translocation. In translocation, chromosome 21 of one of the parents has become attached to another chromosome, usually 15. When the chromosomes of this parent are examined under a microscope, only 45 can be seen, but chromosome 15 is larger than usual because it also contains all of the genes

Table 5-2 Incidence of Down's Syndrome as a Function of Maternal Age

Mother's Age	Incidence of Down's Syndrome
Under 30	One in 1500
30–34	One in 750
35–39	One in 280
40–44	One in 130
Over 45	One in 65

Adapted from Smith and Wilson, 1973.

of chromosome 21. Because the parent is not lacking any genetic material, there is no abnormality manifest in the phenotype. However, when the parent's cells divide to produce gametes, a sperm or ovum may be produced which contains the genetic material of chromosome 21 replicated twice, and thus, if conception occurs with this cell, the result will mimic trisomy 21.

In theory, if one parent is a translocation carrier, one third of the offspring should have Down's syndrome, one third should be unaffected carriers, and one third should have normal chromosomes (One fourth of their conceptions would also be nonviable because they would only have 45 chromosomes.). However, because various selective forces are acting against producing an abnormal infant, the actual probabilities are less than this. If the mother is the carrier, the abnormality occurs about once in six births, and if the father is the carrier, it occurs only once in 20 births. (Smith, 1971).

A third, much rarer type of Down's syndrome is called mosaicism. In mosaicism, the defect occurs after conception. The initial zygote has a normal number of chromosomes, but some time during prenatal development during one of the early cell divisions, an error occurs with one cell receiving 47 chromosomes and the other 45. The cell with only 45 dies, but because chromosomes always reproduce themselves exactly, the one with 47 chromosomes will continue to produce cells with 47 chromosomes. Thus, in the case of a mosaic child, some of the cells have a normal 46 chromosomes and others have the atypical 47. The more normal cells the individual has, the more normal he or she is. Mosaics form a sort of continuum between Down's syndrome and normalcy.

Down's syndrome is by far the most frequent of the organic syndromes of retardation. The incidence is estimated to be about one in 600 live births. It has been estimated that there are about 65,000 people with Down's syndrome in the country (Koch, Fishler, and Melnyk, 1971), and they make up about 10 percent of the population of institutions for the retarded. Anyone who has had any experience at all working with retarded children has certainly run across a number of Down's syndrome children.

The presence of a complete extra chromosome means that there is no specific qualitative defect of metabolism; instead, there seems to be numerous quantitative differences in body chemistry such as an increase in gamma gobulin and a decrease in albumin and calcium in the blood. Thus, there are numerous symptoms that characterize the disorder.

The most obvious symptom is impaired intelligence. The average person with Down's syndrome is in the severely retarded range, with an IQ around 30. However, there is a wide range of intelligence. A few never even learn to walk while there are some who are only mildly retarded. There are occasional reports of children with Down's syndrome in the borderline range.

Buck (1955) describes a case of a man with Down's syndrome who scored a full-scale IQ of 83 on the Wechsler. Another Down's syndrome child has even written a book, *The World of Nigel Hunt,* describing his experiences. While such cases are certainly the exception, it should certainly not be assumed that all children with Down's syndrome will be hopelessly retarded.

One difficulty in determining the average intellectual capabilities of people with Down's syndrome is that the disorder can usually be diagnosed at birth, and, as a result, many children with the disorder were institutionalized when they were very young. In fact, it used to be common medical practice for physicians to advise parents to institutionalize a mongoloid child immediately and forget about it. Placing children in an institution is usually quite detrimental to their intellectual development, and several studies have shown that Down's syndrome children reared at home are more capable than those in institutions.

In addition to mental retardation, there are numerous physical stigmata associated with Down's syndrome. Few cases show all of these symptoms, but many are quite frequent. Perhaps the most obvious is the peculiar Oriental eyes from which the name mongolism is derived. Actually, the structure of the eyes if somewhat different from that of normal Orientals, but the appearance is similar to the layman. There is also a characteristic shape to the skull, small and flattened in the back. Another characteristic feature of Down's syndrome is a large, fissured, protruding tongue. This is one factor contributing to speech problems. People with Down's syndrome tend to be considerably shorter than the general population, many being under five feet at adulthood. Their hands tend to be squared, with short, stubby fingers. The little finger is frequently missing a joint and may bend inward. There is often a space between the big toe and the other toes. There is a characteristic line on the palms of their hands called the simian line.

People with Down's syndrome are quite susceptible to various other disorders. More than a fourth of all children born with Down's syndrome have congenital heart deformities of various types, such as an opening between several chambers. They also have greatly lowered resistance to respiratory infections, and, as a result, a chronic runny nose is a common feature. Until recently, few children with Down's syndrome survived to adulthood because of their increased susceptibility to pneumonia, but with the widespread use of modern antibiotics, their life expectancy has been greatly increased in the past two decades. However, Fabia and Drollette (1970) in a study of 2421 mongoloid children born in Massachusetts from 1950 to 1966 report that only about two-thirds were still alive by age 10. Twenty-eight percent had congenital heart defects, and of these, less than half survived to age 10. Hearing loss and poor vision are also somewhat more frequent among children with Down's syndrome.

Children with Down's syndrome have a reputation for being very cheerful, friendly, good natured, and affectionate. Even Langdon Down described them as being good mimics, "humorous . . . with a lively sense of the ridiculous" (Penrose and Smith, 1966, p. 54). Several researchers have attempted to verify this by surveying ward personnel. For example, Domino, Goldschmidt, and Kaplan (1964) had 12 aides in an institution check personality traits that described 56 different residents, of whom 21 were mongoloids. There was a significant positive correlation between Down's syndrome and a number of desirable personality traits such as unexcitable, content, relaxed, cheerful, good natured, clownish, affectionate, friendly, and warm. People with Down's syndrome were significantly less likely to be described as emotional, nervous, whiny, anxious, restless, and irritable. This research tends to support the stereotype. However, the people with Down's syndrome were being compared to other institutionalized retarded children, many of whom presumably had severe emotional, behavioral, and social problems (these traits tend to characterize institutionalized, low-functioning mentally retarded). In other words, it is probably not the case that mongoloids are more likely to have these traits than are normal children of similar mental age, but they seem like little angels when they are compared to other institutionalized children. Most preschoolers are generally cheerful, affectionate, and good natured, and Down's syndrome children functioning at the same level ought to behave similarly.

Benda (1969), a physician who has studied this disorder for many years, provides a good description of the development of the Down's syndrome child. The whole developmental process is slowed down. Even at birth, the child, although developing for the full nine months, may show characteristics of a less well-developed child such as poor muscle tones. Their motor development from birth on is very much delayed. Many mothers report that their mongoloid baby was "the very best baby we ever had" because it is not restless, seldom cries, and is usually quiet. Children with Down's syndrome seldom sit up before they are one year old, and most do not begin to walk independently until they are three to six years old. Speech development is similarly very much delayed. Many children with Down's syndrome never learn to speak very well. They may pronounce sounds so indistinctly that only their family can understand them. The ages of 6 to 12 are more difficult times, both for the child and for the parent, because the child is more restless, the parents and others are making more demands, and the child is often confused about what is expected of him or her. However, the social development of children with Down's syndrome generally seems to exceed their mental development, often by a considerable margin. Their sexual maturation is usually delayed. Despite the fact that there are characteristic deformities of the genitals, there are reports of women with Down's syndrome conceiving and giving birth. Consistent with predictions, about half these children are normal and half have Down's syndrome. There are no reported cases of men with the disorder fathering children. Although development is slowed down, signs of premature aging are seen, in many cases, even in their twenties.

Other researchers disagree with parts of Benda's description. Fishler, Share, and Koch (1964), Dameron and Lawrence (1963), and Dicks-Mireaux (1972) argue that the development of Down's syndrome children is only slightly delayed during the first few months, and the rate of development becomes progressively slower as the child grows older.

An issue that is important to those providing services for the mentally retarded is to what extent the etiology of children's retardation affects their programming. Is it safe to treat all children functioning at the same level in the same way regardless of whether they have Down's syndrome, an inborn metabolic error, brain damage, or familial retardation, or is it more desirable to establish separate training programs for mongoloids, brain damaged children, and the like? Benda (1969) argues that Down's syndrome children ought to be considered a separate group from other retarded even though all are functioning at the same level. Most other workers in the field take the opposite point of view, and classes for specific etiologies are the exception rather than the rule.

This issue can be experimentally tested by comparing subjects with different etiologies who are matched on MA and IQ. There are only two etiologies that have been investigated in this way to any extent. One is Down's syndrome, and the other is a looser etiology called brain damage, which will be discussed below. Johnson and Olley (1971) have reviewed a number of studies comparing mongoloids to nonmongoloids. They conclude that while a number of studies have found minor differences in psychological functioning between people with Down's syndrome and other retarded people matched on MA, there is no clear pattern to these differences and the similarities between the two are far more striking. For example, Nakamura (1965) individually matched 64 institutionalized adult mongoloids and nonmongoloids on MA, CA, IQ, and sex, and administered the Stanford-Binet to all of them. Of 60 items on the test, on only 4 were there significant differences in percentage passing between the two groups, and there was no pattern or common factor to these 4. A series of studies by Lyle (1959, 1960) suggests that people with Down's syndrome have less verbal ability than nonmongoloids even when nonverbal MAs do not differ between the two groups. But the differences, although statistically significant, are relatively small and might be partially attributable to the characteristic large protruding tongue that limits good articulation. Other studies have found differences between mongoloids and nonmongoloids in such things as tactual discrimination ability and reaction time, but, in general, there is little evidence to support Benda's contention that children with Down's syndrome ought to be educated separately from other children of similar ability.

At the present time, there is no cure for Down's syndrome. Benda and others have suggested treatment with thyroid and pituitary hormones, but these have not generally proved to be successful. However, it might be possible to prevent it in the near future. Physicians are now experimenting with a technique called amniocentesis in which cells are removed from the amniotic sac of the developing fetus during pregnancy. In this way, the child's chromosomes can be examined, and it can be determined whether the child has a chromosome disorder. Thus, Down's syndrome can be detected early in pregnancy, and if the parents desire it, the child can be aborted.

Other Chromosome Disorders

The development in the 1950s of techniques enabling scientists to observe individual chromosomes resulted in the discovery of a number of other syndromes associated with chromosomal aberrations. Edward's syndrome results from trisomy of one of the chromosomes in the 16 to 18 group (also known as the E group). Symptoms include severe mental retardation, a number of peculiar facial features such as low, malformed ears, an elongated skull, and developmental disorders such as feeding difficulties and failure to thrive (Taylor, 1968). The incidence is estimated to be about one in 6700 births, but 90 percent die within a year (Polani, 1969).

Patau's syndrome is similar in many ways. It results from trisomy in the 13 to 15 (D) group of chromosomes, and is associated with a wide variety of severe defects including brain malformations. Other features include peculiar facial characteristics and deformities such as cleft palate and harelip, cardiovascular abnormalities, and deformed limbs. The incidence is about one in 7600 births, but the survival rate is low. Both of these syndromes are more common in offspring of older mothers (Taylor, 1968; Polani, 1969).

The *Cri-du-chat* or Cat Cry syndrome is so named because of the peculiar catlike cry of the infants with this disorder. It is associated with the deletion of one of the arms on a chromosome in the 4 to 5 group. Other symptoms include severe mental retardation and unusual facial features. It is extremely rare, only being found in one in 50,000 to 100,000 births (Polani, 1969).

Sex Chromosome Disorders

Turner's Syndrome. With the exception of Down's syndrome, the only common chromosome aberrations are those associated with the sex chromosomes. The error that produces these is usually nondisjunction. Recall that normal females have two X chromosomes in position 23, and normal males have an X and a Y chromosome. If during the formation of an ovum, nondisjunction occurs in a normal female, one daughter cell would have two X chromosomes, the other would have none. The ovum with no sex chromosomes may be fertilized either by an X bearing or a Y bearing sperm. If the latter occurs, the zygote cannot survive, but if the fertilizing sperm has an X chromosome, the result is a viable individual with only 45 chromosomes, and the sex genotype is XO. This is the only known case where individuals can survive without a full complement of chromosomes. Apparently, all of the chromosomes are essential for life except for the very tiny Y chromosome. This condition is called Turner's syndrome. The resulting individual has the appearance of a female, but the ovaries are either absent or vestigial. As a result, secondary sex characteristics do not develop and the individual is infertile. Other symptoms are occasionally present such as webbing of the neck, short stature, and skeletal abnormalities. However, many cases are so symptom free that the condition is not diagnosed until the teen years. About 20 percent of the cases of Turner's syndrome are mentally retarded. Interestingly, several studies indicate that the mental deficit is largely limited to the nonverbal aspects of intelligence, traditionally the more masculine abilities (Shaffer, 1962; Buckley, 1970).

Klinefelter's Syndrome. Other chromosome aberrations result from the fertilization of the ovum with both X chromosomes in our nondisjunction example. If this ovum is fertilized by a Y-bearing sperm, the result is a zygote with 47 chromosomes and the genotype XXY. This condition is called Klinefelter's syndrome. Individuals with this disorder appear to be males but with a number of feminine characteristics, such as overdeveloped breasts, high voice, hairlessness, small testes, and infertility. Mild or moderate retardation is frequently present, but not always. Klinefelter's syndrome is relatively common; the frequency is estimated to be about one in 400 male births (Kessler and Moos, 1970), and it is estimated that these individuals make up about 1 percent of the institutionalized mentally retarded.

Other Sex Chromosome Disorders. If the XX chromosome is fertilized by an X-bearing sperm, the result will be an XXX individual, which is occasionally referred to as a superfemale. This is a misnomer, because apparently, the presence of too many female chromosomes is detrimental to the development of normal female characteristics. Individuals are frequently sexually undeveloped and occasionally mentally retarded. However, the symptoms are not severe, and presumably many cases go undiagnosed because the family does not suspect that there is anything wrong.

Nondisjunction can also occur in males but results in identical syndromes for the most part (with the exception of an XXX individual). However, there is one syndrome that is limited to males that has just recently been discovered, but that has achieved wide notoriety. This is an XYY male. These individuals tend to be tall; many are over six feet, and there is a good deal of evidence that suggests that they tend to have propensities toward aggressiveness and criminal behavior. Incidence estimates vary widely, but one study of the chromosomes of nearly 12,000 newborns found 17 such XYY individuals, which is an incidence of one in 700 live births. (Hook and Kim, 1970). However, when chromosome studies are done in prison populations, 2 percent or more have been found with this chromosome pattern. The existence of such a syndrome has caused controversy in the legal profession since it is difficult to justify punishing someone for a crime if it can be shown that the person's criminal tendencies are somehow inherited. However, there is some evidence that their crimes are limited to crimes against property rather than violent crimes. It has been suggested that the disorder is not a criminal tendency per se, but rather an inherited inability to control impulses (Kessler and Moos, 1970). Most individuals with the XYY pattern are in the normal range of intelligence, but retardation is more frequent than in the general population.

These four basic syndromes are the most common varieties of sex chromosome aberrations, but there are numerous variants of these. Mosaics of Klinefelter's and Turner's syndromes are fairly common; these are individuals with both normal and abnormal cells caused by the nondisjunction occurring some time after conception. Other variants include people with an XXXY pattern of chromosomes who exhibit characteristics similar to Klinefelter's syndrome, XXYY individuals, and even cases of XXXX females.

Gestational Disorders

The final category of purely organic causes of mental retardation is gestational disorders; that is, mental retardation arising from complications of pregnancy that are not included in any of the above categories. The only important item in this category is prematurity.

Prematurity

Technically, a premature birth is one with a gestation period of less than 37 weeks. However, because it is difficult to determine the time of conception, prematurity is more typically defined as a birth weight of less than 2500 grams (5.5 pounds). Numerous studies have shown a relationship between prematurity and lowered mental capacities. There are two ways in which such research can be done: one can either take a sample of mentally retarded children and examine their birth histories to determine what percentage were born prematurely (the retrospective method) or one can follow a group of premature infants for a number of years and measure their IQs as soon as they become reliably testable. This is called the prospective or longitudinal method. There are numerous examples of both designs in the literature, and most show a relationship between prematurity and mental retardation. For example, Birch et al. (1970), in a retrospective study, examined the perinatal histories of some 100 mentally retarded children in Scotland and found that 24 percent had been born prematurely (defined as a gestation period of less than 38 weeks) while only 7 percent of the overall birth rate in the whole community had been premature. A typical prospective study is one by Knobloch and her associates (Knobloch et al., 1956) who followed up 500 premature infants born in the Baltimore area in the early 1950s and compared them to a control group of full-term infants of similar socioeconomic background. At 40 weeks, all of the children were administered a test of mental and motor development. Only 1 percent of the control group, but 2.8 percent of the premature infants were classified as dull normal, 0.7 percent of the prematures and 0.4 percent of the control infants were classified as borderline defective, and 1.5 percent of the prematures and 1 percent of the control group were considered defective. These differences, although not large, were statistically significant. More importantly, the incidence of lowered intelligence was considerably greater among those infants of extremely low birth weight, defined as less than 1500 grams (3.3 pounds). In this group, 8.8 percent were clearly defective and an additional 10.6 percent were classified as borderline or dull normal. However, 5.3 percent of the extremely low birthweight babies were also in the high average and superior categories. This indicates that many premature babies develop well above average mental abilities. In a later follow-up of these children when they reached school age, Wiener et al. (1968) reported that those whose birth weights were between 1500 and 2000 grams scored an average of 6.2 IQ points lower than the controls. This was the case even though 16 obviously defective children had been excluded from the low birth weight group. Drillien (1964) found an even larger difference in mental development between premature babies and full-term infants. At age four, the mean DQ (Developmental Quotient, roughly equivalent to IQ) of her full-term subjects was 106.7 while the average DQ of those children with birth weights between 1600 and 2000 grams (3.5 to 4.5 pounds) was 10 points lower, and the average DQ of 40 extremely low birth weight children was only 80.2.

A general summary statement of this type of research is that moderately low birth weight is associated with a slight decrement in mental abilities, and severe low birth weight is associated with a more drastic lowering of intelligence. It is important to remember, however, that this does not necessarily mean that prematurity causes diminished mental abilities. It is also possible that children who are not developing properly are more likely to be born with lowered birth weight; in other words, lowered intelligence causes prematurity rather than the reverse. Investigating the relationship between low birth weight and diminished cognitive capacities is further complicated by the fact that prematurity is far more common among the lower socioeconomic classes. For example, Rider et al. (1955) reported that the prematurity rate among the most advantaged tenth of whites in the city of Baltimore was 5.0 percent, while it was 7.6 percent in the lowest tenth. However, the prematurity rate was 11.4 percent for the nonwhite population. This strikingly greater prematurity rate among nonwhites has been reported in other studies also. While a simple racial explanation cannot be rejected at this time, it is more likely that the difference is accounted for by the far inferior economic, medical, and nutritional conditions to which the nonwhite elements of the population are exposed in our society. Birch and Gussow (1970), in summarizing a number of prematurity studies, conclude that the effects of prematurity on mental ability is largely limited to the lower socioeconomic classes. Premature babies born to advantaged families show a negligible decrease in intelligence when compared to full-term infants of similar background, while premature children born to disadvantaged families are lower in mental ability, even when compared to full-term children of similar background. Apparently the advantaged family can somehow overcome the negative effects of prematurity better than a disadvantaged family can.

The Importance of Organic Factors in the Etiology of Mental Retardation

It is clear that deficits in intelligence can be caused by a bewildering array of conditions. However, even though medical science has made tremendous progress in identifying these conditions, it is still the case that no definite cause can be found for most retardation. Most of the clear syndromes described above are relatively rare, and many of the more common medical causes of retardation such as prematurity or birth injury do not result in unique clinical pictures which can be readily identified. Table 5-3 summarizes the etiologies of 13,978 children who had been diagnosed as mentally retarded in federally funded clinics in fiscal year 1972. While these figures are not entirely representative of the mentally retarded population of the United States, they give a good picture of how frequent various etiologies are relative to other syndromes. The most striking thing about this table is the high percentage of cases for which the cause is unknown. Fully one third of the diagnosed cases of mental retardation had no evidence of organic ab-

Table 5-3 Medical Classification of New Patients Classified as Mentally Retarded in Federally Funded Mental Retardation Clinics, Fiscal Year 1972

	Number	Percentage
Total mentally retarded	13,978	100.0
Phenylketonuria (PKU)	94	0.7
Other disorders of protein metabolism	28	0.2
Cerebral lipidosis, infantile (Tay-Sachs Dis.)	15	0.1
Other disorders of lipid metabolism	35	0.3
Galactosemia	9	0.1
Other disorders of carbohydrate metabolism	53	0.4
Hypothyroidism	57	0.4
Hurler's syndrome	24	0.2
Other disorders of metabolism, growth, or nutrition	165	1.2
Neurofibromatosis	75	0.5
Tuberous sclerosis	80	0.6
Other new growths	30	0.2
Down's syndrome (mongolism)	1,087	7.8
Congenital cerebral defect associated with primary cranial anomaly (mostly hydrocephaly and microcephaly)	355	2.5
Congenital cerebral defect of undetermined cause	1,177	8.4
Kernicterus	107	0.8
Other maternal intoxications	49	0.4
Prenatal infection	296	2.1
Toxemia of pregnancy	184	1.3
Prenatal injury	196	1.4
Other prenatal causes	1,137	8.2
Prematurity	737	5.3
Mechanical injury at birth	289	2.1
Anoxia at birth	735	5.3
Postnatal cerebral infection	450	3.2
Postnatal injury	350	2.5
Postimmunization encephalopathy	25	0.2
Other postnatal intoxications	82	0.6
Unknown cause with structural reaction	1,408	10.1
Unknown cause—functional reaction alone manifest	4,649	33.3

From DHEW, *Children Served in Mental Retardation Clinics, Fiscal Years, 1970–1972.*

normalities at all, and this is certainly an underestimation because many functionally retarded people never go to clinics for the mentally retarded. An additional 18 percent of the cases consisted of those with apparent organic impairment for which no cause could be determined (the categories of congenital cerebral defect and unknown cause with structural reaction). The specific syndromes make up only a small proportion of the overall population of the mentally retarded.

Summary

A distinction is frequently made between two broad categories of mentally retarded people. One group consists of those people for whom there is evidence of organic abnormalities that result in diminished mental abilities. This group is called the organically retarded. The second group consists of those individuals for whom there is no apparent biological or medical cause for their diminished mental abilities. These people are sometimes referred to as the culturally retarded, the familially retarded, or the functionally retarded.

The following are the important categories of organic causes of mental retardation.

Prenatal Infections. There are a variety of microorganisms that can infect the developing embryo or fetus and cause permanent abnormalities, including mental retardation. Among these are rubella (German measles), syphilis, cytomegalovirus, and toxoplasmosis.

Postnatal Infections. There are several types of microorganisms which, if they infect a growing child, can result in brain damage and mental retardation. The two best known of these are encephalitis and meningitis.

Intoxications. There are several types of poisons that can cause brain injury and mental retardation. Among these are maternal antibodies that have developed to the Rh factor in the blood of the developing fetus, various drugs which the mother may take during pregnancy, and radiation. Other maternal conditions such as a disorder called toxemia of pregnancy can also lead to toxic conditions in the child. After birth, mental retardation can also result from the child ingesting lead.

Perinatal Complications. There are a number of complications of the birth process itself that can result in brain damage and mental retardation. For example, if the infant's oxygen supply is cut off for more than a few minutes, the resulting anoxia will cause brain injury. Similarly, it is possible for the brain to suffer a mechanical injury of some sort during the birth process.

Postnatal Trauma. Certain types of brain injuries suffered after birth can result in mental retardation. One injury of this type that has received a good deal of attention lately is child abuse.

Inherited Metabolic Disorders. Occasionally an individual is born with an inherited inability to metabolize certain substances, and the result can be mental retardation. One of the best known of these is a disorder called PKU, which is an inability to metabolize an amino acid. The condition can now be detected at birth and treated with a special diet. Another such condition is galactosemia, an inability to metabolize milk sugar. This can also be treated with a special diet. Both of these are transmitted by a recessive gene.

Disorders of Lipid Metabolism. There are a number of rare disorders that result from an inability to properly metabolize fats. The best known of these is Tay-Sachs disease, which always results in severe mental retardation and an early death.

Hypothyroidism. Hypothyroidism, formerly called cretinism, results from an abnormally low level of thyroid hormone. The condition is often present at birth, and it can result from a variety of different causes. If not treated it can result in diminished mental abilities, but with treatment by thyroid medication, it does not usually present a problem.

Malnutrition. Deficient diet, if it is severe and if it occurs either prior to birth or shortly after birth, can result in permanent brain damage and mental retardation.

Postnatal Gross Brain Disease. There are a number of rare diseases that effect the brain after birth. The only two that are at all common are tuberous sclerosis and von Recklinghausen's disease. These two are somewhat unique in that they are transmitted by a dominant gene and thus cannot skip a generation.

Cranial Malformations. There are a number of congenital conditions, usually of unknown cause, which are characterized by deformities in the skull or the spine, and these can result in mental retardation. Hydrocephaly results from the inability of the cerebrospinal fluid to drain properly, thus resulting in tremendous pressure on the skull and brain. It can sometimes be treated with surgery. Hydrocephaly is often accompanied by spina bifida, an opening in the spine that can cause paralysis of the lower limbs. Another type of cranial anomaly is microcephaly, which is characterized by an unusually small head.

Chromosome Aberrations. A number of disorders result from the presence of an extra chromosome. The most important of these as far as numbers are concerned is Down's syndrome, known colloquially as mongolism, which results from an extra chromosome 21. Among the characteristics of Down's syndrome are lowered intelligence (mean IQ in the 30s), the characteristic eye shape, short stubby fingers, and a large tongue. The only other chromosome aberrations that are not extremely rare are those involving the sex chromosomes. These include Klinefelter's syndrome (XXY) and Turner's syndrome (XO). The former is a phenotypic male and the latter is a phenotypic female. Both are frequently characterized by mild mental retardation.

Prematurity. Children who are born prematurely or who have a birth weight of less than 2500 grams have a greater probability of being mentally retarded. Such prematurity is far more common among lower-income groups and among racial minorities than it is among middle-class whites, and presumably is caused by inadequate nutrition and poor medical care.

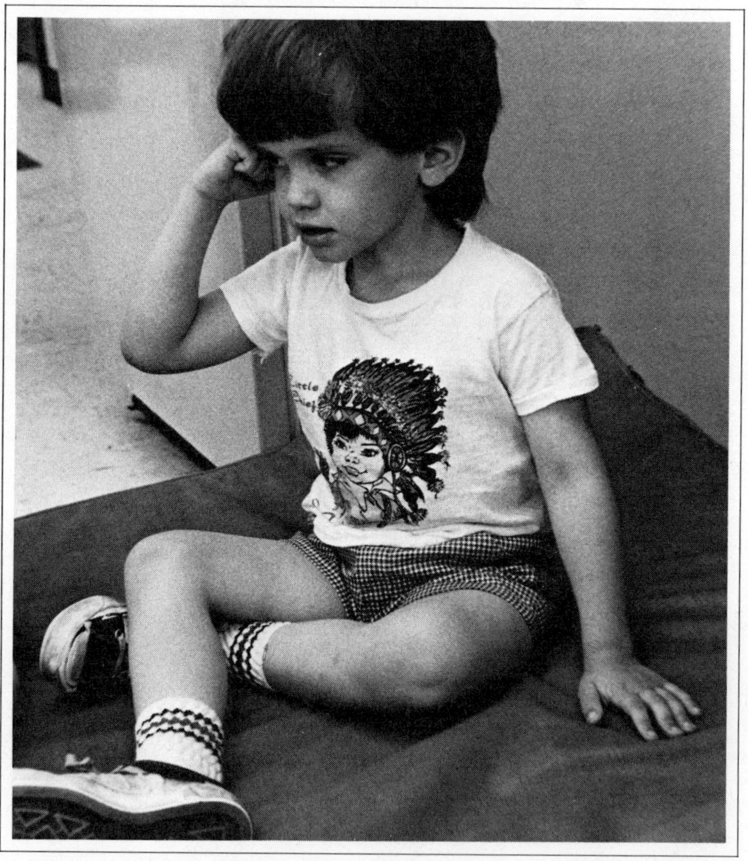

6

Brain Damage and Related Conditions

A distinction that was commonly made in the past but that is now considered to be obsolete is the distinction between endogenous and exogenous mental retardation. Endogenous retardation refers to retardation that originates from conception, and the largest group of endogenously retarded people are the familially mentally retarded, those people who are at the lower end of the normal curve as far as intelligence is concerned and whose diminished mental abilities are presumably inherited. Exogenous retardation refers to those cases whose development started out normally and then was interfered with in some way, usually by an external agent or condition that resulted in damage to the nervous system. Thus, a rough synonym for exogenous retardation is brain damaged, although this label has fallen out of favor with educators and psychologists. The distinction between endogenous and exogenous retardation may seem to be somewhat trivial, but several theorists (e.g., Strauss and Lehtinen, 1947) have suggested that children with brain damage have thought and behavior patterns that are qualitatively different from endogenously retarded and normal children.

This chapter investigates the concept of brain damage, reviewing its causes, its diagnosis, and its relationship to mental retardation. Then it discusses a number of consequences of brain damage besides diminished mental abilities. This section includes a brief review of conditions like cerebral palsy and epilepsy that, although they do not cause mental retardation directly, are often found in retarded populations. Then it discusses several conditions that are often believed to be caused by some sort of brain dysfunction, although the causal link has not been proved. These include hyperactivity and learning disabilities.

Brain Damage

The term brain damage refers to the physical destruction of brain tissue or brain cells. Such nervous system damage has a wide variety of causes, and thus there are numerous different types of brain damage. Most brain damage in children is not confined to one area of the brain but is diffuse; many cells throughout the brain are either killed or else their metabolism is interfered with so that they do not function properly.

Causes of Brain Damage

Any condition that can result in injury to a normally developing brain causes brain damage. Thus, the majority of the conditions discussed in the previous chapter are causes of brain damage. This includes prenatal and postnatal infections, toxic conditions, some types of metabolic and nutritional disorders such as PKU, endocrine disorders such as hypothyroidism, gross brain diseases such as tuberous sclerosis, the various cranial anomalies such as hydrocephaly, and prematurity. In fact the only major category of disorders discussed in the previous chapter that is not generally considered to be a cuase of brain damage is the chromosome disorders such as Down's syndrome since these result in malformations of the nervous system starting at conception. Notice that PKU, even though it is a genetic disorder, results in brain damage and exogenous retardation because the brain develops normally during the embryo and fetal periods of development, and then is slowly poisoned by the by-products of abnormal metabolism after birth.

Thus, each of these conditions can result not only in mental retardation, but also in a variety of other conditions such as cerebral palsy, epilepsy, and perhaps learning disabilities.

Diagnosis of Brain Damage

Because a physician cannot usually examine a child's brain directly, brain damage must often be inferred from the child's functioning and behavior. There are some conditions, such as epilepsy and cerebral palsy, that always indicate brain dysfunction, but if such conditions are not present, neurological impairment may be very difficult to diagnose, particularly if the damage is subtle. A physician who suspects brain impairment would test a wide variety of functions. For example, abnormal functioning of certain reflexes such as the knee jerk suggests a neurological problem. Poor coordination can indicate brain impairment, and the physician may test this by asking the child to place his or her heel on the opposite knee and slide it down the shin or by asking the child to close his or her eyes and touch a finger to the nose. Abnormal muscle tone, either too rigid (hypertonic) or too flaccid (hypotonic), can also indicate a nervous system dysfunction. A physician specializing in neurology may have more sophisticated tools. The physician may take a skull X ray, which can indicate certain kinds of abnormalities such as tumors or can actually take a sample of the electrical waves of the brain with a device called an electroencephalograph (EEG), which amplifies small electrical currents from the skull and translates them into pen tracings on moving paper. An expert can frequently learn a good deal about a brain's functioning by studying its EEG.

A number of psychologists have attempted to construct tests that will indicate brain damage. Typical of such work is a test battery developed by Halstead, which includes the following tests (Reitan, 1966).

1. *Category Test.* The subject must discover a common principle that distinguishes correct from wrong answers by testing hypotheses.
2. *Critical Flicker Frequency.* A strobe light flickers at a progressively faster rate until the subject indicates that he or she no longer sees flickering, and the light appears continuous.
3. *Tactual Performance Test.* The subject fits various shaped forms into a formboard while blindfolded, then the board and blindfold are removed and the subject must draw the board from memory.
4. *Rhythm Test.* The subject hears a series of 30 pairs of rhythmic beats and, in each case, must indicate whether the two members of the pair were the same or not.
5. *Speech Sounds Perception Test.* The subject hears 60 spoken nonsense sounds and, in each case, must indicate on a sheet of paper which sound was heard.
6. *Finger Oscillation Test.* A test of how fast the subject can tap with a finger.
7. *Time Sense Test.* The subject observes a hand on a clock and must stop the hand after it has gone around 10 times. After a number of such trials, the subject is required to estimate a comparable amount of time with the clock not available.

Research has shown that adult subjects with known brain damage generally do more poorly on this battery of tests than do similar subjects with no history of brain damage, and thus, if a person without certain brain damage does poorly, neurological impairment might be suspected.

Brain Damage and Mental Retardation

Many people assume that brain damage and mental retardation are approximate synonyms, but this is certainly not the case. Many people who are obviously retarded show no signs of brain damage or other organic impairment, and many people with obvious brain damage manifest little or no impairment in intelligence. There are cases of people with extensive brain damage who have well above average mental abilities. For example, Kennedy and Ramirez (1964) describe the case of a 7-year-old boy with massive nervous tissue destruction as indicated by a pneumoencephalogram (a type of skull X-ray). Although the boy was spastic, he was considered quite intelligent and well behaved. He had an excellent school record and a tested IQ of 137. Hebb (1939) described a 15-year-old boy who had had three different brain operations to remove infected tissue. His left frontal lobe was almost completely useless, and there was some atrophy of the right frontal lobe. Yet, four months after the last operation, he had a tested IQ of 110.

However, these cases are exceptions. There is clearly a relationship between brain damage and diminished mental abilities, and, for the most part, those individuals with *extensive* brain damage show impaired cognitive capacities. However, many individuals with mild brain dysfunction or injury may be of normal intelligence although there may be other manifestations of the dysfunction.

A Continuum of Reproductive Casualty

Knobloch and her associates (e.g., Pasamanick and Knobloch, 1966) have suggested that brain damage, rather than being either present or absent as it is usually conceptualized, should be considered to be a continuum, with perhaps more than half the population having some sort of brain damage. They have labeled this a continuum of reproductive casualty. At one extreme of this continuum is death from extensive nerve damage. Other infants have severe brain damage and are severely mentally retarded or have severe cerebral palsy. Still others have only moderate brain damage and may be only mildly retarded. A great many children have only minimal brain damage. These are the children who are hyperactive and who have learning disabilities. There are also presumably children whose brain damage is so slight that it is never detected.

Conditions Other than Mental Retardations that Are Associated with Brain Damage

There are a number of conditions besides mental retardation which are either definitely caused by or widely assumed to be caused by brain damage. These conditions include epilepsy, cerebral palsy, hyperkinesis, perceptual problems, and learning disabilities. These conditions, although clearly distinct from mental retardation, are frequently found among the mentally retarded or else are closely enough related to mental retardation to warrant discussion in a book such as this.

Epilepsy

Like mental retardation, the term epilepsy does not refer to a unitary condition but includes a variety of similar symptoms. Epilepsy is a general term used to describe a condition of recurrent seizures or convulsions. There are a number of different kinds of epileptic seizures and a wide variety of different causes. Until recently, it was poorly understood and thus very much feared. As recently as the 1960s, many states prohibited epileptics from marrying, driving a car, or working in certain kinds of jobs, and compulsory sterilization laws were common (Barrow and Fabing, 1966). Job discrimination has probably been more widespread for epileptics than for any other handicapped group.

It is difficult to estimate the prevalence of epilepsy because defining it is often difficult. Almost anyone can be induced to have a seizure if conditions are right. Isolated convulsions associated with fever occur occasionally among children, but this is not usually considered to be a type of epilepsy because the seizures are not recurrent. The most widely cited figure for the incidence of true epilepsy is about 5 per 1000 births (Telford and Sawrey, 1972). Epilepsy is considerably more common among males than females, and children are far more likely to have seizures than are adults. In fact, there are many cases of children whose seizures cease when they reach the teen years. Because it is caused by brain disorders, it is far more frequent among the mentally retarded. Epileptics are three to four times more likely to be retarded than are nonepileptics (Boshes and Gibbs, 1972), and in any large population of severely retarded people, as many as a third or more may be epileptic (Illingsworth, 1959). Epilepsy is seldom if ever the cause of the retardation. The two are found together frequently because they have the same cause. It is important to remember, however, that the vast majority of epileptics are of normal intelligence.

The classic seizure that most people associate with epilepsy is called a grand mal seizure. A grand mal seizure is characterized by the individual abruptly losing consciousness and falling to the ground as all of the muscles tighten up. After a few seconds of this tonic stage, the person begins to thrash around violently. This phase, called the clonic stage, is distinguished by rapid, violent, uncontrolled movements. This stage can be quite dangerous, as the person may injure himself or herself as he bangs into walls, furniture, or the floor, and may bite the tongue or lips. This stage is frequently characterized by frothing at the mouth, and the whole episode has a frightening appearance to observers. After several minutes of the clonic stage, the individual lapses into a comalike sleep which may last for several hours. When the person awakens, he or she typically has no recollection of the seizure, although he or she knows that one has occurred.

Grand mal seizures are the most familiar type, but another common variety of seizure is called petit mal. This is far less serious and is characterized by only a brief lapse of consciousness that may last a few seconds. The child may blink the eyes rhythmically or experience a sudden jerking or loss of posture and may drop what he or she is doing, but there is none of the violent thrashing around which is so typical of grand mal seizures. Petit mal seizures are far more frequent among children and tend to clear up with age. Although people suffering from grand mal seizures are more common than are those with petit mal, some children with petit mal seizures may have up to 200 per day. However, many go unnoticed because of their mildness.

There are a number of rarer types of epileptic disorders. A Jacksonian seizure is characterized by a twitch or jerk that starts at one location in the body such as a limb or a side of the face, and it gradually spreads to other parts. This type of seizure sometimes enlarges to encompass the whole body and thus becomes a grand mal seizure. On the other hand, the seizure may be entirely localized to one part of the body.

The terms psychomotor seizure is a general term that encompasses a variety of conditions not characterized by convulsions or blackouts. The individual may suffer distortions of perception such as a *déja vu* experience or may engage in incoherent muttering or bizarre behavior such as buttoning and unbuttoning the shirt. The person appears to be in a sort of trance and, although not losing consciousness, generally will not remember his or her actions. This type of seizure, although it is relatively rare, is partially responsible for the prejudice that some people still have against epileptics because occasionally a psychomotor seizure will be characterized by uncontrollable rage or even criminal acts such as assault. It is sometimes difficult to distinguish between a seizure-induced violent act and other types of emotional disturbance.

Epileptic seizures result from the normal electrical activity of the brain going out of control. The immediate cause of this is always some sort of brain dysfunction, and thus the etiology of epilepsy is the same as for many other types of brain damage. It is found more frequently among those cases with a history of birth complications, prematurity, lead poisoning, encephalitis, and physical injury. The epilepsy generally begins in a specific region where damage has occurred. The seizure does not originate from the dead cells, but frequently, a region of malfunctioning cells will develop around the site of an injury, and this type of cell is likely to induce a seizure. The EEG is often used to determine the location of the origin of the epilepsy, but it is not always reliable because many individuals with a clear history of seizures have a normal EEG, and many normal, seizure-free people have an epilepticlike EEG.

A distinction is sometimes made between two types of epilepsy, ideopathic and secondary. Secondary or symptomatic epilepsy can be traced to a specific cause, such as physical injury or lead poisoning, while the term ideopathic epilepsy describes those cases of epilepsy where there is no apparennt brain damage. There seems to be a hereditary component to ideopathic epilepsy since some cases have a history of seizures in the family.

There are certain kinds of environmental conditions that seem to induce epileptic seizures. Seizures are more common when the person is overtired or under stress. Even things like the weather or a woman's menstrual cycle are correlated with the rate of epileptic seizures. Occasionally, flickering lights can trigger a seizure. Some children can apparently voluntarily induce a seizure. On the other hand, focusing attention on a task seems to reduce the possibility of petit mal seizures.

A number of drugs have been successful in reducing the frequency of epileptic seizures, and, as a result, epilepsy is not nearly as serious a problem now as it used to be. The two most common anticonvulsant drugs are phenobarbital and Dilantin. The former is a mild barbituate that has been in use for more than 60 years. It is quite safe in moderate doses, but it can occasionally make people drowsy. It can also produce irritability in some hyperactive children. While it is not truly addictive, sudden withdrawal of the drug can induce seizures. Dilantin is more effective in reducing seizures and does not have the sedative properties of phenobarbital, but there are a number of annoying side effects. Children on Dilantin will sometimes show unusual hair growth, a skin rash, or excessive growth of the gums over the teeth.

Antiepileptic medication must be individualized since cases differ widely in their reaction to the drugs. However, seizures can be effectively controlled, usually eliminated completely, in about 85 percent of the cases with some combination of these or other similar drugs. A much rarer treatment, which is used only in intractable cases, is surgical removal of the diseased brain tissue.

Even serious convulsions are not generally dangerous if proper precautions are taken. Boshes and Gibbs (1972) list the following steps to take if a child has a seizure:

1. KEEP CALM. The person is not in pain, is not suffering, and is not in danger.
2. DO NOT be frightened if near an individual with seizures, for they are not catching.
3. DO NOT attempt to stop the attack once it has started. DO NOT try to revive the patient, but let the seizure run its course, which usually takes a few minutes.
4. EASE the person to the floor, loosen tight clothing, but DO NOT restrain his or her movements.
5. TURN the person's face to the side to permit release of saliva and make certain that breathing is not obstructed. A coat may be placed under the head.
6. DO NOT force open the clenched jaws. DO NOT force anything between the person's teeth. NEVER place a finger in the mouth.
7. DO NOT give the individual anything to drink.
8. STAY with the person until all movement has ceased and stand by until the person has recovered consciousness fully and is no longer confused. A small child may be carried to a rest room, and a larger individual may be allowed to lie until able to talk. If the person is tired, permit him or her to rest, and when he or she feels better, encourage him or her to go about his or her regular activities.
9. DO NOT be frightened if the person with a seizure may appear not to be breathing for a while or breathing poorly.
10. CAREFULLY OBSERVE the details of the attack so this can be reported subsequently to the person's family or physician.
11. If the person is a child, notify the parents. If no one is available, you may call proper authorities. If the attack is an initial one, you may call a physician (Boshes and Gibbs, 1972, p. 151).

Cerebral Palsy

Cerebral palsy is defined as a motor impairment such as paralysis, weakness, or incoordination that results from a brain dysfunction. Thus, by definition, all children with cerebral palsy are brain damaged. Like mental retardation and epilepsy, cerebral palsy is not a unitary condition but is a general term encompassing a variety of symptoms.

There are a number of different types. The most common is called spasticity. Spasticity results from injury to the motor cortex or the pyramidal tracts of the brain and the result is a loss of coordinated muscle movement. More technically, spasticity refers to an exaggerated contraction to muscles that are stretched. Thus, when the person tries to perform a movement such as raising an arm, as soon as the arm muscles begin to stretch, they contract reflexively. The result is jerky, uncoordinated movements. The person's muscles become excessively rigid, and voluntary movements can be made only with difficulty. A similar condition is called rigidity, when there is increased resistance to passive movements of the limbs. Athetosis is the second important category of cerebral palsy. It results from brain damage to the extrapyramidal system and the basal ganglia, and is characterized by involuntary, slow, writhing movements of the involved limbs. These uncontrollable movements increase when the person tries to control them or when attempting a voluntary act, but, interestingly, they are not present when the person is asleep.

The third common type of cerebral palsy is ataxia. Ataxia results from damage to the cerebellum and is characterized by difficulties in balance. The person walks as if intoxicated and speech is frequently slurred. There are a number of other rarer types of cerebral palsy, and sometimes several types are found in the same person.

There is tremendous variability in the degree of impairment of cerebral palsied people. Some cases are very minimally impaired, and their condition results in little more than slightly lessened coordination or increased clumsiness. At the opposite extreme are individuals so impaired that they are unable to do anything for themselves; they do not have enough control of their limbs to even feed themselves. Most cases lie somewhere between these two extremes. Many cerebral palsied people have the additional handicap of impaired speech. If the articulatory muscles are affected, they may have difficulty communicating their needs to others.

There is considerable variability in estimates of the incidence of cerebral palsy, but Kirk (1972), after summarizing several studies, concluded that the most accurate estimate is one to two per thousand births. Estimates of the percentages of different types of cerebral palsy are even more variable, reflecting the difficulty in making an accurate diagnosis. For example, a study by Hansen (1960) found that 78.5 percent of cerebral palsied children were spastic and only 9.3 percent athetoid, while a study of Phelps (1948) found only 40 percent of cerebral palsied cases to be spastic and 40 percent to be athetoid.

Because cerebral palsy is caused by brain damage, it is usually found in conjunction with other handicaps associated with neurological impairment such as sensory loss, perceptual disorders, epilepsy, and learning disabilities. For example, of 1265 cases of cerebral palsy studied by Hopkins, Bice, and Colton (1954), 369 or 29.2 percent had a history of seizures. In the same group, 21.4 percent had visual impairments and 68 percent had speech impairments.

Accurate assessment of the intellectual functioning of cerebral palsied children and adults is often difficult, particularly in severe cases where the individual's repertoire of responses is very limited. However, it is generally assumed that the average IQ of cerebral palsied children is considerably below 100, and that approximately half of all cerebral palsied children and adults are also mentally retarded. For example, in the survey of Hopkins, Bice, and Colton, 49 percent of their cerebral palsied children had IQs below 70 and only 6.6 percent had IQs above 110. However, this does not mean that there are no unusually intelligent cerebral palsied people. There is a novelist in England who is so severely impaired that he is forced to type with his toes, but nonetheless has written several widely selling books.

Severe cerebral palsy is perhaps the most devastating of any handicap. Many people seem almost relieved to hear that a cerebral palsied child is also retarded because the child will be less aware of the cruel affliction. Many such children are confined to wheelchairs for their entire lives and can never hope to even take care of their basic needs such as dressing and feeding. Some are too severely handicapped to be productively employed. Fortunately, however, as a result of changing attitudes and expanded programs of training and rehabilitation, most victims of severe cerebral palsy can look forward to a more productive and meaningful life than was the case a few years ago.

Hyperkinesis

Hyperkinesis is a poorly defined collection of behavioral traits that are frequently found together. Symptoms include hyperactivity, distractibility, short attention span, impulsivity, and emotional lability. There is little doubt that there are a great many children who fit this general description, but there is considerable debate regarding whether it constitutes a genuine syndrome and even more debate concerning its etiology. Some authors (e.g., Strauss and Lehtinen, 1947) argue that it is always a result of brain injury. A widely used name for the syndrome is minimal brain dysfunction (Wender, 1971). However, there are many children who fit the classical description of hyperkinesis but show no other indications of brain damage. Marwit and Stenner (1972) have proposed that there might be two separate syndromes that appear similar—one caused by brain dysfunction, the other purely psychological.

Almost everyone is aware of children who fit the general description of a hyperkinetic child. This is a child who is continually on the go and who usually cannot sit still for more than a few minutes. While all children tend to be quite active, the hyperkinetic child is particularly distinguished by aimless activity. There is little apparent pattern to the constant motion, and the child flits from one thing to another on an apparently random basis. The behavior has been described as driven, meaning that the child has little control over it.

Most children who are hyperkinetic seem to have been this way since birth. Their mothers describe them as difficult even as infants; they are continually crying and colicky, they do not feed well and their sleep is irregular. As soon as they are able to walk, the problems become worse; these children are continually getting into everything in the house and need to be continually watched to prevent them from doing considerable damage. The problem reaches a peak in the elementary school years, when the child will not sit long enough to do any school work and is a constant annoyance to the other children and the teacher.

In addition to being hyperactive, these children seem to have a very short attention span and they are easily distracted. They are continually focusing on irrelevant stimuli in the room rather than concentrating on one task. Strauss and Lehtinen (1947) have proposed that such children ought to be taught in a minimally stimulating classroom, or even in individual booths in order that there be as few distractions as possible, but research has not shown that these children learn more in such an environment (Somerville, Warnberg, and Bost, 1973).

A third problem of hyperkinetic children is their emotional lability. They become angry or aggressive at seemingly minor provocations. Their tolerance of frustration is very limited, and they overrespond emotionally to everyday situations, either crying inappropriately, being excessively elated, or engaging in violent tantrums for no apparent reason. They are also frequently characterized as being excessively aggressive toward other children.

Because the syndrome is so hard to define, it is difficult to get reliable prevalence figures, but everyone agrees that it is very common. Stewart et al. (1966) reported the prevalence of the "hyperactivity syndrome" to be about 4 percent among a group of St. Louis elementary school children, and Huessy (1967) found the prevalence of hyperkinesis to be about 10 percent. There is probably at least one and frequently several hyperactive children in most classes in the nation. Hyperkinetic children clearly form the largest diagnostic category among children referred for psychiatric help

(Wender, 1971). The syndrome is far more prevalent among boys than it is among girls. The male-to-female ratios reported range from three or four to one up to nine to one or more (Wender, 1971). All of the syndromes discussed so far, including mental retardation itself, are found more frequently in males than in females, but hyperkinesis favors boys to a much greater extent than do any of the others. Needless to say, interpretations of this sex ratio range from purely biological to purely psychological.

The hyperkinetic syndrome usually dissipates as the child gets older. Many of these children improve markedly as they move into adolescence. However, in severe cases, the symptoms may persist, or even develop into a more serious disorder such as psychosis (Menkes, Rowe, and Menkes, 1967).

There is a major controversy surrounding the treatment of hyperactivity with drugs. For reasons that are presently unknown, stimulants such as amphetamines (known colloquially as speed), which cause adults to be more active, have the opposite effect on hyperkinetic children and seem to calm them down. This enables them to concentrate better and in some cases improves their school performance. Frequently, there is a dramatic change in children's behavior as soon as they are put on such a drug, and they immediately regress back to their old ways if they skip taking their pills for as little as a single day. As a result, such drugs are being prescribed for an increasing number of hyperactive children, in many cases based on the recommendation of the child's teacher. The *Journal of Learning Disabilities* (1974) reports that the use of such "pep" pills for the treatment of hyperactivity was up 55 percent in the previous two years, and that about 600,000 children in the United States, nearly 2 percent of the total school population, were receiving some kind of drug treatment for hyperactivity. The controversy centers around the fact that drugs that are known to be dangerous and addictive in adults are being given so indiscriminately to children, particularly when the reason for the drug treatment is such a vague diagnosis as hyperkinesis. It is feared that many teachers are using drugs as an excuse to control unruly children rather than making a sincere effort to try to teach the child. Other people argue that the underlying cause of most hyperactivity ought to be treated rather than just the symptoms. For example, there is evidence that hyperactivity can be produced by allergies, particularly to certain food additives (Havard, 1973), as well as by various other chemical imbalances (Walker, 1974).

Perceptual Disorders

Another characteristic symptom of brain dysfunction is perceptual disorders. This type of disturbance received particular attention from one of the pioneers in research on brain damage, A.A. Strauss. One such disorder is left-right inversions. For example, a child might mistake a "b" for a "d" or the word "was" for the word "saw." Another sort of perceptual disturbance particularly emphasized by Strauss was figure-ground difficulties, the ability to distinguish an object from its background. Some children are likely to attend to irrelevant details of a picture rather than to the main subject. For example, a child shown a picture of a girl standing in front of a group of trees might say, "it's a tree" or "it's a button."

A large number of tests have been developed to diagnose perceptual disorders, and these are frequently used as general tests of brain damage. Strauss and Lehtinen (1947) used a marble board test, two identical boards with rows of holes in them. The experimenter or tester makes a pattern with marbles on one of the boards and the subject tries to copy the pattern on the other. A number of studies indicate that children with brain injuries do not do as well on such tasks as do unimpaired children. The most widely used perceptual test is called the Bender Visual Motor Gestalt Test. This consists of a number of patterns on cards, and the subject is asked simply to copy them on a sheet of paper. There are developmental norms, and if a child is not performing up to his or her age level on this test, perceptual disturbances and possible brain dysfunction are indicated.

Learning Disabilities

The term learning disabilities has become very widely used in the past few years, but there is little consensus on what the term refers to. In its broadest sense, it includes all those children who are having trouble in school. It is also used as a synonym for minimal brain dysfunction and, thus, includes the syndrome of hyperkinesis described above. Usually, however, the term is used in a somewhat narrower sense. A typical definition which captures the way the term is most widely used is that of Kirk and Bateman (1962).

> *A learning disability refers to a retardation, disorder, or delayed development in one or more of the processes of speech, language, reading, writing, arithmetic, or other school subjects resulting from a psychological handicap caused by a possible cerebral dysfunction and/or emotional or behavioral disturbances. It is not the result of mental retardation, sensory deprivation, or cultural or instructional factors (Kirk and Bateman, 1962, p. 73).*

Children are diagnosed as learning disabled if they are not mentally retarded and have no vision or hearing problems and are not culturally deprived but still have difficulty with certain basic subjects in school. A frequently used criterion for diagnosis is that children are considered to be learning disabled if in a certain subject they are more than one year behind what would be expected from their mental age. Since the beginning of formal education, teachers have had students who have done poorly in one subject or another, yet do not seem to fit into any of the standard categories of exceptional children. Thus, there was a real need for a new diagnostic category, and this accounts in part for the popularity of the term. Research and writing on learning disabilities has grown geometrically in the past decade. As recently as 1962, there were no published articles indexed under "learning disabilities" in the *Psychological Abstracts,* a compendium of all articles written in the field. In 1967, there were only 12 articles listed, but by 1970, the number of articles listed under learning disabilities was over 100, and there were 174 articles listed in 1972 (Black, 1974). Classes, both public and private, have sprung up in numerous communities to service children with learning disabilities, and an increasing number of state and local governments are providing funds for such children.

By definition, learning disabilities and mental retardation are mutually exclusive. Technically, a child diagnosed as mentally retarded cannot also be diagnosed as learning disabled. This is somewhat misleading, however, since retarded children can have an unusual deficit in some subject or activity relative to their mental age. For example, a retarded child with a mental age of nine years whose overall academic functioning is at the third-grade level may be functioning at the first-grade level in mathematical ability, and this is certainly a type of learning disability. More and more, learning disabilities are being considered as a sort of middle ground between normalcy and mental retardation. That is, the term includes children whose learning is clearly behind the average child of like age, but not far enough behind to be labeled mentally retarded. There is some evidence that political motives may be involved in diagnosing a child as having a learning disability. Franks (1971) found that white, middle-class children who are having school difficulties are more likely to be assigned the less stigmatizing label of learning disabled, while black children were more likely to be labeled mentally retarded.

An assumption that is made either explicitly or implicitly by many researchers is that most learning disabilities are caused by neurological dysfunction rather than by purely psychological processes. The evidence for this comes from the fact that many children with learning disabilities, particularly those with more severe disorders, also show other signs of brain dysfunction such as hyperactivity or abnormal EEG or atypical reflexes, but there are just as many learning disabled children who show no other signs of brain dysfunction. Thus, the question of the etiology of learning disabilities is still unanswered. Most likely, there are a number of qualitatively different types of learning disabilities with different causes. Some result from specific brain lesions while others have nonorganic origins.

The term learning disability is extremely general, and there are a number of different terms that are used to refer to specific types of learning disabilities. For example, the term dyslexia refers to a specific disability in reading. An older term for dyslexia is word blindness, and this phrase characterizes the nature of the disorder. Although the individual's visual acuity is adequate, there is difficulty recognizing words. The person may make inversion errors of the type described in the previous section such as mistaking "b" for "d" and "was" for "saw." Other children may only attend to the first few letters of a word or only to the first and last letter. Still other children have unusual difficulty extracting meaning from what they read. They can read aloud with few problems but have no comprehension. It is impossible to arrive at an accurate figure for the prevalence of dyslexia because it is so poorly defined. As many as a third of all schoolchildren have reading difficulties of one sort or another, but it is impossible to say how many of these have specific dyslexia. The prognosis for dyslexic children, at least in milder cases, is fairly good, and most such children eventually develop adequate reading skills.

Other terms are occasionally used to refer to other kinds of learning disabilities. The term dyscalculia refers to a specific difficulty with mathematics, although like dyslexia, there are a number of different manifestations (Kosc, 1974). Dysgraphia refers to a condition where the child has particular difficulty in writing skills. Either the child cannot form the letters properly or there is unusual difficulty in written expression. The term agnosia refers to a condition where the individual has unusual difficulty in identifying or using information from a particular sensory channel. An example of auditory agnosia would be a person with intact hearing who hears keys jangling but cannot identify what the sound is until seeing the keys. Tactile agnosia refers to a condition where the individual cannot identify things by feel. Apraxia is an inability to perform certain motor skills when the motor system is intact. An example would be a child with normal coordination who is unusually delayed in learning to tie shoes.

Another major category of learning disability is aphasia (dysphasia). Aphasia refers to any sort of difficulty or delay in language or verbal skills. As with other learning disabilities, there are numerous manifestations. In many cases, the child's language skills are simply somewhat delayed. Expressive aphasia refers to conditions where the individual can understand spoken language, but cannot speak it properly, even though the articulatory apparatus is apparently intact. This person is unable to choose the correct words or form them into proper sentences. Thus, speech is slow and halting. Receptive aphasia refers to conditions where the individual has difficulty understanding spoken language, even though hearing is intact. Many sorts of language disorders such as these tend to clear up with age. Aphasia tends to be far more serious among adults who have suffered brain damage, usually as a result of stroke. In these cases, aphasia tends to be a far more permanent condition.

It is easy to see why learning disability is such a poorly defined area. It is often difficult to identify exactly what a child's problem is when the child is having difficulty in school. It is usually more desirable to pinpoint a child's difficulty than it is to decide on the correct way to label the behavior, and, as a result, many of these labels are not widely used except in extreme cases. There are also varying degrees of learning disabilities, and it is rare to find classic cases of one type such as those usually described in textbooks.

Because of the difficulties in diagnosis, good research on the incidence of learning disabilities is very rare. Estimates range as high as one third of the school age population (Ilg and Ames, 1967, cited in Tarnopol, 1969), and this could easily be true if all children with any difficulty in learning are included. At the opposite extreme is Gallagher (1969), who reported that between 1 and 3 percent of the nation's school population suffer from learning disabilities serious enough to require educational intervention beyond the usual classroom activity.

The Current Status of Brain Damage

There is considerable debate regarding the question of whether brain damage represents a valid diagnostic category or even whether it is necessary to try to determine whether brain damage has occurred. At one extreme are such theorists as Goldstein (1942) and Strauss and Lehtinen (1947), who argue that there are certain symptoms that occur to a greater or lesser extent in all cases of brain damage, regardless of the nature of the injury. These include more concrete thinking, perceptual disorders, and catastrophic emotional reactions. A number of people such as Delacato (1963), Kephart (1971), and Cruickshank et al. (1961) have proposed specific educational and therapeutic techniques for brain injured children based on this theory. Even today, one can find a number of schools and classes, mostly privately run, designed to accommodate brain injured children.

Opponents to this approach argue that there is no one set of symptoms that characterize brain injured people. Brain injury can result in an almost infinite variety of different symptoms. It is quite likely that brain damage is a continuum, and that almost everyone has suffered injury to the brain to some degree. Ross (1968) argues that attempting to determine if a given child has suffered brain injury is largely a waste of time except in the rare case where the injury is progressive, for example, when the damage is getting worse as a result of a tumor. A diagnosis of nonprogressive brain injury contributes nothing to a person's therapy or education, and the label of brain injury can have frightening implications for the child's parents since it has such a connotation of irreversibility and hopelessness. Others (Sarason and Doris, 1969) argue that brain damage cannot be used as an explanatory concept because of the diversity of signs associated with it. The current trend in this debate is toward this latter position. Children who in past years would have received a label of minimal brain dysfunction or some similar term are now diagnosed as having a learning disability. The learning disability may very well be due to organic causes, but whether the disability is organic or not does not effect treatment or therapy, and as a result, there is no need to make a firm diagnosis.

Summary

A good deal of mental retardation results from a loosely defined condition called brain damage. Such retardation is called exogenous because it results from interference in normal development as a result of external agents. Almost all of the conditions mentioned in Chapter 5 can cause brain damage, and thus there are a wide variety of different types and degrees. It is important to remember that brain damage and mental retardation are not synonyms. Many people with brain damage have normal intelligence, and many people who are obviously retarded show no sign of brain damage.

There are a number of conditions besides mental retardation that are presumably caused by brain damage or brain dysfunction, and they are found far more frequently among retarded populations than in the general population. Epilepsy is a condition characterized by temporary blackouts or convulsions. There are a number of different types. A grand mal seizure is characterized by violent thrashing and convulsions. A petit mal seizure is a brief blackout. Most epilepsy can be effectively controlled with drugs. Cerebral palsy is a general term for motor disturbances resulting from brain damage. There are a number of different types and the severity of the condition varies widely. About half of the people with cerebral palsy are also mentally retarded. Hyperkinesis is a condition characterized by hyperactivity, particularly a large amount of aimless activity, short attention span, distractibility, and emotional lability. It is believed to be caused by minimal brain damage, but there is considerable disagreement on this point. The standard treatment for hyperkinesis is stimulant drugs, which have the paradoxical effect of slowing down hyperactive children. Perceptual problems are also widely assumed to result from brain dysfunction. All of the above conditions are frequently found among the exogenously retarded.

One last condition that is widely assumed to result from minimal brain dysfunction is learning disabilities. This term refers to a variety of conditions in which the child has unusual difficulty learning one particular subject. By definition, a child who is retarded cannot be diagnosed as learning disabled, but this is distinctly misleading since many retarded children have a great deal more difficulty learning some subjects than others. Learning disabilities represent a sort of middle ground between mental retardation and normalcy, and there is an increasing tendency to label slow-learning children as learning disabled rather than retarded because of the less stigmatizing connotations.

The term brain damage has fallen out of favor as a diagnostic label among educators and psychologists because of its implication of hopelessness and because of its wide variety of different symptoms. Also, a diagnosis of brain damage contributes little to a child's program. Nevertheless, it is an important cause of diminished mental abilities.

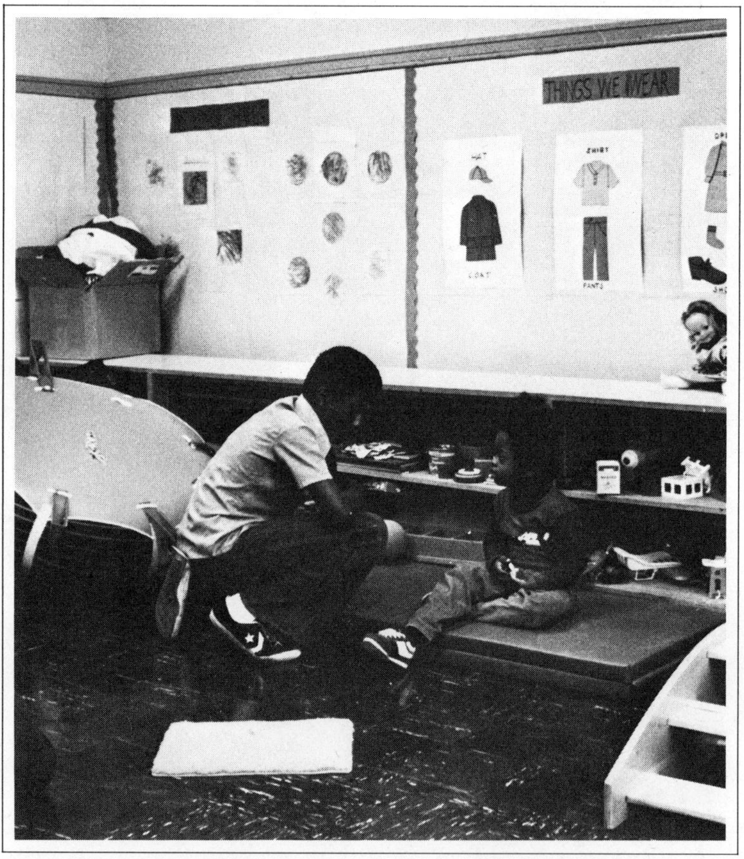
THINGS WE WEAR

7

Poverty, Race, and Mental Retardation

A distinction has been made between two different kinds of mentally retarded people. One group, described in the previous chapter, consists of those who have some sort of organic impairment such as brain damage, which is responsible for their diminished intellectual abilities. These people tend to have IQs below 50 and are found in approximately equal proportions in all levels of society. The second, much larger group, consists of those people who are functioning at a mentally retarded level but who have nothing physically wrong with them. Their nervous system is intact, and their physical appearance does not differ from the general population. This second group, the functionally retarded, is larger than the first and its members come almost exclusively from the lower strata of society. Racial minorities are overrepresented. The retardation of the functionally retarded is almost always mild rather than moderate, severe, or profound, and it presumably derives not from biological factors, but rather from psychological and social conditions. It has been widely accepted since the 1930s that how a child is raised can have important effects on that child's intellectual abilities, and thus, a major cause of retardation, the most important as far as numbers are concerned, is that many children are reared in environments not conducive to doing well on intelligence tests, in school, and in life. This chapter is concerned with those aspects of the child's family and cultural environment that seem to have an effect on mental capacities, school success, and general adaptiveness.

The Effects of Socioeconomic Status and Race on Mental Functioning

The Effects of Socioeconomic Status

The United States is theoretically a classless society, but it is clear that there are large differences in opportunity for education and vocational success resulting from differences in family background. Sociologists use the concept of socioeconomic status (SES) to refer to these differences. A person's socioeconomic status is determined by a number of characteristics such as income, occupation, amount of education, and residence. With rare exception, these variables are highly related to each other; that is, those people with the highest incomes tend to have more education, tend to be in high-status occupations, and are likely to live in the most desirable neighborhoods. Similarly, those people living below the poverty line tend to be poorly educated and are almost universally either unemployed or in the lowest-level jobs and live in the poorest neighborhoods. In this chapter, social status is divided into only two categories. One category will be labeled low SES. Synonyms for low SES are poor, disadvantaged, or underprivileged. Everyone else will be considered high SES or middle class or advantaged (there are so few people in the United States who consider themselves upper class that they can be combined with the middle class).

One of the most consistent findings in the research with IQ tests is that children from low SES families tend to achieve lower IQ scores than do children from high SES families. For example, Table 7-1 shows the average IQs of children from different family backgrounds as reported by McNemar

Table 7-1 Mean IQs of Children According to Fathers' Occupations

	Fathers' Occupational Classification	Chronological Ages			
		2–5½	6–9	10–14	15–18
I	Professional	114.8	114.9	117.5	116.4
II	Semiprofessional and managerial	112.4	107.3	112.2	116.7
III	Clerical, skilled trades, and retail business	108.0	104.9	107.4	109.6
IV	Rural owners	97.8	94.6	92.4	94.3
V	Semiskilled, minor clerical and business	104.3	104.6	103.4	106.7
VI	Slightly skilled	97.2	100.0	100.6	96.2
VII	Day labor, urban and rural	93.8	96.0	97.2	97.6

From Q. McNemar, *The Revision of the Stanford-Binet Scale,* Copyright © 1942 by Houghton-Mifflin Co., Boston. Reprinted with permission of the publisher.

(1942) in the standardization of the 1937 Stanford-Binet. Averaging across ages, children of professional men had an average IQ of 116 while children of day laborers had an average IQ of only 96 and children of farm owners had an average IQ of only 95. Thus, there is a difference of some 20 IQ points between the typical child in the most advantaged group and the typical child in the least advantaged group. Notice also that the difference is almost as large among preschoolers as it is among high school students. Jencks et al. (1972) estimate that the correlation between SES and IQ is about .35. This relationship is true not only in the United States, but also in most other countries of the world (Jensen, 1969).

The Effects of Ethnic Background

Discussion of racial differences, particularly with regard to such a value laden concept as intelligence, is a very emotional issue. However, differences between blacks and whites on tests of mental abilities are of such a magnitude and are found in such a variety of situations that they cannot be ignored. Perhaps the most thorough study of black IQ in America is that of Kennedy, Van de Riet, and White (1963). They administered the Stanford-Binet to 1800 black school children in five southern states in an attempt to gather normative data. They found an average IQ of only 80.7 for black children in their sample, nearly 20 points below the average for whites. This might be an underestimation of black IQ nationwide, since all of the children were from the South where IQs tend to be lower than for northern children, but the general conclusion that blacks score considerably below whites on IQ tests is unchallenged. An interesting finding of the study was that black IQ seemed to drop with increasing age. While the 6 year olds had an average IQ of 84.4, the 9 year olds had an average IQ of only 80.1, and the 12 year olds had an average IQ of only 75.5.

Audrey Shuey (1966) reviewed more than 380 different studies in which blacks and whites were compared on some type of mental test and reported that virtually all of them found that blacks scored far below whites. The average difference seems to be about 15 IQ points. There has been a long and bitter debate regarding the interpretation of these findings. Certainly, some of the differences can be accounted for by the fact that blacks have been at the very bottom of the social ladder for many generations. The U. S. Bureau of the Census reports that in 1973, the median income of black families was $7270 compared to $12,600 for white families. Thus, on the average, black families earn only 58 percent of what white families earn. This ratio has been relatively constant for many years. Twenty-eight percent of black families were below the poverty line. The unemployment rate for blacks has traditionally been about twice the white rate.

These figures tell only a part of the story. For generations, black people have been subjected to extremes of personal degradation. They have been so looked down on by the vast majority of whites that they were almost considered an inferior species. They weren't allowed to use the same bathrooms, they were forced by law to sit in a separate section on public transportation, they were not permitted to use most public facilities such as restaurants or hotels, and they were required to attend different schools. There was blatant job discrimination that relegated blacks to the most menial and lowest-paying jobs that few whites would take. With the passage of the 1964 civil rights legislation, most of the more flagrant abuses were made illegal, but public attitudes change slowly, and both blacks and whites still retain many of their old attitudes toward themselves and each other.

Other ethnic minorities have received similar treatment. Hispano-Americans, primarily Mexican Americans and Puerto Ricans, in addition to facing many of the same problems of prejudice and discrimination, also had to contend with a language problem. If one speaks English only poorly, it is going to be extremely difficult to learn anything in school, get a job, or even apply for welfare.

However, even when black children and white children are matched on social background to the extent that this is possible (it is reasonable to assume that a black child is at a social disadvantage even when compared to a white child whose family is making the same income), there are still differences in test performance between the two groups, although the differences are somewhat reduced. For example, Deutsch and Brown (1964) measured the IQs of 543 school children, both black and white, at three different levels of SES. The results are shown in Figure 7-1. This graph shows that the effects of SES and race seem to exert their effect on test performance independent of each other. There is about a 10-point difference between blacks and whites at each SES level, but the effect of SES level on blacks is just as strong as it is for whites. Black children in the higher SES category score about 12 points higher than black children in the lowest level.

Blacks have also traditionally had difficulty in school. Their deficit in academic performance was best documented by a government project in the 1960s called the Coleman Report (Coleman et al., 1966). The U.S. Office of Education surveyed more than 645,000 pupils in 4000 public schools and collected an enormous variety of educational data. Among other things, they administered an achievement test to all of the pupils in certain grades. This test was designed to have a mean of 50 and a standard deviation of 10 for each grade. The results are shown in Table 7-2. It is clear that black first graders lag behind white first grade children by a whole standard deviation and that this deficit in academic achievement becomes even larger by

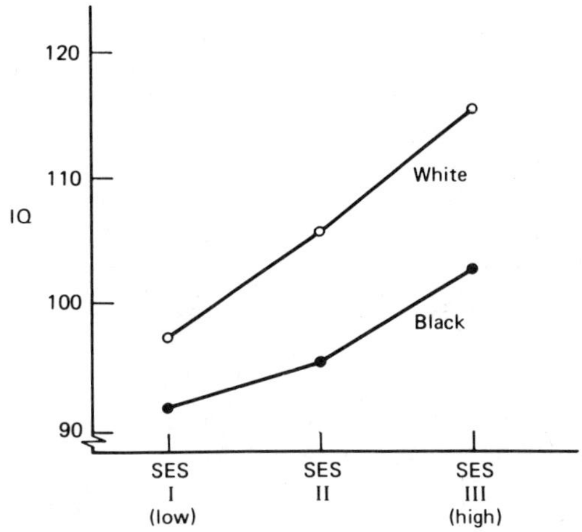

Figure 7-1 IQ as a function of SES and race. Adapted from Deutsch and Brown, 1964.

grade 12 even though many of the lowest-achieving blacks have dropped out of school. The average black high school senior is roughly three years behind his white counterpart in verbal ability and reading and more than five years behind in mathematical skills. This table also shows the achievement levels of other ethnic monorities, and it can be seen that with the exception of orientals, all racial minorities have far lower school achievement than do whites.

Table 7-2 Nationwide Median Test Scores for 1st- and 12th-Grade Pupils, Fall 1965

	Racial or Ethnic Group					
Test	Puerto Ricans	Indian Americans	Mexican-Americans	Oriental Americans	Negro	Majority
1st grade						
Nonverbal	45.8	53.0	50.1	56.6	43.4	54.1
Verbal	44.9	47.8	46.5	51.6	45.4	53.2
12th grade						
Nonverbal	43.3	47.1	45.0	51.6	40.9	52.0
Verbal	43.1	43.7	43.8	49.6	40.9	52.1
Reading	42.6	44.3	44.2	48.8	42.2	51.9
Mathematics	43.7	45.9	45.5	51.3	41.8	51.8
General information	41.7	44.7	43.3	49.0	40.6	52.2
Average of the 5 tests	43.1	45.1	44.4	50.1	41.1	52.0

From Coleman et al., 1966.

The Nature of SES and Racial Differences

Unless one assumes, as few people do these days, that intelligence is a unitary ability, it is reasonable to assume that minorities and poor children might show more of a weakness on some abilities than on others. A study by Lesser, Fifer, and Clark (1965) investigated this question. They developed tests to measure verbal ability, reasoning, numerical skills, and space conceptualization, and administered these four tests to a total of 320 six- and seven-year-old children. These children were equally divided among four ethnic groups, Chinese, Jewish, black, and Puerto Rican, and half of each group was lower class, half middle class. Figure 7-2 shows the results. Two conclusions are apparent. First, each ethnic group appears to have a characteristic pattern of abilities. For example, Jewish children are strong in verbal abilities relative to the other three, while Chinese children are relatively weak in verbal skills. Black children manifest a particular weakness in numerical skills (recall that the Coleman Report found that black children had more of a deficit in mathematical achievement than in verbal achievement). The second conclusion is that social class differences do not alter this basic pattern of abilities; low SES seems to be associated with about the same amount of deficit on all four tests for each group.

A number of researchers have attempted to develop an intelligence test that would not favor middle-class children. For example, Eells et al. (1951) administered a number of standard intelligence tests to nearly 5000 children ages 9, 10, 13, and 14 of various SES levels in an attempt to determine what kinds of test questions favor the middle class and what kind do not. Unfortunately, nearly two thirds of the test items at the 10-year level and about 90 percent of the items at the 14-year level favored middle-class children at a statistically significant level. There was some tendency for the items that favored middle-class children to be more verbal in nature, and the items that showed the least SES difference tended to be nonverbal, but there were numerous exceptions. This group attempted to construct a culture fair test of intelligence called the Eells Davis Games, but this test showed just as much of a middle-class bias as did more traditional tests, even though it was largely nonverbal. In fact, others have found that black children actually seem to do better on traditional verbal, culturally loaded tests than they do on so-called culture fair tests such as the Raven Matrices or the Leiter International Performance Scale (Higgins and Sivers, 1958; Costello and Dickie, 1971).

Another type of culture fair test derives from the theory of Jean Piaget. His theory will be discussed in some detail in a later chapter, but, for the moment, it is sufficient to say that he has postulated a series of stages of cognitive development that all children go through in the same order, re-

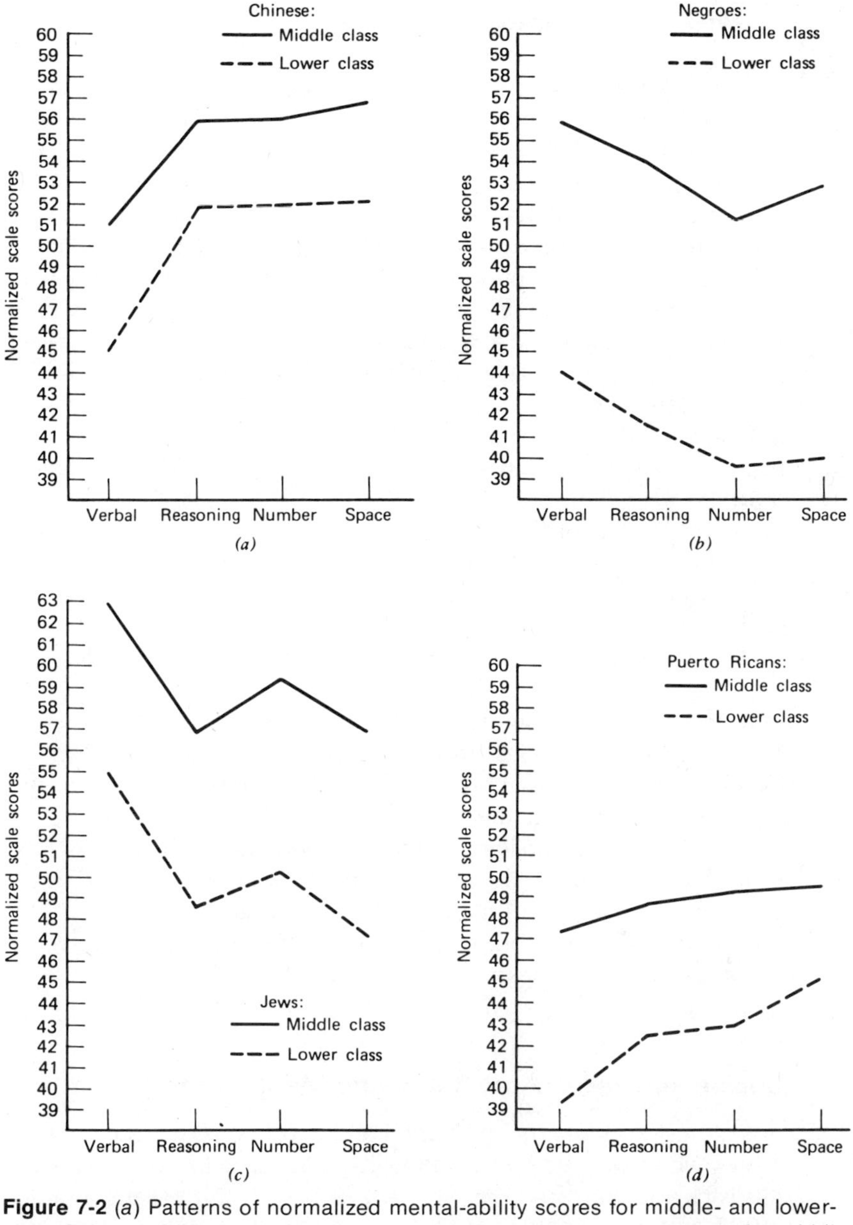

Figure 7-2 (*a*) Patterns of normalized mental-ability scores for middle- and lower-class Chinese children. (*b*) Patterns of normalized mental-ability scores for middle- and lower-class Negro children. (*c*) Patterns of normalized mental-ability scores for middle- and lower-class Jewish children. (*d*) Patterns of normalized mental-ability scores for middle- and lower-class Puerto Rican children. From Gerald Lesser and Susan Stodolsky, Learning patterns in the disadvantaged, *Harvard Educational Review* **37,** Fall 1967. Copyright © 1967 by President and Fellows of Harvard College. Reprinted with permission.

gardless of their cultural background. Gaudia (1972) tested lower-class children of three racial groups, white, black, and American Indian, on the Conservation Concept Diagnostic Kit, which assesses Piagetian development. Gaudia found that the black children in the sample were significantly below the whites, while differences between white and Indian children were slight. All three groups were lower-class children and scored below national norms.

Thus, the poor test performance of poor and minority children does not seem to be limited to certain areas, although deficits seem to be greater in tests which measure the ability to abstract. To date, no one has developed a valid test of mental abilities on which poor and black children do as well as middle class whites.

These test differences between SES levels and between ethnic groups are not present during the first two years of life but apparently develop during the third year. The best demonstration of this is Bayley's (1965) standardization of her Infant Scales. She administered a mental and a motor test to 1409 infants between 1 and 15 months old, both black and white, and of various backgrounds. She found no differences at any of these ages between boys and girls or between firstborns and later siblings. The educational level of the parents, presumably a measure of SES, did not correlate with test performance, and there were no differences on the mental scale between black and white children. However, black children were significantly superior to whites on the motor scale. What this means is that the black children in her sample sat alone, stood unsupported, and walked at a younger age than did the white children. The fact that there are no differences in mental abilities between Negro and white babies under two years has been found in other studies. Golden and Birns (1968) administered the Cattell Infant Intelligence Scale and a Piagetian test to black children under two years old and found no effect of SES. However, when the same children were tested a year later, there were clear SES differences (Golden, Birns, Bridger, and Moss, 1971).

Socioeconomic Status, Race, and Mental Retardation

It is almost an tautology that any condition that is associated with lower IQ scores would also be associated with an increase in mental retardation, and this is clearly the case both with low SES and with racial minorities. Mercer (1973) in her prevalence study on mental retardation in Riverside, California, analyzed the mentally retarded by social status and race. Social status was measured by place of residence. While 40 percent of the overall population lived in low-status housing districts, 59 percent of the mentally retarded came from these districts. There was an even larger difference as a result of race. Whites of European descent (Anglos) constituted 82 percent of the population of the community, but only 54 percent of the mentally retarded population was Anglo. Mexican-Americans composed 9.5 percent of the population, but 32 percent of the mentally retarded were from this group. Blacks constituted 7 percent of the community population, but 11 percent of the mentally retarded population. Thus, there were only two thirds as many Anglos as would be predicted if mental retardation were distributed evenly among all groups. However, there were more than three times as many Mexican-Americans and 57 percent more blacks than would be expected. Other studies have found racial minorities to be overrepresented in special classes for the retarded. In some inner cities, the problem is so serious that special classes result in a form of de facto segregation.

There is a growing reluctance to label these children of poverty mentally retarded. While many of them have tested IQs in the 60s, it is clear that most of them show no impairment in many aspects of adaptive behavior. For the most part, these children are socially adept; they have no trouble learning their way around the community or dealing with other people. On the other hand, most white middle-class children with IQs in the 60s show definite impairments in adaptive behavior. However, if we include academic skills such as reading or arithemetic under the rubric of adaptive behavior, then these children show deficiencies, and one frequent justification for placing many of these children in special classes is that they are largely unable to benefit from a regular classroom situation.

The Concept of Cultural Deprivation

It is safe to say that this issue of the relationship between social conditions, race, and school failure has occupied the attention of more scholars, researchers, and educators than has any other single issue in the 1960s and 1970s. It is also safe to say that despite the massive amounts of research and millions of words that have been written on the subject, the solution to the problem of school failure is not much closer now than it was 10 years ago, and the rate of school failure among blacks, Hispano-Americans, and the poor in general is just as great now as it ever was.

At the risk of oversimplifying the issue, it is possible to divide writers on this problem into three general camps, depending on how the issue is conceptualized and how it is explained. The first view, represented by such people as Bereiter and Engelmann (1966), Deutsch (1967), and Klaus and Gray (1968), says that there are important cognitive and verbal deficits in the poor and racial minorities, and that these deficiencies can be traced to deficits in the children's early environment. This is the cultural deprivation hypothesis. An important implication is that the cognitive deficits and resulting school failure can be largely alleviated by establishing compensatory education programs such as the widely publicized Head Start classes of the late 1960s.

The second camp is characterized by such people as Jensen (1969, 1973) and Herrnstein (1973). They argue that the differences between SES levels and between races on test performance and in school achievement are due in large part to genetic factors.

The third group, which includes such writers as Cole and Bruner (1971), Ginsburg (1972), and Baratz and Baratz, (1970) says that there are no significant cognitive or intellectual deficits among the poor or racial minorities; instead, their language and style of thinking is different. The schools and the mental tests are biased in favor of white, middle-class culture, and as a result, they detect a deficit when in fact there is none. This viewpoint has become very popular in the past few years.

This book does not advocate one position over the others. Each theory is presented in as positive a light as possible, but some of the more frequent criticisms will also be presented. As is usually the case with such controversies, each approach has certain merits, and the long-run solution to the debate will almost certainly be a synthesis of two or all three of these positions.

The Cultural Deprivation Hypothesis

The term cultural deprivation does not have a precise meaning. It refers, on one hand, to all of the circumstances associated with poverty, such as dilapidated housing, overcrowding, broken families, and a general lack of the cultural amenities. However, poverty by itself does not cause poor performance on mental tests or inferior school achievement. Thus, the word is also used to refer to those circumstances associated with poverty that seem to contribute to poor achievement. This includes such things as poor health, poor parental child-rearing practices, lack of adequate exposure to appropriate stimulation, and a general feeling of helplessness.

Poor Physical and Medical Care. Chapter 6 discussed a large number of conditions in the child's pre- and postnatal environment that have been linked to lowered intelligence. Birch and Gussow (1970) have documented in considerable detail how most of these conditions are found far more frequently among the poorest groups in society, racial minorities in particular. For example, prematurity is more than twice as frequent among blacks as it is among whites in this country. Lead poisoning from eating paint chips is almost exclusively a condition associated with poverty, first because poor children are more likely to eat paint chips in the first place, and second, because newer, more expensive homes do not have lead-based paint on the walls. Inadequate nutrition is also a condition found almost exclusively among the poor. The poor are less likely to receive adequate medical care at all stages of the life cycle, and this contributes to a higher rate of infant mortality as well as a higher rate of birth defects and other conditions associated with brain damage. Poor mothers are less likely to be innoculated against rubella. Thus, it is certain that at least a part of the SES differences in mental abilities can be accounted for by poor medical conditions.

Psychosocial Environment. However, more attention has been focused on the psychological environment as an important cause of school failure. Some writers have speculated that a major source of the impaired mental abilities was sensory deprivation. Poor children have few toys to play with, there are fewer objects of any kind in their homes, and poor families seldom take their children on trips to places like the zoo or to museums to expose them to new things (Deutsch, 1967). Others have stressed that poor children are overstimulated by so much going on in a crowded apartment in a noisy city, and as a result, they learn to ignore most stimuli in their environment (Klaus and Gray, 1968). However, neither of these contentions is supported by specific research findings.

A good deal of attention has been focused on the child-rearing patterns of poor families, particularly in the preschool years since this seems to be the time when differences originate. It seems that middle-class mothers spend a good deal of time preparing their children for success in school by developing in them a positive attitude toward academic achievement and by exposing the child to the kinds of stimulation that are conducive to academic success. Some mothers seem to spend a good deal of time talking to their children, reading to them, and explaining things to them, and these children seem to be the ones who do best in school. This teaching, whether it be deliberate or incidental, has been referred to as the middle-class curriculum.

Language Habits. The particular aspect of this middle-class curriculum that has received the most attention is language habits. The classic theorizing was done by Basil Bernstein (1961), an English sociologist. He postulated two kinds of language codes, a restricted code and an elaborated code. A restricted code is characterized by short sentences with a limited number of sentence forms and vocabulary, and its purpose is to convey information when there is a large body of shared knowledge, and thus, there is a reduced need for elaborate communication. The focus is on the concrete and the here-and-now rather than on universal principles. Restricted codes are frequently used between husbands and wives who can communicate a good deal of information with few words. It is also more characteristic of the lower class.

While everyone uses restricted codes from time to time, middle-class families are more likely to use an elaborated code, one with more complex sentence structure, larger vocabulary, and so forth, which is designed to organize meaning and facilitate symbolic activity. Thus, middle-class mothers are more likely to explain to their children why certain activities are prohibited, while lower-class mothers are more likely to simply outlaw the behavior. The following two conversations between a mother and a child on a bus illustrate the difference between a restricted code and an elaborated code.

Restricted code:

Mother: Hold on tight.
Child: Why?
Mother: Hold on tight.
Child: Why?
Mother: You'll fall.
Child: Why?
Mother: I told you to hold on tight, didn't I?

Elaborated code:

Mother: Hold on tightly, darling.
Child: Why?
Mother: If you don't, you will be thrown forward and you'll fall.
Child: Why?
Mother: Because if the bus suddenly stops, you'll jerk forward onto the seat in front.
Child: Why?
Mother: Now, darling, hold on tightly and don't make such a fuss (Bernstein, 1967, p. 97).

These language differences are considered to be particularly important because many people assume that language is an important facilitator of thought. Language provides the symbols that are needed for more abstract kinds of thinking, and thus, some people have speculated that children exposed primarily to a more restricted language code would necessarily have to have more restricted and less abstract thought processes. The importance of language to thinking has been the subject of considerable debate. At one extreme is B.L. Whorf (1956) who argued that one's native tongue structured all of one's thought processes, and indeed determined one's entire outlook on the world. At the other extreme is Hans Furth (1966), who argues that we don't think in a language at all, but that our thought involves some sort of abstract code that is fairly universal regardless of what language we happen to speak. The most reasonable approach is an in-between position, that language, while not essential for thinking, is an important mediator of thought and certainly determines the kinds of things that we think about. Insofar as this is true, if many low-SES children are exposed to a limited kind of language, their thinking processes could also be limited. Similarly, if a middle-class family uses many abstract words, this could encourage their children to think more abstractly.

Child-Rearing Style. A number of research projects have addressed themselves to SES differences in language habits and general child-rearing style. Hess and Shipman (1965) sought to test some of Bernstein's assertions. In particular, they hypothesized that the central quality involved in the effects of cultural deprivation is a lack of cognitive meaning in the mother-child interactions. They speculated that many families of culturally deprived children disciplined their offspring in an authoritarian manner and offered their children few alternatives relative to middle-class families. This leads to problem-solving strategies that are impulsive rather than reflective, that deal with the immediate rather than the future, and that are disconnected rather than sequential. Disciplining would be oriented toward role norms. Examples would be, "You do this because I say so" or "Girls don't act like that." On the other hand, in families of more advantaged children, control is effected by appealing to the individual characteristics of those involved or by appealing to rational explanation. An example would be, "Would you please keep quiet for a minute because I want to talk on the phone and can't hear with you banging like that."

Hess and Shipman (1965) located 163 Negro mothers of four year olds of four different social levels, upper middle class, upper lower class, lower lower class, and on welfare with father not present. These mothers were interviewed in their homes and their behavior observed in a laboratory setting in which they taught their child simple games. There were large differences between the middle-class mothers and the three kinds of lower-class mothers in the manner in which they interacted with their children. In terms of total verbal output, the typical middle-class mother said more than 60 percent more than did the lower-class mothers. In addition, they tended to use longer sentences, more complex sentences, and more abstract words. Confirming their hypothesis, the middle-class mothers tended to use more rational and person-oriented means of control, while the lower-class mothers appealed to authority. For example, all mothers were asked, "Suppose your child were starting school tomorrow for the first time. What would you tell him?" A middle-class mother answered, "First of all, I would remind her that she was going to school to learn, that her teacher would take my place, and that she would be expected to follow instructions. Also, that her time was to be spent mostly in the classroom with other children, and that any questions or any problems that she might have, she could consult with her teacher for assistance." A second mother responded like this. "Well, John, it's time to go to school now. You have to know how to behave. The first day at school, you should be a good boy and should do just what the teacher tells you to do'' (Hess and Shipman, 1965, p. 877). Thus, the first mother was informative, emphasized the personal relationship between teacher and child, and emphasized that school was for learning. The second mother emphasized unquestioning obedience to the teacher. It is easy to imagine how these differences in maternal teaching style over a long period of time could result in large differences in the way in which children face the world. The child of the status-oriented mother would learn to be passive and unquestioning while the child of a person-oriented mother would learn to solve problems rationally and to give explanations for his or her behavior.

A similar study was done by Bee, VanErgen, Streisguth, Nyman, and Leckie (1969). They observed lower- and middle-class mothers interacting with their preschoolers. The middle-class mothers were almost all white while the lower-class mothers were predominantly black. The results were similar to those reported by Hess and Shipman. Regardless of the situation, the middle-class mothers used more verbal instruction, used longer and more complex sentences, and used less criticism. On a problem-solving task in which mothers were asked to teach their child, the lower-class mothers were more likely to intrude physically, while the middle-class mothers were more likely to ask leading questions.

A third example of research into the relationship between child-rearing practices and the later competence of the child is the Harvard Preschool Project directed by Burton White (White and Watts, 1973). They were concerned with the problem of how to structure the experiences of a preschooler to maximize the development of competence. Instead of defining competence with the usual measures of mental development, they observed a large number of six year olds and, from these, selected those whom they considered to be the most competent and the least competent. From intensive observation of these children, they developed a checklist of competencies that included such behaviors as getting and maintaining the attention of adults in socially acceptable ways, using adults as resources, expressing both hostility and affection toward others, achieving linguistic competence, attaining the ability to note discrepancies, and achieving the ability to carry out multistep activities.

Further observation suggested that these differences in competence were largely nonexistent in one year olds, but were clearly present in three year olds. In fact, in many ways, competent three year olds were more similar to competent six year olds than they were to incompetent three year olds. Thus, White concluded that the crucial differences in experience that produce competence or incompetence must occur during the second year of life.

The next step was to identify a number of one and two year olds who were predicted to become either very competent or very incompetent based on observation of older brothers and sisters. A total of 31 children were intensively observed over a two-year period. A trained observer actually went into the homes of these children on numerous occasions and recorded the children's streams of experience as they went about their daily activities. To facilitate this, a complicated checklist was developed with which all of the child's experiences could be categorized.

There were some clear differences between mothers of competent children and mothers of incompetent children in the way that the mothers interacted with their children. Competent children experienced much more interaction with their mothers than did incompetent children, and mothers of competent children spent a higher proportion of this time in activities that were highly intellectual, such as naming things or showing the child how things work. This difference was present as early as 12 to 15 months after birth, and the difference increased as the children grew older. When the child is less than two years old, mothers of both types of children encourage about twice as many activities as they discourage. However, once the child enters the "terrible twos" and becomes much more active, the mothers of competent children encourage about three times as many activities as they discourage, while the mothers of incompetent children double the number of times in which they discourage the child's behavior. In other words, the mothers of incompetent children are far more restrictive.

Each of these three studies and a number of others have shown that there are differences in child-rearing style between low- and high-SES families. Lower-class parents use less language and tend to discipline by appeal to authority rather than by logical explanations. It is impossible to say conclusively that these differences in child-rearing patterns directly produce differences in mental abilities since observing a correlation between two variables does not imply that one causes the other, but this could well be an important contributing factor to the generally poorer school performance and higher incidence of metal retardation among the lower classes.

Family Structure. Another dimension of cultural deprivation is family disorganization. For various reasons, family structure is less stable among the most disadvantaged members of the population, particularly among blacks. It has been argued that their history of slavery encouraged a tradition of weak family bonds, since slave owners frequently broke up families. Also, if a man cannot provide for his family because he cannot get a job, he is more likely to abandon them. The welfare laws are frequently designed to encourage the father to leave home, since that is the only way that the mother and children can get aid. Whatever the reason, there is an alarmingly high rate of father absence among the poor and minorities. The U. S. Bureau of the Census (1973) reports that only 56 percent of black children live with both parents.

While there is by no means universal agreement, a good deal of research suggests that father absence has the effect of lowering mental performance in children. Deutsch and Brown (1964), in studying the effects of SES and race on intelligence, found that when they matched children on other variables, the IQs of children with father present tended to be higher than the IQs of children with absent fathers. Similarly, Santrock (1972) found that father absence lowered IQ and achievement test performance of children, more so among boys than among girls. He also found that when the father was absent due to divorce, desertion, or separation, the deficit was greater among boys whose father had left when the boy was very young, but if the father was absent because of death, the deficit was greatest when the death had occurred during the boy's early school years.

Motivation. Perhaps the most devasting effect of being raised in conditions of poverty surrounded by relative affluence is its effect on motivation, personality, and general world outlook. People reared under such conditions develop a sense of resignation and helplessness, a feeling that they have little control over their lives and that what happens to them depends not on their own actions but is determined by the actions of others such as the welfare bureaucracy or by chance. Middle-class children, on the other hand, learn at a young age that they can have an effect on their world through their own actions. This difference has been documented in numerous studies. Rotter (Battle and Rotter, 1963) has labeled this dimension locus of control. People who believe that their own actions determine what happens to them have an internal locus of control while those who believe that events are largely a matter of fate have an external locus of control. Battle and Rotter (1963) administered a children's version of a scale measuring locus of control to school children of different SES levels and found a tendency for low SES children to have a more external locus of control than middle-class children. Stephens and Delys (1973) found similar SES differences in locus of control in children as young as three and four.

It is not difficult to imagine how locus of control could have an important effect on school performance. If people have little faith that their actions are important in determining success, there is no need to try very hard. The effect of locus of control on school performance was clearly documented in the Coleman et al. study (1966) described above. They asked students whether they agreed with a number of statements pertaining to locus of control, such as "Good luck is more important than hard work for success" or "People like me don't have much of a chance to be successful in life." They found that blacks more often than whites were likely to agree with these statements, and, more importantly, locus of control was an extremely important predictor of academic achievement, more important even than the child's background. Students with an internal locus of control consistently outperformed externals. However, this observation must not be taken as proof that external locus of control leads to poor performance. It is just as likely that poor school performance leads to an external locus of control. Students who work hard and still do poorly might decide that their actions have little effect on their achievements.

Schooling. The role of the schools as a determinant of the failure of so many poor and minority children has been the subject of considerable controversy. Americans have always had tremendous faith in education as a vehicle for social equality and justice, and it is disturbing that such a significant portion of the population seems to be largely unable to benefit from the present school system. On one level, schools are not at all responsible for SES differences in mental ability, since there are distinct differences in mental ability between children of different social classes and children of different ethnic backgrounds long before they first set foot in a school. For various reasons, middle-class children arrive for their first day of school better prepared for academic success than do their lower-class and minority counterparts. On the other hand, it is obvious that the schools are not meeting the needs of many of the poor and black children of the nation. Too many of these children learn little in school, are bored by it, and spend more time getting into trouble than they do working.

For years, it has been generally accepted that the schools attended predominantly by blacks were inferior in physical plant, academic facilities, and other amenities. The Coleman study (1966), however, in surveying the facilities of more than 4000 schools found little difference between predominantly black and predominantly white schools in such factors as the age of the building or the presence of a library, laboratories, an auditorium, or other physical features usually considered to be important for learning. While some schools have far better facilities than others, there is no consistent trend for blacks to attend schools with poorer facilities than whites. In fact, the opposite seems more and more to be the case; that is, schools attended predominantly by low SES and minority children are getting more money relative to white, middle-class schools. Gittell (1971) reported that the New York City schools that received more than $1100 per pupil per year had reading and arithmetic achievement scores five to seven months below scores of students in New York City schools receiving less than $600 per pupil per year. In a statewide survey in Georgia, Osborne (1973) found a correlation of +.47 between per capita expenditure and percentage of nonwhite students, indicating that more money is being spent on black schools than on white schools.

However, merely because facilities are similar does not mean that all children are receiving the same education. For example, Deutsch (1967) observed that 50 to 80 percent of the classroom time in an all-black school was devoted to disciplining the children compared to only 30 percent of the time in an all-white school of comparable SES. One aspect of the school environment that has received particular attention is the role of teacher expectancies on school performance. It is reasonable to assume that if a teacher expects certain children to fail, these children are more likely to do poorly. A classic experiment by Rosenthal and Jacobson (1968) is frequently cited. They administered an IQ test to the children of a school, and then told the teachers that on the basis of the test results, certain of their children (actually selected randomly) would be expected to bloom that year and do better than they had done previously. At the end of the year, the IQ test was readministered. The children in the first and second grades who had been designated "spurters" gained significantly more in reading and arithmetic achievement and in IQ than did the other children. There were no significant differences between spurters and nonspurters in the other four grades. Since the only difference between spurters and nonspurters was the fact that the teachers expected them to do better, this expectancy must have caused the difference. However, the expectancy effect was rather small, and most other attempts to demonstrate expectancy effects have failied (Elashoff and Snow, 1971).

The precise mechanism by which teacher expectancies might effect learning has been described by Rist (1970). He observed a kindergarten class in an all-black urban ghetto school. On the eighth day of school, the teacher made permanent seating assignments. Children could be assigned to one of three tables, table 1 for the fast learners table 2 for the average learners, and table 3 for the slow learners. Since these assignments were made on the eighth day of kindergarten, they could not possibly have been made on the basis of any reliable or objective evidence of learning potential, and thus, were based largely on subjective opinion. Not surprisingly, the children at the fast learner table were generally neat and clean, while the children at table 3 were sloppily dressed and frequently smelled of urine. There were no children with parents on welfare at the first table, but 4 of the 10 children at table 3 were on it. The teacher almost invariably stood by the first table and made her remarks to them. In fact, the children at the last table had trouble seeing the blackboard. Whenever the teacher had to select a student for a special project such as show and tell or acting a part in a skit, she would select someone from table 1 rather than from the others. At the end of the year, the teacher made the following comment on her children:

> *It seems to me that some of the children at table 2 and most all of the children at table 3 at times seem to have no idea of what was going on in the classroom and were off in another world all by themselves. It just appears that some can do it and some cannot. I don't think that it is the teaching that affects those that cannot do it, but some are basically just low achievers* (*Rist 1970, p. 425*).

It should certainly not be concluded that this example is typical of what goes on in schools serving predominantly disadvantaged children. It is to be hoped that this is an extreme example, but it is instructive nonetheless, because it serves as a warning to potential teachers.

While the educational system has been harshly criticized for its failure to educate everyone to an adequate level, there is little agreement regarding what to do about the problem. Some people have suggested relatively open classrooms, others have suggested highly structured programmed learning. Some people feel that the answer is to bus black pupils to suburban schools, others advocate having black teachers and administrators for black students, since the white, middle-class teacher cannot understand ghetto children. A detailed discussion of educational practices for slow and retarded children will be deferred to later chapters.

Advocates of the cultural deprivation hypothesis have universally favored programs of compensatory education of one kind or another such as the Head Start programs of the 1960s. The assumption behind compensatory education is that the families are not doing an adequate job of preparing their children for school and, therefore, it is necessary to set up preschool programs to systematically teach the things that most middle-class children learn casually from their parents. An important assumption is that the proper time to expose children to this stimulation is in the preschool period since many of the effects of deprivation seem to be difficult to reverse once the child is in school. In other words, events in early years are more important in determining one's level of intellectual functioning than what happens later on. There is a good deal of animal research indicating that this is the case, and Bloom (1964) determined on the basis of correlations with IQs at later ages that 50 percent of one's intelligence is determined by age four. However, there is also scattered evidence contradicting this assumption. For example, Davis (1947) described a case of a child who spent the first six years of her life locked in an attic. When she was found, her IQ was estimated to be 25, but within three years, she was functioning at her age level.

The Genetic Hypothesis

The cultural deprivation hypothesis is based on the assumption that most children have about the same intellectual potential at birth, and that differences in mental abilities are due primarily to differences in the environment. As we have seen, there are enough differences between the environments of slow learners and fast learners to make this a reasonable hypothesis. However, an alternative theory is that children are born with wide differences in intellectual potential due to differences in heredity. Chapter 2 reviewed a considerable amount of research that suggested that this might be the case; that is, that intelligence test performance has a high heritability. For example, identical twins who are reared in different homes tend to be very similar in their intelligence test performance, while biologically unrelated children who are raised in the same home by the same parents tend not to be very similar in intelligence test performance, suggesting that differences in genes are more important than are differences in environment in determining intellectual capabilities. However, it is important to remember that even though many differences in intelligence can be attributed to differences in heredity, intellectual level can still be considerably modified by one's upbringing.

If most differences in intelligence were due to differences in genes, then it would follow logically that children from high-SES families would tend to do better on intelligence tests than children from low-SES families. In other words, those people with more intellectual potential would be likely to move into the higher social levels because they would tend to get more education and because our society tends to reward intellectual accomplishments. Similarly, those people with less intelligence would be likely to fall in social standing. Therefore, high-SES families are likely to have more of the genes that predispose one to have superior intellectual abilities, and thus, their offspring are likely to be more intelligent.

Jensen (1969) has carried this argument one step further and suggested that the fact that blacks show such poor performance on such a wide variety of different kinds of mental tests and under such a wide variety of conditions cannot be entirely explained away by environmental factors, and therefore there must be genetic differences in intellectual potential between blacks and whites. This conclusion, and Jensen himself, have been severely attacked on a wide variety of grounds. Some of the attacks have been more emotional than rational, and some people have misquoted him and attributed ideas to him that he has never argued, such as the idea of fixed intelligence, but other criticisms must be taken more seriously.

One type of attack is that racial differences in intelligence ought not to be discussed because of the social and political ramifications. For example, Brazziel (1969) cites a legal case in the South in which Jensen was quoted in support of racial segregation. However, to say that certain subjects are not appropriate for scientific research is counter to a long tradition of scientific inquiry and academic freedom.

Others have pointed out that Jensen has used within-group findings to explain between-group differences. He has concluded that the heritability of intelligence for the white population is .81, and concludes from this that the same is true of the black population. This is not necessarily true, since heritability only applies to a specific population and may be radically different between populations. It is also possible that the 15 point difference in IQ between black and white children can be accounted for entirely by environmental factors such as motivational differences, cultural differences, and so forth, even though heritability is high. The strongest argument against Jensen's theory, however, is the fact that blacks have been living in such decrepit conditions for so long that it is impossible to say what their level of intelligence would be if they had been exposed to a more advantageous environment. It is clearly the case that when black children move to a more stimulating environment their IQ goes up. Jensen counters this argument by pointing out that most American Indian children are raised in conditions even worse than those of blacks, yet their IQs are higher.

Do Low SES and Minority Children Actually Have a Deficit?

During the 1960s, it was widely accepted that there was a genuine deficit in the cognitive functioning, language skills, and learning ability of children from poor families and racial minorities, but in recent years, this assertion has been widely challenged. The argument is that black children or children from other minorities have been raised in a very different subculture from white, middle-class children, and they only appear to have a deficit because they are being measured with a yardstick from a foreign culture. Just as no one says that Parisian children are culturally deprived because they don't speak English, it is equally wrong to say that a black child is culturally deprived because he speaks a different dialect of English. Supporters of this view place particular emphasis on the strengths of the black culture in America, and they study this black culture, not as a degraded form of white society, but as a separate culture, just as anthropologists would study the social patterns of a newly discovered non-Western culture. A principle that is widely accepted in anthropology is the principle of cultural relativity, which states that each culture must be judged according to its own values rather than be measured by the values of Western man. The opposite of cultural relativity is ethnocentrism, evaluating everyone's behavior according to the standards of one's own culture. Much of the research on black people up through the 1960s had an ethnocentric bias in that black people's speech, behavior, and social patterns were compared to white, middle-class standards. Because black culture differs from white culture in a number of ways, it was not surprising that it was judged inferior by white standards. Thus, it was logical to talk about "inadequate mothering," or "deprived environments," or "language deficits," and these various deficiencies were the justification for most of the compensatory education programs of the 1960s (Baratz and Baratz, 1970).

This argument can be most clearly understood by considering the language of black children. Their dialect can be described in two ways; one way is to assume that Standard American English, the kind of English described in grammar books, is correct and then count the errors that black children make. There are a number of characteristic deviations of black dialects from the grammar books. For example, black children are more likely to use slang words such as "ain't," they are more likely to use double negatives such as "I don't want no more milk," and there are numerous articulation errors such as "birfday" instead of "birthday." There is little question that if the grammar book is the standard, many black children speak poorly.

However, there is nothing sacred about the grammar books. "Ain't" is only wrong because it is not used by educated people. An alternative way of viewing black language is as a separate dialect, just as English spoken on one side of the Atlantic differs from English spoken on the other. Both are acceptable; they are just different. Viewed in this way, it is apparent that black children speak a highly structured, colorful language. Labov (1970) has attempted to describe the grammar of Negro Nonstandard English (NNE). For example, in NNE, it is permissible to construct a sentence "They mine," deleting the verb completely, while in Standard English, it is permissible to form a contraction "They're mine" but not acceptable to eliminate the verb completely.

Justification for this viewpoint comes from a tenet of modern linguistics that there is no such thing as a primitive language. Around the turn of the century, it was fashionable for anthropologists to try to find primitive languages in order to get an idea of how man originally learned to speak, but even the most primitive cultures spoke a language as complex as any of the so-called advanced languages such as English. Thus, there is no way to create a hierarchy of languages with some being more developed than others; all languages are equally well developed.

How does one account for the fact that many black children seem to have such a limited verbal output? One important norm of black culture that is transmitted to very young children is a suspicion of whites (Gay and Abrahams, 1973). Young children develop a defensive strategy when dealing with white adult strangers in which they say as little as possible. This is demonstrated in the following interview of Leon, an eight-year-old black boy, recorded by Labov (1970).

Interviewer: What if you saw somebody kickin' somebody else on the ground, or was using a stick, what would you do if you saw that?

Leon: Mmmm.

Int.: If it was supposed to be a fair fight—

Leon: I don't know.

Int.: You don't know? Would you do anything? . . . huh? I can't hear you.

Leon: No.
Int.: Did you ever see somebody got beat up real bad?
Leon: . . . Nope . . .
Int.: Well—uh—did you ever get into a fight with a guy?
Leon: Nope.
Int.: That was bigger than you?
Leon: Nope.
Int.: You never been in a fight?
Leon: Nope.
Int.: Nobody ever pick on you?
Leon: Nope.
Int.: Nobody ever hit you?
Leon: Nope.
Int.: How come?
Leon: Ah 'on' know.
Int.: Didn't you ever hit somebody?
Leon: Nope.
Int: (Incredulously) You never hit nobody?
Leon: Mhm. (Labov, 1970, p. 159.)

Based on this interview it would be easy to conclude that this child had a language deficit. Later, however, the same interviewer was able to break down the child's defensive barriers, and Leon proved to be just as verbal as any other eight year old, speaking in Negro dialect, of course.

However, there are other phenomena besides language that require explanation. For example, why do black children consistently do so poorly on intelligence tests? Part of the explanation lies in the supposed cultural bias of the tests. For example, one of the questions on the WISC is "What are you supposed to do if you find someone's wallet or pocket book in a store?" The correct answer, trying to find the rightful owner, reflects middle-class values. However, a child from a poor family may have seen one of his parents find and keep some money and thus he would answer to keep it, which gets no credit. This child is not necessarily less intelligent, he has simply learned different values. However, such cultural bias does not account for all of the differences, since black children do as badly or worse on completely culture-free questions, such as matching block designs.

Zigler and Butterfield (1968) have stressed motivational differences between middle-class and lower-class children. There is no logical reason why children should strive to do well on intelligence tests since they are seldom rewarded for correct answers or even told that they were correct. Middle-class children have learned that correctness for its own sake is good, but poor children may not have learned this, and, thus, their only goal in taking a test might be to get away from the test situation as quickly as possible. The best way to do this is to answer "I don't know" to all the questions. Zigler and Butterfield tested this hypothesis by administering the Stanford-Binet twice to a number of preschoolers from poor neighborhoods. Some of them were administered the test in the standard fashion in both instances, others were given the standard administration the first time, but in the second administration, the tester deviated from the standard procedure in order to optimize performance. This did not include giving the child the correct answers, but they were given extra encouragement, and the order of the items was changed so that the children would have lots of success experiences. The children in the optimizing condition gained 10.2 IQ points, while the children in the standard administration group gained only 4.2 points. This suggests that many low-SES children are not performing up to their true potential on regular administrations of the tests.

Other people have been concerned with the race of the tester. If distrust of whites is a norm of the black culture, it is reasonable to assume that a black child might do better with a black tester than with a white tester. The results of research on this issue are conflicting. A review of this issue by Sattler (1970) reported that while a few studies find an effect of the race of the tester on performance, most do not. In a recent study, Quay (1974) administered the Stanford-Binet to black school children in Negro dialect (the tester was black). For example, in verbal absurdities problems, instead of asking "What is foolish about that?" as the test manual prescribes, the tester asked "Why don't dat make no sense?" However, she found no difference in test performance between different kinds of administration.

Advocates of the no deficit position have been extremely critical of the concept of compensatory education (Baratz and Baratz, 1970; Ginsburg, 1972). They argue that the concept of compensatory education is based on the false assumption that children from poor families and racial minorities are deficient and thus need special training, when in fact there is no deficiency. Because there is no deficiency, the blame for school failure of so many of these children must be placed squarely on the schools themselves. The schools are white, middle-class institutions run by white, middle-class teachers and administrators who have no understanding of the black subculture. In the past few years, many educators have been making tremendous strides toward a policy of cultural pluralism, an acceptance of the fact that the cultural background of each child, whether it be black or white, Spanish speaking or English speaking, Christian, Jewish, or Moslem, has innate worth and must be valued. In other words, the schools must now attempt to teach children according to their own family backgrounds rather than assume that all children will fit into the mold of the white middle class. Thus, reading primers have been written describing events in the life of the poor and the black as well as the white culture. Some children are even being taught to read in black dialect rather than in standard English.

This policy of cultural pluralism has important implications for special classes for the mentally retarded. The U.S. Office of Civil Rights has issued guidelines for assigning children to special classes that stipulate that children can only be placed in a special class after their family and cultural background have been given close scrutiny to assure that no child will be stigmatized as mentally retarded solely because of cultural background. This will certainly mean that in future years, the total number of children in special classes for the retarded will decrease.

Implications for the Treatment of Mental Retardation

The position that one takes on this issue has some important implications for the study of and the treatment of mental retardation. Children from poor families, particularly minority children, have always been very much overrepresented in special programs for the retarded, and it is vitally important that a decision be made regarding whether this represents an appropriate placement for most of them. Each of the three hypotheses described previously tends to deal with this problem from a somewhat different point of view. If one assumes that poor and minority children fail in school primarily because they lack appropriate stimulation and because their family life does not provide good language models, good thinking skills, and positive attitudes toward school, then the appropriate solution to the problem is a massive dose of compensatory education. Much of government policy at all levels has been in this direction. In addition to the tremendous variety of preschool programs that have been organized for this type of child, schools that serve predominantly poor and minority children are likely to receive extra funds, have extra reading personnel, and are likely to have a variety of experimental programs to test new ways of teaching. If one accepts the view that a poor environment can produce intellectual deficits just as permanent and just as severe as can organic impairment, then it is not inconsistent to find poor and minority children very much overrepresented in special programs for the retarded. This overrepresentation does not reflect anything wrong with the screening process or the labeling process or the educational process, although it is certainly an indication of some major flaws in the structure of society.

Advocates of the genetic hypothesis, such as Jensen (1969) or Herrnstein (1973), are far less attracted to compensatory education on the grounds that it will not be successful. Indeed, Jensen began his controversial 1969 article with the statement that "Compensatory education has been tried, and it apparently has failed." One of the principal objections to this theory is that it is pessimistic and undemocratic; the genetic theory implies that with the present state of technology, there is nothing much that can be done for the problem of school failure.

The genetic theory would predict that poor children would be over-represented in special classes for the retarded. In fact, the concept of familial retardation, mental retardation running in families for many generations, has a long history.

The last viewpoint, the cultural difference hypothesis, is beginning to have major impact on the provision of services to the retarded. Unlike the other two theories, this viewpoint emphasizes that the actual diagnostic process by which children are assigned to special programs is biased because the tests used and the schools themselves are a reflection of middle-class ethnocentricity. Advocates of this position argue that there is no logical reason to assume that there will be more retarded people among one cultural group than another, and the fact that there are such large differences in the prevalence of children in special classes between different groups is proof of the bias inherent in the labeling process. It has been suggested that the best way to overcome this problem is to consider an equal proportion of each ethnic group to be mentally retarded. For example, California has mandated that different norms must be used in the testing of each ethnic group.

On at least one level, this is an illogical policy. Children should be assigned to special programs not because they are retarded but because they are able to benefit from such a special program, and if for whatever reason, a greater proportion of children from one ethnic group than from another require special programming, then these children are only being penalized by being excluded from such a program.

Summary

One of the biggest problems facing the United States today is the fact that a significant proportion of its children, particularly those from poor families and from racial minorities, are largely unable to benefit from the present educational system. At least some of these children have been labeled mentally retarded. There are three theories concerning why children raised in poverty have such a dismal record of school achievement. The most widely accepted theory is a version of the cultural deprivation hypothesis. This approach states that there are certain aspects of parental child-rearing style and the general environment of poverty that predispose these children to failure. Their parents do not provide positive role models, they do not provide good language models, and the culture is oriented toward acting on the basis of impulse and emotion rather than on reason. As a result, these children do not learn acceptable language habits and they do not develop good thinking skills. There is a good deal of research documenting the fact that the child-rearing styles of low-income mothers tend to be oriented toward obedience rather than toward reason.

A second theory is that one's intellectual potential is determined to a considerable extent by one's heredity. People with weaker intellectual abilities tend to be found in the lower-income groups, and they pass this propensity toward lower intelligence on to their offspring. This theory is not widely supported today, partially for political reasons and partially because evidence has accumulated indicating that how one is reared can have a considerable effect upon one's mental abilities.

The third theory suggests that children of low-income and minority families do not in fact have any kind of intellectual deficit. They only appear to have a deficit because they are being measured with a white, middle-class yardstick. The schools are white, middle-class institutions run by white, middle-class teachers and administrators who reinforce the kinds of behaviors and personalities produced by the white middle class. Poor children and black children do poorly on measures of language ability because they speak a different dialect of English that, to some extent, uses different rules of grammar and different vocabulary. Similarly, they do poorly on intelligence tests because these tests measure the kinds of skills learned in a white, middle-class culture to the exclusion of knowledge inherent to other subcultures. Advocates of this approach are opposed to any kind of compensatory education because it is unnecessary and because it is based on the ethnocentric assumption that white, middle-class life-styles, language habits, and child-rearing styles are superior to those of other cultures.

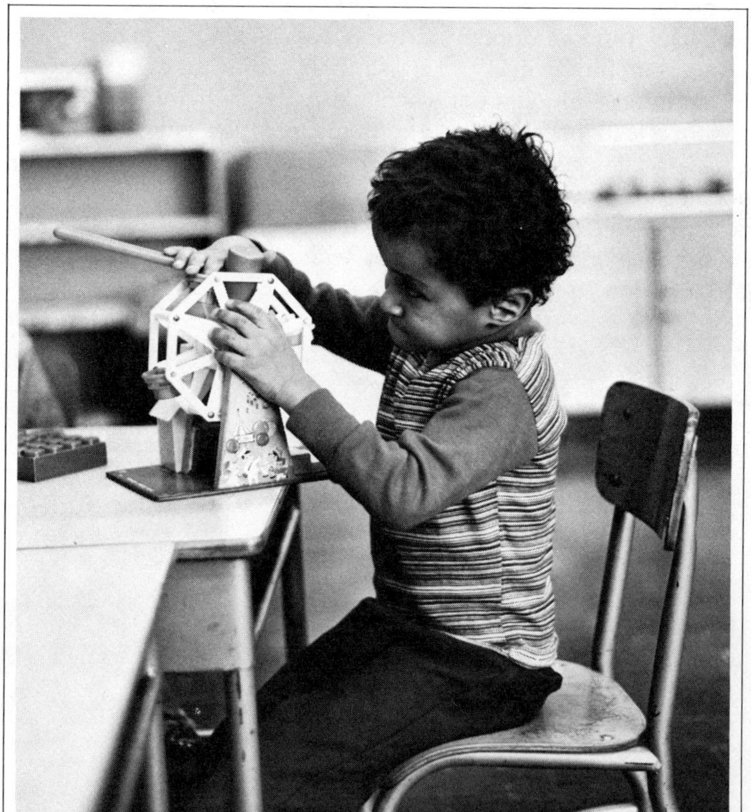

8

Learning and Memory in the Mentally Retarded

The most basic feature that distinguishes the mentally retarded is some sort of weakness, slowness, or deficiency in basic cognitive skills such as learning, thinking, verbal skills, and the like. Because of the importance of these processes to a thorough understanding of mental retardation, Chapters 8, 9, and 10 discuss these basic cognitive processes. This chapter discusses research on learning and memory, Chapter 9 covers language and language acquisition, and Chapter 10 discusses Piaget's theory of cognitive development and its applications to the mentally retarded. First, however, it is necessary to consider various kinds of research designs and what kinds of questions such research can answer.

Research Designs and Strategies

Experimental research with the retarded can be divided into two basic types: experiments that compare retarded subjects to nonretarded subjects on a variable or process and research that uses retarded subjects only. These two designs are addressed to somewhat different questions.

Research Comparing Retarded to Nonretarded Subjects

Research studies in which retarded and nonretarded subjects are compared on some process are asking the question, "In what way do retarded people differ from nonretarded people?" In a sense, this approach is trying to determine the fundamental nature of mental retardation, to develop a theory of retardation, so to speak. Unless we assume that the retardation label is applied to people on an entirely capricious basis, this is a reasonable question.

Zigler (1969) has distinguished two types of theories of mental retardation: developmental theories and defect theories. A developmental theory postulates that a retarded person goes through the same developmental stages that a normal person does, but the retarded child goes through the stages more slowly and does not reach the same final level. In order to have a valid developmental theory, it is necessary to have a good understanding of normal cognitive development. By far the best example of such a theory is that of Piaget, whose approach is discussed in Chapter 10. Insofar as a developmental theory is correct, when a retarded person is compared to a younger nonretarded person who is at the same stage of development, mental functioning and capabilities ought to be the same in both people. As a result, the type of experimental design that tests a developmental theory involves comparing a group of retarded children to a group of normal IQ children matched on mental age, and if no differences are found in mental performance between the two groups, the developmental theory is supported.

A defect theory is one that postulates that retarded people are characterized not so much by delayed development per se but by a specific defect in one or more mental processes. It is often implied that other mental processes are relatively intact. Heal (1970) has suggested that defect theorists might prefer the term mentally deficient to mentally retarded. A number of such defect theories have been proposed. For example, the Russian psychologist Luria (1963) has proposed that retarded children have a particular defect in using verbal mediation and inner language to guide thought and behavior. Ellis (1963) has proposed that retarded people have a particular defect in their memory trace. In particular, he suggested that nervous system damage results in a more rapid decay of memories. Spitz (1966) suggested that the particular defect of the retarded lies in their inability to organize stimulus information. Heal and Johnson (1970) presented a good deal of evidence indicating that retarded people have particular difficulty in the inhibition of responses. Brown (1974) suggested that retarded people have particular difficulty in using strategies such as rehearsal to aid learning and memory.

There is some disagreement regarding the appropriate type of nonretarded comparison group to use to demonstrate such a defect. For example, suppose a researcher suspects that retarded people have a particular defect in short-term memory as measured by digit span (how many digits the individual can recall after hearing them read once). The researcher administers a digit span test to a number of retarded children who have an average IQ of 60 an average chronological age of 10 years, and thus an average mental age of 6 years. To what kind of nonretarded people does the researcher compare them to demonstrate that they have a defect? The more obvious type of experimental design is to compare them to children of average IQ who are the same age, a CA-matched group. This strategy is reasonable because children are labeled retarded because they do not perform as well as typical children of their same age. However, one would expect to find a fairly large difference between these two groups on practically any mental task, and it would not be a striking finding to discover that normal 10 year olds could remember a span of six digits, while the retarded children could only remember four digits. This type of experimental design frequently produces the most interesting results when processes are discovered on which retarded and nonretarded subjects of the same age do not differ. Ellis (1969) has provided some good justifications for such CA-matched control groups.

Many researchers elect to compare retarded children to MA-matched nonretarded children as was the case in experimental tests of the developmental theory. In this case, our researcher would compare the performance of 10-year-old retarded subjects to the performance of 6-year-old children of normal IQ. Even though these two groups of children have achieved the same average total score on an intelligence test, it is reasonable to expect that retarded children are not entirely comparable to normal children of the same stage of development. After all, the two groups have reached the same developmental level by different means. The retarded subjects, with their greater experience, would be likely to do relatively better on those tasks that require more experience, while the younger normal children would be expected to score relatively higher on tasks that tap general learning rate (Heal and Johnson, 1970). In other words, it is likely that the condition of low IQ imparts some deficit to intellectual functioning beyond the fact that development is slowed down, and a mentally retarded child is not entirely comparable to a normal child of similar mental age.

The ideal experimental design is one in which retarded people are compared to two different groups of nonretarded controls, one group matched on CA and the other matched on MA. In this way, the effects of both developmental stage and of IQ can be determined independently for a given process (if one makes the assumption that CA independent of MA has no effect). An excellent example of such a design is the research by Harter (1965), described later in this chapter.

Difficulties with Retarded-Normal Comparisons

There are three precautions that must be considered in evaluating research that compares retarded and nonretarded subjects. The first is that differences in performance between retarded and nonretarded people on a learning or memory task might be due to motivational or emotional differences rather than cognitive differences. Zigler (1966) has presented some strong evidence supporting such a position. He advocates the developmental theory, which suggests that a retarded child is equivalent in mental functioning to a nonretarded child of the same developmental stage, that is, the same MA. Thus, any research that finds differences between retarded and nonretarded people matched on MA is a potential embarrassment to his theory. Numerous studies have found such differences, but Zigler postulates that most of these differences can be attributed to noncognitive processes. For example, much of the research with retarded people has used institutionalized subjects. The reason for this is that institutions tend to be centers for research with the retarded, and institutions provide a readily available pool of retarded subjects for research purposes. However, individuals who have spent time in institutions have often experienced a good deal of neglect, and as a result, they crave attention from other people more than do noninstitutionalized individuals. Thus, it is reasonable to assume that an institutionalized retarded child would have different motives in an experimental situation than would a noninstitutionalized child. For example, the institutionalized child might be more willing to please the experimenter or make an attempt to prolong the experimental session as long as possible in order to maintain social contact. Thus, if the research is investigating how long it takes a subject to learn a certain task and the retarded subject takes longer than a nonretarded subject, it might be a mistake to conclude that the retarded child has deficient learning ability. A similar problem involves the expectancy of success in retarded people. Most retarded people have had fewer success experiences and more failure experiences than a nonretarded child, and, as a result, the retarded are probably more likely to expect to fail when they undertake a new learning project. A person who expects to fail is more likely to fail, and this factor could also make retarded individuals appear to have a learning deficit when, in fact, none exists.

A second difficulty is that any research that compares retarded to nonretarded people makes the implicit assumption that the retarded and the nonretarded form two distinct groups, and that each group is relatively homogeneous. A major theme of this book is that exactly the opposite is the case. Mental retardation is on a continuum with normalcy, and there are considerable differences between retarded people. Thus, it makes no sense to expect that a common defect would be found that would characterize all retarded people and distinguish them from the nonretarded. However, this does not mean that retardate-normal comparisons are worthless; it is fruitful to think of such comparisons as research into the nature of IQ differences rather than as comparing two homogeneous groups of people. In other words, it would be just as fruitful, although it is seldom done, to compare individuals with IQs of 90 to those with IQs of 120 as it would be to compare individuals with IQs of 70 to those of IQ of 100.

A related problem concerns the etiology of the retardation. While it might be true that the cause of the diminished mental abilities is irrelevant to mental processes, this is by no means obvious. There is no reason to assume that a child with Down's syndrome who has an IQ of 40 should have the same defects or style of cognitive functioning as an individual who has suffered brain damage at birth whose IQ also happens to be 40. It makes more sense to talk about a specific defect for Down's syndrome or for brain damage than it does to talk about a specific defect for retardation. However, in most studies of basic processes in the retarded, etiology is ignored. The only exception to this is that many researchers make a distinction between organic and nonorganic retardation and develop a defect theory that only includes one of these two. However, this implies that people can be easily divided into two groups, those with brain damage and those without, but the recent research on learning disabilities and minimal brain dysfunction has suggested that brain damage is on a continuum just as IQ is. It is reasonable to assume that a great many children, perhaps more than half, have suffered some sort of brain damage at some point in their life, even though the effects may be very subtle or even indetectable.

Retardate Research without a Nonretarded Comparison Group

A good deal of the basic experimental research with the retarded does not use a nonretarded comparison group. From a practical point of view, if one is interested in determining the most effective teaching techniques for use with retarded children, there is no need to compare retarded to nonretarded people. Researchers can simply manipulate whatever variables they feel are important and in this way discover how to facilitate various kinds of learning in the retarded. It is also possible to make general statements about learning processes in the retarded based on such research, but it is not possible to draw any conclusions about how retarded people differ from normal.

However, it is probably the case that most learning processes in the mentally retarded are not very different from learning in people of normal IQ. There are very few exceptions to the generalization that whatever facilitates learning in mentally retarded subjects will also facilitate learning in other kinds of people and vice versa. Thus, such research can be thought of as investigating the process of learning or memory in the general sense. While it may seem strange to study general laws of learning by using retarded subjects, recall that much of what is known about learning is derived from research with rats and pigeons. One might prefer to use retarded rather than nonretarded subjects for a variety of reasons. For example, some learning processes occur too rapidly in nonretarded people to be easily studied, and thus research with people of low IQ gives the experimentalist an opportunity to study learning "in slow motion." One example of this type of approach is the attentional model of Zeaman and House (1963) to be described shortly. They have developed a theory of retardate learning based almost entirely on research with retarded subjects only, with little attempt to compare retarded to nonretarded subjects. However, it is assumed that their theory applies equally well to similar learning in other kinds of subjects.

Learning in the Retarded

Probably the most widespread conception of a retarded person is that of an individual who has a defect in learning or at least one who is a slow learner. This conception, although generally true, is somewhat misleading. The term learning encompasses so many different processes that the statement that the retarded have a learning deficit is too general to be of much use. In the first place, there are many different kinds of learning. Retarded people seem to have a great deal of difficulty with some kinds of learning, but they show little or no apparent deficits with other kinds of learning. Second, any research on learning must necessarily involve numerous other processes also; perception, memory, motivation, and mediation, to name a few. If an experiment finds that it takes retarded people more trials to learn a particular task than it does for nonretarded subjects, it cannot necessarily be assumed that the difficulty was with the rate of learning. For example, Zeaman and House (1963) have found strong evidence that rate of learning by itself is not an important variable in accounting for differences in the outcome of learning experiments between retarded and nonretarded subjects, but instead, the differences can be attributed to attention processes.

A third difficulty with describing a retarded child as a slow learner is that this characterization suggests that if a retarded child is merely given many more trials to learn something, the retarded child can learn as well as a nonretarded child. For example, Kolstoe (1970) suggests that if a child has an IQ of 50, this means that the learning rate is half that of a normal child, and thus, if the retarded child were kept in school for twice as long, for 24 years instead of 12, the retarded child could complete a full school program through the high school level. However, it is obvious to anyone who has worked with retarded children that there are many skills that cannot be taught to a retarded child simply by giving twice as many exposures as a normal child requires. For these reasons, the statement that a retarded child is predominantly a slow learner is too much of an oversimplification to be of much use. Like the term intelligence, the term learning is fine for a chapter title, but certainly does not refer to a single unitary process.

Classical Conditioning

Much of the research on learning has focused on the very simple kind of learning called conditioning. Conditioning involves pairing a specific response to a specific stimulus or stimulus situation. There are two basic kinds of conditioning paradigms. One is called classical conditioning or respondent conditioning, the other is called operant or instrumental conditioning. The best-known experiment demonstrating classical conditioning was done by Pavlov (1927). He prepared a dog by making a small surgical opening in the dog's cheek so that he could collect and measure the dog's saliva. The dog was then put in a restraining harness in the laboratory. Pavlov struck a tuning fork that produced a tone, and then he presented a small amount of meat powder to the dog. The dog's natural response to the meat powder was to begin to salivate. At first, when the tuning fork was sounded, the dog did nothing, but after a number of such trials, he began to salivate to the sound of the tuning fork prior to the presentation of the food. Thus, learning had occurred.

Any classical conditioning experiment involves four components. There must be an unconditioned stimulus (UCS) that produces an unconditioned response (UCR). In the case of Pavlov's dog, the UCS was the meat powder and the UCR was salivation. These are called unconditioned because the animal does not have to learn them. Dogs will naturally begin to salivate to food without any special training. The UCS must be paired with a neutral stimulus, the conditioned stimulus (CS). At first, the CS elicits no response (which is why it is called neutral) but after a number of pairings, the CS also begins to elicit the same response or a fraction of it, but in this case, the response is called the conditioned response (CR).

A number of researchers have done experiments that compare the performance of subjects of different IQ and MA levels on simple classical conditioning. The experiment by Baumeister, Beedle, and Urquhart (1964) is typical. Their subjects consisted of 40 institutionalized adult retardates with an average IQ of 49 and 29 nonretarded adults recruited from university faculty and students. The UCS was a very mild shock applied to the wrist. Such a shock produces a change in the electrical resistance of the skin, which is called the galvanic skin response, usually abbreviated GSR. Thus, the UCR was the GSR. The CS was a one-second tone. Each subject first received 10 preconditioning trials in which they simply heard the tone unpaired with any other events. This was followed by 20 paired trials in which the tone was followed by a shock. The interval between the CS and the UCS was 0 for some subjects, 0.5 seconds for others, and 1 second for others. The dependent variable in the experiment was the number of GSRs given in response to the tone. There was no difference in this between the retarded subjects and the nonretarded subjects. Most other research comparing retarded and nonretarded subjects on simple classical conditioning has reached the same conclusion, that there is no difference in learning between subjects of low IQ and subjects of average intelligence (Zeaman and House, 1966). Thus, the generalization that retarded subjects are poorer learners than nonretarded subjects must be qualified.

Operant Conditioning

With few exceptions, little research is now being done with classical conditioning. However, the opposite is true for the second important type of conditioning, operant conditioning or instrumental learning. Operant conditioning is the name given to changes in behavior that result from rewards and punishments. The classical experiment on operant conditioning was done by Skinner (1938). He put a hungry rat in a box with a bar at one end (this type of apparatus is commonly called a Skinner box, although Skinner objects to this label). The rat sniffed around exploring the box, and, by accident, he pressed the bar. The bar was hooked up so that when it was pressed, a food pellet dropped into the box. The rat ate the food and continued exploring. After a while, he pressed the bar again and received another food pellet. After the rat had had a number of these experiences, the frequency of his pressing the bar increased until he was pressing the bar almost continuously.

The underlying pattern behind all operant conditioning is that an organism learns to perform a behavior in order to get a reward, or, more precisely, a reinforcement. Organisms tend to repeat those behaviors that are reinforced and tend not to repeat those behaviors that are not reinforced. It is easy to think of examples of operant conditioning in everyday life. A toddler throws his first temper tantrum, perhaps in imitation of another child. His mother runs over to him, picks him up, comforts him, and otherwise provides him with lots of reinforcement. Because the child is being reinforced for temper tantrum behavior, the frequency of temper tantrums will increase. Very soon, if the mother does not change her ways, her child may start having one or more tantrums a day.

Operant conditioning forms the basis of the technique of training and therapy known as behavior modification, and as a result of its usefulness in applied settings, the amount of research in this area has burgeoned in the past few years. However, most of the research has been directed toward applied problems rather than trying to answer theoretical questions about retardate learning processes, and as a result, this research is presented in later chapters.

Discrimination Learning

One variant of operant conditioning that has received a considerable amount of theoretical attention is discrimination learning. In its simplest form, discrimination learning involves placing two stimuli in front of the subject and allowing the subject to select one of the two. If the subject selects the correct one, he or she gets a reinforcement such as a piece of candy, and if the subject chooses the wrong one, he or she gets nothing. The dependent variable in such research is generally either the number of trials that it takes the subject to reach a preset criterion such as 10 correct in a row or the number of errors made before reaching the criterion. Discrimination learning is a useful experimental paradigm because there are numerous variants on this procedure and a large number of ways to make the problems easier or more difficult.

Discrimination learning was originally conceived as a measure of perceptual abilities, but it has evolved into a method of study concept learning and problem solving. The easiest kinds of problems are called junk discriminations because the subjects are simply required to distinguish between two everyday objects, for example, a comb and an ashtray. The experimenter arbitrarily selects one to be correct, for example, the comb, and thus, the reinforcement is always under the comb and never under the ashtray. The positions of the two stimuli are randomly alternated. More common than junk stimuli are geometric forms. These are convenient because the experimenter has precise control over the number of relevant and irrelevant dimensions. A dimension is a characteristic such as shape, color, or size that can be systematically varied. Usually, there are two levels of a given dimension in a given problem, and one dimension is relevant while all the others are irrelevant. Figure 8-1 shows a number of trials in a typical problem with color as the relevant dimension and form and position as irrelevant dimensions. Color is said to be relevant because the color of the object determines whether it is correct or wrong. In this case, red is always rewarded and blue never. Shape and position are irrelevant dimensions because which stimulus is correct does not depend on them. The two levels of the shape dimension—square and circle—are each rewarded half the time. Similarly, position is irrelevant because a strategy of always going left or always going right would be reinforced only half the time.

Zeaman and House (1966) reviewed the research on simple discrimination learning with retarded subjects. They found 18 studies that compared

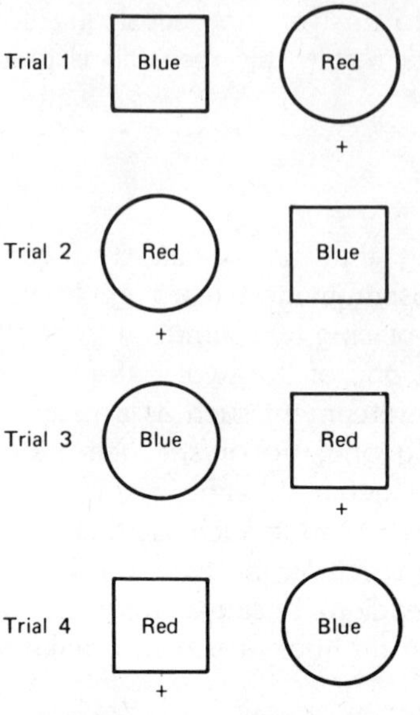

Figure 8-1 A discrimination problem.

retarded subjects to normal subjects matched on mental age. Of these 18 studies, 12 found that the subjects of average IQ were superior to the retarded subjects, and 9 found no reliable difference in performance between the two groups. Three of the studies report differences between retarded and normal subjects with some types of learning but not with others, which explains why the figures don't add up. It is a frequent occurrence in psychological research that a number of studies supposedly measuring the same process find opposite results. This is usually becuse two experiments are seldom exact replications of each other, and apparently minor differences in procedure can occasionally make major differences in result. For example, retarded children can solve a form discrimination problem much faster when the forms are cut out of board rather than when they are simply drawn onto a two dimensional surface. Zeaman and House analyzed these 18 studies more closely to determine what factors seemed to differentiate the different results, and they concluded that one possibility was that if the discrimination was more difficult, the nonretarded children seemed to outperform the retarded while if the problem were easy, there was no difference between the two groups.

Several recent studies have tested this hypothesis. Gruen and Berg (1973) compared mildly and moderately retarded adolescents to younger children of normal intelligence matched on MA. They varied the level of difficulty of the discrimination learning problem by varying the number of irrelevant dimensions. Some subjects had a problem with two irrelevant dimensions and some had a problem with three irrelevant dimensions. Learning criterion was 10 correct in a row. As expected, the problem with three irrelevant dimensions was more difficult than the problem with only two irrelevant dimensions for both groups, and, more importantly, there were no differences in learning performance between the two IQ groups on the easy problem, but the nonretarded children tended to do better than the retarded children on the more difficult problem, a result that supports the hypothesis that retardate-normal differences will only be found on more difficult problems.

Zeaman and House (1963) examined the shape of the learning curve for individual subjects. A learning curve is a graph of the probability of the subject making a correct response on various trials. They found that subjects who take a long time to reach criterion remain at chance until just before they reach solution; they are selecting the correct and wrong stimuli with equal probability. Then, rather abruptly, their performance on the problem becomes almost perfect. It appears that no learning at all occurs until a point just prior to solution. In order to explain this finding, they have developed a two-stage theory of discrimination learning in which subjects solve such problems by chaining two responses together. The first response is covert and involves the subjects' selecting one of the dimensions to look at. This is called an observing response or an attention response. The second response is overt and involves the subjects actually choosing one of the two values revealed by the observing response. In other words, the first response might be the decision to attend to the shape dimension. Once this decision is made, the subjects must decide whether to select the circle or the square. When the subjects are rewarded for their choice, both the attentional response and the instrumental response are reinforced, and thus, the probability of their choosing them again is increased. Apparently, subjects of low IQ and low mental age have little difficulty learning the second, instrumental response, but they have difficulty attending to the relevant dimension. Thus, it is technically incorrect to characterize mentally retarded subjects as slow learners in discrimination learning since their rate of learning, once they are attending to the relevant dimension, is as fast as that of normal children. What distinguishes the slow child is that he or she spends many trials attending to the wrong dimension.

This theory can be tested by shifting the subjects to a new problem once they have learned the old one. There are two basic types of shift problems, those in which the same dimension that was relevant in the original problem remains relevant in the new problem, and those in which a new dimension is made relevant. A reversal shift is an example of the former type. In a reversal shift, the same stimuli are used but the previously negative stimulus is now rewarded. For example, in Figure 8-1, the relevant dimension is color and the correct stimulus cue is red. In a reversal problem, once the subjects have reached criterion on the first problem they are switched to a new problem with blue as the correct stimulus. Reversal shifts are complicated by the fact that the subjects have already learned never to select the negative cue that has suddenly been made positive, and thus, a better type of shift problem in which the same dimension remains relevant involves introducing new values of the same dimensions in the shift problem. For example, in the problem in which the two colors were red and blue, the shift problem might use green and yellow, with one of these two arbitrarily selected to be correct. This type of shift is usually called an intradimensional shift. An extradimensional shift is a shift problem in which the subject is switched to a problem in which a different dimension is made relevant. For example, once the subjects had learned to select the red stimulus and not the blue one, they could be shifted to a problem where the triangle was always rewarded and the star never. These shift problems are important tests of the Zeaman and House (1963) theory because if subjects have already learned which dimension is correct, they ought to learn intradimensional shift problems faster than extradimensional shifts because the same dimension is relevant in both. Numerous experiments have investigated this question, and all have reported that intradimensional shifts are learned faster than extradimensional shifts (Shepp and Turrisi, 1966). Typical is the experiment by House and Zeaman (1962). Their subjects were two groups of institutionalized retarded children, one with low MA (four to six years) and other with higher MA (six to eight years). All of their subjects learned an initial problem with one relevant dimension (either form or color) and one irrelevant dimension (again, either form or color, position was always irrelevant). Following training to a criterion, one third of the subjects in each of the two MA groups were shifted to a reversal problem in which the same stimuli were used and the same dimension was relevant, but the previously positive cue was made negative and the previously negative cue became positive. Another third received an intradimensional shift with new stimuli, but the same dimension relevant, and another third of each group received an extradimensional shift, with new stimuli and a different dimension relevant. Both MA groups learned the reversal shift and the intradimensional shift at the same rate, and the extradimensional shift learning was slower for all groups.

This theory is presumably applicable to the learning of both retarded and nonretarded subjects, and since the actual learning rate does not appear to differ between subjects of different mental levels, it is difficult for this theory to account for the large differences in performance on discrimination learning tasks between retarded and nonretarded that are sometimes observed.

One implication is that retarded subjects do not have a learning deficit but an attentional deficit; they spend a much longer time attending to irrelevant dimensions before learning. Further support for this comes from the observation that many retarded subjects appear to adopt a position strategy, always selecting the right-hand stimulus or always the left-hand stimulus, and thus ignoring the relevant attributes. In fact, if position is made the relevant dimension (e.g., the left-hand stimulus is always rewarded, the right-hand stimulus never) young children and children of low IQ will actually solve discrimination learning problems faster than older and higher IQ subjects (Milgram and Furth, 1964).

However, such an explanation obviously cannot account for most of the differences in learning performance that are found between children of differing MAs and IQs. One prediction of the theory that has not been substantiated by experimental research is that retarded and nonretarded children ought to do equally well on intradimensional shifts because both have been trained to attend to the relevant dimension. However, Lobb and Stogdill (1975) found that retarded children do more poorly than MA-matched nonretarded children on the intradimensional shift problem as well as on original learning.

In a revision of the theory, Fisher and Zeaman (1973) have suggested other possible deficits that can account for the poor performance of retarded subjects besides the observation that they attend to the wrong dimension. One possibility might be that retarded subjects have more difficulty remembering the specific responses and rewards. Another difference might be in the breadth of attention, how many dimensions a subject can observe on any one trial. If higher functioning subjects are able to look at several dimensions simultaneously, they could clearly solve this type of problem faster. This assumption was substantiated in an experiment by Ullman (1974). He used three types of subjects, nonretarded children, mildly retarded children, and moderately retarded children, all matched on mental age. Each subject was shown a series of single stimuli, which could vary on five different dimensions. After each one, they were asked to pick out the stimulus they had seen from an array of 32. They were scored on the number of dimensions that were the same in the stimulus object and the object that the subject selected. That is, if a subject selected the correct object, the one identical in every way to the one they had seen, he received a score of 5 because he was able to attend to and remember all five dimensions. If a subject selected a stimulus that was only different from the sample on one dimension, he received a score of 4, because he was able to attend to and remember four of the five dimensions. There was no difference in performance between the nonretarded children and the mildly retarded children, but the performance of the moderately retarded subjects was significantly inferior, suggesting that subjects of lower IQ are not able to attend to as many aspects of a stimulus as are children of higher IQ, even though they are matched on mental age.

Learning Set

One variant of discrimination learning that deserves special attention is learning to learn, or learning set. Learning set refers to the improvement in performance that is observed over a number of similar problems. For example, in a series of junk stimuli problems, a given subject might make 20 errors before learning always to choose the comb and never the ashtray. However, when given a second problem with the two stimuli being a tin can and a block, the subject might make only 10 errors before solving the problem. On the third problem, distinguishing between a pencil and a toy truck, the subject might make only 3 errors, and after several more such problems, the subject might reach a point where he or she would make, at the most, 1 error on a problem. This improvement in performance over problems is called learning set. The classic study of learning set as a function of IQ and MA was done by Harter (1965). She selected subjects at three different IQ levels—70, 100, and 130—at each of three different MA levels—five, seven, and nine years—thus making nine different groups of subjects. Each subject learned a series of two choice object discriminations. The results are shown in Table 8-1. The dependent variable was the improvement in performance over trials. She concluded that both MA and IQ exerted independent effects on learning set formation; that is, as MA increased, learning set performance improved, but even when MA was held constant, as IQ increased, learning set performance increased. For example, consider the three groups of subjects with a mental age of seven years. The youngest subjects reached criterion after only 16 problems, while the oldest subjects took 38 problems before they reached criterion.

Table 8-1 Trials to Criterion in Learning Set Problems

	MA		
IQ	5	7	9
130	19 (CA 3.8)	16 (CA 5.4)	11 (CA 8.5)
100	31 (CA 5)	24 (CA 7)	18 (CA 9)
70	52 (CA 7)	38 (CA 10)	18 (CA 12.9)

Adapted from Harter, 1965.

Verbal Mediation

Another aspect of discrimination learning that has received a great deal of experimental attention is the role of verbal mediation. The term verbal mediation refers to the use of inner speech as an aid to solving problems. It is reasonable to assume that many older children say to themselves "Red is correct" or some similar phrase as they try to solve a discrimination learning problem, and this inner speech helps them to solve the problem. One of the most widely cited of the defect theories of mental retardation is that retarded children are unable to use verbal mediation as well as nonretarded children of the same mental age, and this explains why they tend to do more poorly on many tasks (Luria, 1961). Partial support for this theory comes from the fact that when retarded subjects are actively encouraged to verbalize aloud what the correct strategy is, their performance on discrimination learning problems improves dramatically. For example, Lobb and Childs (1973) measured discrimination learning in a group of retarded children and a group of nonretarded children matched on mental age. Half of each group was asked to say aloud what their choice was, while the others merely had to make a choice. Of the retarded subjects who were asked to verbalize, 85 percent reached criterion, while of those who were not asked to verbalize, only 15 percent reached criterion. However, the effect was similar for the nonretarded children, which indicates that verbal mediation training was equally effective for both groups. Evidence that retarded children have a particular deficit in verbal mediation comes from experiments where subjects are asked to verbalize the solution to a problem after they have solved it, and several such studies report that retarded children are less able to verbalize the correct solution than are nonretarded children (e.g., Klugh and Janssen, 1966).

Paired Associate Learning

Another type of learning that has received an enormous amount of attention by researchers in mental retardation is paired associate (PA) learning. In paired associate learning, a stimulus word is presented and the subject must learn to give a certain word in response. The stimulus and response words can be presented to the subject either in written form, orally, or with pictures. With retarded subjects, the latter mode of presentation is the most frequent. The response words are usually linked with the stimulus words on a random basis in order that the task represent rote memory rather than any kind of reasoning process, and generally, the order of stimuli is changed from trial to trial. An experiment by Ring and Palermo (1961) is typical. Their subjects were 42 children divided into three groups according to age and IQ. Group I was made up of 14 mildly retarded children with a mean IQ of 76 and an average chronological age of 14. Group II was made up of 14 normal youngsters matched to the retarded children on chronological age, that is, they were also about 14 years old. Group III consisted of 14 younger children matched to the retarded children on mental age. Their average age was 12 years. Each of the subjects was required to learn a list of eight paired associates. The stimuli and responses were both drawings of everyday objects that all of the children could readily identify. For example, one pair consisted of the stimulus CLOCK and the response LEAF. On the initial run through the list, each subject was shown the stimulus picture together with the response picture, and on all subsequent trials, the stimulus was presented alone and the subject was asked to name the response that went with it. Regardless of whether the subject was right or wrong, the response picture was also shown so that each subject could eventually learn the list. The order of presentation of stimuli varied from trial to trial. The dependent variable was the total number of correct responses in 15 runs through the list (subjects who had three successive errorless trials were stopped and it was assumed that they would get all the rest correct). There were no statistically significant differences between the three groups, although the older nonretarded children made slightly more correct responses than the other two groups. Thus, this experiment concluded that retarded children do not differ from nonretarded children on paired associate learning.

Zeaman and House (1966), in their review of the relationship of IQ to learning, found 10 studies that compared retarded subjects to MA-matched normal subjects. Of these 10, 7 found no differences between the two groups, while 3 reported that nonretarded subjects were superior to retarded subjects. After closer analysis, the authors concluded that the larger the difference in IQ between the retarded and the nonretarded subjects, the more likely that a difference between the two would be found, although there were several exceptions. Lipman (1963), reviewing the same material, concluded that retarded subjects were more likely to show a deficit if the stimulus material was less meaningful.

A more relevant question than simply finding retardate-normal difference in some task is attempting to account for these differences. When the paired associate learning paradigm was originally developed, it was considered to be a simple process of connecting a stimulus to a response by rote. At that time, it was widely assumed that all thinking could be characterized by such associations. However, more recent research has revealed that the process of learning which words go with which stimuli is far from a simple process of association or rote memory; there are a large number of different processes involved. The subjects must select a relevant portion of the stimulus, they must learn the appropriate responses and integrate them into units if necessary and, they must learn the actual associations. The majority of the research on paired association learning with the retarded has involved the process of mediation. When college students learn paired associates, they generally develop elaborate mediating strategies called mnemonics, which greatly facilitate learning. With the example given above of learning the response CLOCK to the stimulus LEAF, a subject might picture a clock sitting on top of a leaf or think of a sentence such as "The clock was on the leaf," and such strategies act as an aid to learning. Retarded subjects are less likely to do this, and a number of researchers have suggested that the process of learning in the retarded could be greatly facilitated if they could be taught to mediate.

The classic study of mediation in the paired associate learning of retarded subjects was done by Jensen and Rohwer (1963). Their subjects were mildly retarded (average IQ 55) adults, and their materials were everyday objects randomly paired up. The stimulus member of each pair was attached to the outside of a box, while the response member was placed inside the box. There were six such pairs, each with its own box, and the subjects were asked to learn what was inside each box when shown the stimulus attached to the lid. Half of the subjects were given special training. They were asked to repeat a sentence that contained both the stimulus and response words. For example, in one case, the stimulus was CUP and the response was GLASSES, and the sentence was "The CUP wore GLASSES." The results of the experiment were quite dramatic; those subjects who had been given the sentences learned the list in an average of 3.5 trials, while those subjects who had not been given this tool took 16.3 trials to learn the list.

The discovery of such a powerful technique to aid learning in the retarded stimulated a great deal of research into the question of what kinds of mediators were most effective. Davidson (1964), in a design similar to that of Jensen and Rohwer, found that joining the stimulus item to the response item with a simple preposition (e.g., glasses on cup) was as effective as asking a subject to repeat a whole sentence. Turnure (1971) reported that placing the two items together in a two sentence paragraph was more effective than merely providing the subject with a sentence as an aid to recall. Rohwer and Lynch (1968) found that showing subjects pictures depicting the stimulus and response items interacting could act as an effective mediator, and that a brief movie on which the two items were engaged in a short action episode (e.g., a sequence showing a DOG walking to a GATE and closing it) was even more effective. A general summary of this research is that almost any kind of elaboration of the stimulus-response connection will facilitate learning, but more complex elaborations such as reading a paragraph containing the two items or showing a film depicting the two items interacting are more effective than simpler elaborations.

Another type of mediation can be studied in a chaining paradigm. According to association theory, if an association is formed between a stimulus A and a response B, and another association is formed between a stimulus B (the same as the above response) and a response C, then the presence of these two associations ought to facilitate the learning of the association A-C. The mediator in this case is B. For example, if a student is trying to learn the Spanish word for ocean, which is *mar,* there is no obvious connection between these two items (ocean and *mar*), but if the subject can think of a mediating item that will connect them, learning will be easier. For example, the word marine is an associate of ocean and could act as a stimulus to produce *mar.* Such chaining paradigms have been found to be helpful in the learning of paired associates by normal adults (Horton and Kjeldergaard, 1961).

Borkowski and Johnson (1968) employed such a chaining paradigm with retarded subjects. Their subjects learned three PA lists, and the dependent variable was the learning performance on the final list. The responses for the first list made up the stimuli of the second list, and the third list consisted of the stimuli from the first list paired with the responses from the second list. For example, one item was as follows: the first list pair was GIRL-DRESS, the second list pair was DRESS-YELLOW, and the third list pair was GIRL-YELLOW. With the mediation, the retarded subjects performed as well as the MA matched nonretarded controls, but without the mediation, the retarded subjects were considerably worse than the nonretarded subjects. Thus one interpretation of these results is that mediation helps retarded subjects more than nonretarded subjects, perhaps because nonretarded subjects are more capable of providing their own mediators.

It is clear from this research that retarded subjects are capable of using experimenter-supplied mediators to facilitate learning of paired associates. However, there is little research addressed to the question of whether low IQ subjects are less able to use mediators thar. are nonretarded subjects. Flavell, Beach, and Chinsky (1966) have distinguished two kinds of mediational deficiencies; a production deficiency refers to the situation where the subject is unable to generate an appropriate mediator, even though one is potentially available. A control deficiency refers to a situation where the subject can generate a mediator, but, for some reason, the mediator is unable to facilitate learning. There is little question that retarded subjects do not have a control deficiency. When they are provided with an appropriate mediator, they are able to use it to improve performance. However, it is quite possible that many retarded subjects have a production deficiency. When nonretarded subjects, particularly older ones, are asked to learn paired associates, even though there is no apparent connection between them, they will spontaneously generate a mediator or mnemonic. Perhaps retarded subjects are less likely to do this. Evidence for this theory comes from the experiment by Borkowski and Johnson (1968) in which they found that providing retarded subjects with mediators brought their learning performance up to the level of the MA-matched nonretarded subjects, while providing the nonretarded subjects with mediators had a much smaller effect.

Milgram and Reidel (1969) addressed themselves to this question by asking subjects, both retarded and MA-matched nonretarded, to generate their own mediating sentences aloud; that is, they were asked to make up sentences that contained both the stimulus and response words. Their responses were graded according to several criteria. There were some clear differences between the sentences of the retarded and the nonretarded. At older MA levels (seven and nine), the number of sentences that did not contain both words was negligible for the nonretarded subjects, while a number of retarded subjects gave such responses. The sentences were graded into three levels of context according to the nature of the relationship expressed in the sentence. A sentence was given a score of 1 if the relationship between the two words was simply positional, such as "The TELEPHONE was in the BARN." A sentence was given two points if the sentence expressed a meaningful interaction, such as "The SNOWMAN was holding the FLAG." A sentence was given a score of 3 if it expressed a novel relationship or one that was optimally appropriate, such as "The TELEPHONE was in the BARN so that the cows could call other cows." The nonretarded subjects at all three MA levels received higher scores than did the retarded subjects. In other words, retarded children, on the average, are unable to generate mediating sentences as elaborate or appropriate as are nonretarded children of the same mental age. This is clear evidence of a type of production deficiency. Martin et al. (1968) reported similar results. They administered a PA task to retarded and nonretarded subjects and then asked them to describe whatever mediational strategy, if any, they had been using. Retarded subjects were more likely to report that they were using a very low-level strategy such as rote rehearsal, or else nothing at all.

Memory Processes in the Retarded

The past decade has seen an increase in research in memory processes with the retarded accompanied by a shift in the way that these memory processes have been conceptualized. The older research tended to view memory as essentially a passive process with the subject learning and memorizing material by rote simply by being exposed to it. The newer research views the subject as an active processor of information, someone who transforms raw stimulus information into meaningful elements to facilitate storage. One example of this trend has already been seen in the increased attention being paid to mediating processes in paired associate learning. However, this shift has had its most profound effect on the study of memory.

A number of different information processing models and theories have been proposed (Atkinson and Shiffrin, 1965; Waugh and Norman, 1965). The assumption of each of these models is that information passes through several different types of storage, and each type of storage has different characteristics. Information is first encoded in a sensory register, sometimes referred to as iconic memory (Neisser, 1967), which simply provides a very brief (usually less than a second) memory trace of the physical features of the stimulus. This information is quickly lost unless it is transferred into short-term memory (STM). STM has very limited storage capacity and can only hold a few items at a time. This is where individuals place a phone number that they have looked up and are about to dial. Items in STM are lost fairly rapidly, but they can be maintained through a process of rehearsal. As the individuals walk across the room to the telephone, they repeat the number over and over again to themselves, and this activity keeps it from being forgotten. It is also possible to maintain items in STM more efficiently by elaboration; this is, by using mnemonic devices to make the material more meaningful or by chunking, combining several items together into a single unit. For example, it is easier to remember the list 6, 8, 3, 9, 2, 1, 7, 4 by rehearsing it as 68, 39, 21, 74, than it is by rehearsing it as eight digits. Some items in STM are transferred into long-term memory (LTM), where material is stored for long periods of time out of consciousness. It is generally assumed that nothing is ever forgotten from LTM, although a particular piece of information may not be available (retrievable) at a particular time. LTM is unlimited in capacity; an infinite amount of information can be stored in it without any information ever being bumped out. This is unlike STM, which can only hold a few items at a time.

Short-Term Memory

Most of the research on memory has focused on STM. One of the classic defect theories of mental retardation is that of Ellis (1963) who proposed that retarded subjects have a particular defect in their short-term memory because memory traces fade more rapidly when the nervous system is not intact. Evidence for this theory comes from a variety of memory studies indicating that retarded subjects did not perform as well as nonretarded subjects matched on CA.

However, more recent research has indicated that Ellis' 1963 theory is an oversimplification, and a series of studies by Ellis (1970) based on an information processing approach has substantially modified the earlier theory. The basic task used by Ellis (1970) is as follows: his apparatus consisted of a panel with a horizontal row of nine openings and a tenth opening above this row. A series of slide projectors mounted behind the panel projected digits or letters onto these openings. The subject saw a row of nine digits, presented one at a time from left to right, followed by a tenth digit shown in the opening above the row. This tenth digit was called the probe and was the same as one of the nine digits shown previously. The subject's task was to indicate in which of the nine openings the digit that was the same as the probe appeared.

Ellis interpreted his data in terms of an information processing model that differs somewhat from the more typical one in that he distinguished two types of STM, primary memory and secondary memory. Primary memory can retain only two or three items at best and only for a very brief period of time, while secondary memory can retain several more items and over a longer period of time if the subject rehearses them.

In one experiment, retarded young adults with a mean IQ of 61 were compared with college students of the same age. In some trials, there was a two-second delay between presentation of each item in the row, in other cases, there was no delay. The former condition is called spaced, the latter is called massed. The dependent variable was the percentage of items correct in each position. The results are shown in Figure 8-2. There were a number of interesting conclusions. The first is that there was no difference in performance between the retarded and the nonretarded subjects when the item to be recalled was in the last position. Presumably, performance on the last item before the probe is a reflection of primary memory because the item was presented within the past few seconds. Thus, this research suggests that retarded people have no particular deficit in their primary memory. However, there were large differences between the retarded subjects and the college students on the other items. Performance on these items is presumably a function of secondary memory and requires rehearsal for good performance. Spacing the items resulted in a considerable improvement for the nonretarded subjects but had no apparent effect on the performance of the retarded people. Since spacing affords more of an opportunity for rehearsal, it is likely that the crucial difference between the two groups is the use of rehearsal strategies. Further research tended to support this hypothesis. To summarize, if STM is represented as two separate processes (primary memory and secondary memory), the former being essentially passive but with rapid decay, the latter requiring active rehearsal on the part of the subject, retarded subjects have no unusual difficulty with primary memory—memory for events within the past few seconds—but they have a considerable deficit in secondary memory—memory that requires active rehearsal—and it is

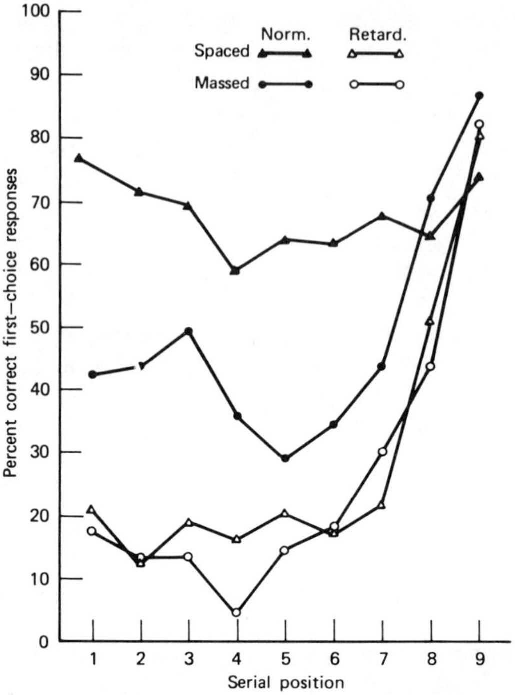

Figure 8-2 Performance of normals and retardates under massed (0.0-second interval) and spaced (2.0-second interval) conditions on the nine-position task. From N. R. Ellis. Memory processes in retardates and normals. In N. R. Ellis (Ed.), *International review of research in mental retardation,* Vol. 4. New York: Academic Press, 1970. Copyright © 1970 by Academic Press. Reprinted by permission of the publisher and the author.

presumed that the main reason why they show such a deficit is that they fail to rehearse.

This basic conclusion has been substantiated in a variety of other research projects. Belmont and Butterfield (1971), using an apparatus and procedure similar to that used by Ellis (1970), permitted retarded and normal adolescents to proceed at their own rate through the initial list of six items. The nonretarded subjects spent progressively more time at each position. They spent more time studying the second item than the first, more time studying the third item than the second, and so on. Such a pattern is consistent with active rehearsal. If, on each trial, the subjects are rehearsing each item that they have seen so far, as the total of items increases, rehearsal time would get progressively longer. The retarded subjects showed no such pattern, and, in fact, there was some tendency for their study time to decrease through the list. As in the Ellis research, the nonretarded subjects' performance was superior to that of the retarded subjects except for the last two items, where there was no difference between the two groups.

In the second part of the same research, some subjects in each of the two groups were instructed not to rehearse; they were told to simply read each letter aloud once as it appeared and then go on to the next one. Other subjects were instructed to actively rehearse aloud by going passively through the first four items of the six-item list, then pausing and rehearsing these four items aloud three times, then going on to the last two. Other subjects in each group were permitted to use whatever strategy they chose, just as before. Their results were entirely consistent with the theory that normal subjects rehearse and retarded subjects do not. When the nonretarded subjects were instructed not to rehearse, their performance dropped considerably. When the retarded subjects were explicitly shown how to rehearse and asked to do it aloud, their performance improved.

Rehearsal of items to be remembered is one example of what are called control processes in information processing models, those processes that are voluntary and that determine what information is stored and where it is stored. Other examples of control processes include the mnemonic tools described in the previous section, attention to certain stimuli while ignoring other stimuli, chunking or grouping items to facilitate memory, and the like. A synonym for these control processes is strategies. Retarded people seem to be generally deficient in the use of such strategies, and this deficiency contributes to their poor learning performance. Three examples have been provided so far. The first is the discovery by Zeaman and House (1963) that in discrimination learning problems, the actual learning rate is similar for retarded and nonretarded subjects, but retarded subjects persist in attending to inappropriate characteristics of the stimulus long after they have been shown to be wrong, and thus, it takes them many more trials to reach the criterion. The second example is the use of mediators described in the section on paired associate learning. The third example is the failure of retarded subjects to use rehearsal strategies in learning a series of digits or letters. A number of other examples of the same principle have also been found. For example, when subjects are asked to learn a list of words without the order being important, a task known as free recall, older subjects of normal intelligence tend to group the words in some way, often by category if this is appropriate, in order to facilitate recall. This process is called associative clustering. Retarded subjects to not do this as much, and as a result, their free recall performance is hindered (Spitz, 1966). Brown (1974) reviewed much of the research in strategic behavior in the retarded and found overwhelming evidence that retarded people have a deficit in such control processes. The only difficulty with this area is that there is very little research comparing retarded subjects to nonretarded subjects matched on MA; almost all of the research used CA matched controls.

Recognition Memory

If the deficit in the memory of retarded subjects is due primarily to their inadequate rehearsal strategies, there ought to be little or no difference in performance between retarded and nonretarded subjects in memory tasks where rehearsal strategies are not possible. One such task is recognition memory for pictures. The general procedure is to show subjects a large number of pictures, often several hundred, and then show the subject a series of pairs of pictures. In each case, one of the pairs was in the original set and the other one was not, and the subjects must identify which of the two pictures they had seen before. Normal adult subjects do remarkably well at this. When all the subjects have to do is identify whether they have seen a picture before, apparently the memory capacity is nearly infinite (Shepard, 1967). This task is different from many other memory tasks in that no rehearsal or other types of strategy is necessary for good performance, and, as a result, one might predict that retarded subjects would show little or no deficit in recognition memory. Several studies have shown that this is the case (Martin, 1970; Brown, 1972). The performance of retarded subjects is nearly as good as that of normal adults, most getting more than 95 percent correct.

Long-Term Memory

Once an item has been stored in long-term memory, no rehearsal or other organizational strategy is necessary to maintain it, and, as a result, it is predicted that the long-term memory—memory over a period of hours, days, and weeks—of retarded subjects would also not differ from nonretarded subjects. Research in this area is difficult to do because it is necessary to equate the two groups of subjects on original learning, but what little research has been done in this area tends to confirm the prediction that retarded people show no deficit in long-term memory relative to nonretarded subjects (Belmont, 1966).

Teaching Retarded Subjects to Use Strategies

If the deficits that retarded subjects show in learning and memory tasks are attributable largely to their poorer use of strategies and tools to aid recall, then it should be possible to train some of these strategies in retarded subjects and thus facilitate their learning. It has been shown in numerous experiments (Jensen and Rohwer, 1963; Belmont and Butterfield, 1971) that if retarded subjects are explicitly provided with mediators, or if they are specifically instructed to rehearse, then their performance improves, but it is desirable to get them to use these strategies spontaneously. A number of researchers have attempted to teach the use of such strategies, and the results, although far from consistent, seem to indicate that retarded subjects can benefit from such training. For example, Butterfield, Wambold, and Belmont (1973) attempted to teach retarded subjects to use a type of rehearsal strategy in the serial learning problem used by Ellis (1970) and by Belmont and Butterfield (1972). The aim was to teach retarded adolescents to memorize a six-item list of letters. The approach that these researchers used was to encourage the subjects to actively rehearse the first three items after the third one, then go quickly through the last three items passively and expose the probe as quickly as possible. Presumably, the last three items would still be in primary memory while the first three items would be in secondary memory because they had been actively rehearsed. In their first attempt, they simply taught subjects to rehearse the first three items. They found that although this improved performance somewhat, performance was still not satisfactory and many subjects who were actively rehearsing apparently could not use this rehearsal to improve their performance. As a result, they broke the task down into eight separate component steps and attempted to train each step individually. The eight steps were as follows. (1) Use the passive system to construct a rehearsable group of the first three letters. (2) Transfer those letters to the active store by rehearsing them. (3) Stop attending to those first three letters while exposing and attending to, but not rehearsing, the last three letters. (4) Expose the probe letter immediately after attending to the sixth letter. (5) Immediately, search the entire contents of the passive memory story. (6) Respond at once if the probe is found in the passive store. (7) If not found, search the active store serially. (8) Terminate the search by responding when the probe item is located. These researchers found that when subjects were taught not only how to rehearse, but also how to retrieve items from store as in the above steps, that the memory performance of retarded subjects could be improved considerably and that this improvement carried over to new blocks of trials.

A number of research projects have systematically tried to teach retarded subjects to generate their own mediators to aid in paired associate learning. The research by Burger and Blackman (1976) is typical. Their subjects were mildly retarded children who were asked to learn lists of nine paired associates. In the pretest list, before any training in the use of mediators, the subjects took about 13 trials through the list before they were able to get them all right. Some of the subjects were then given training a week later in how to use mediators. They were shown a picture of the two items interacting and were given a sentence which used the two items. With this kind of assistance, it took them only slightly over three trials on the average to learn a nine-pair list. This drastic improvement was consistent with other research described above (e.g., Jensen and Rohwer, 1963). A week later, they were asked to learn a third list, and this time, they were asked to generate their own mediating sentences and images. Again, their performance was very good. In the fourth week, they were simply instructed to learn a list of pairs, without any special encouragement to use mediators. It was obvious that they were using mediators, however, because it took these subjects an average of only 4.67 trials to learn the nine-item list, while it took a control group who had had no instruction in how to use mediators more than 10 trials. In other words, once they had been taught how to use mediators and had been encouraged to generate their own, these retarded subjects were able to transfer this instruction to new situations. Other researchers (Wanshura and Borkowski, 1975; Turnure and Thurlow, 1973) have shown the same thing.

However, it is one thing to show that it is possible to teach retarded children to use mediators in a paired associate task or to teach them to rehearse in a serial learning task, but, at the moment, it is doubtful that there is very much generalization to totally new situations. In other words, if retarded children were required to learn their addition tables after having been taught to rehearse in a program such as that of Butterfield et al. (1973), they would probably not spontaneously start to rehearse if they had not done so before, and thus such a program is likely to have limited effectiveness.

Level I versus Level II Intelligence

One of the conclusions that we can draw from the research on learning and memory in the retarded is that there is often little difference between retarded and nonretarded subjects when the material to be learned is very simple, but when the learning becomes more complex, more difficult, or more abstract, retarded individuals seem to be at a disadvantage relative to nonretarded people. This is frequently true even when the two groups are matched on mental age.

Jensen (1970) has developed a theory of retardation that attempts to account for much of these data. His theory applies only to the cultural familial retarded, the group that we have labeled the functionally or nonorganically retarded. He distinguishes between two different levels of intelligence. Level I is called associative ability and refers to the ability to learn simple associations or connections. Much of our everyday learning is associative in nature in that it consists largely of noting simple connections between events or between actions and consequences. A good test of Level I ability is digit span, asking the subject to repeat back a string of digits. Level II is called cognitive ability and can be considered a capacity for understanding complex relations. It is best measured by highly abstract tests such as the Raven's Matrices. Most general intelligence tests are measuring both levels of intelligence to some extent. Many mildly retarded children whose retardation does not have an organic basis have a deficit in Level II functioning but not in Level I functioning. This accounts for the somewhat paradoxical finding that many low-SES children who do poorly in school and on intelligence tests have no difficulty learning their way around the neighborhood or otherwise functioning effectively in most nonacademic situations. Because they have little or no deficit in associative learning, and most adaptive behavior skills require mostly associative learning, they do not show a deficit.

Evidence for this theory comes from a variety of sources. When low-SES children are tested on a simple trial and error task that involves only Level I ability, a wide range of abilities is found; many of these children who are considered EMR perform as well or better than children of much higher IQ. This is entirely consistent with the numerous studies cited above which found little difference between retarded and normal subjects on very simple learning tasks such as classical conditioning and simple discrimination learning or in rote memory tasks such as paired associate learning. Studies that did find differences in simple learning rate as a function of IQ can be accounted for by the fact that they have also included organically retarded subjects who show a deficit in Level I as well as Level II functioning.

This theory is obviously an oversimplification of a very complex problem. However, it is difficult to take issue with one important conclusion, that retarded children have relatively less difficulty learning simple associations than they do learning more complex and abstract concepts. To the extent that this is true, Jensen (1970) argues that much of our effort in special education is misguided. Current educational practices deemphasize teaching specific facts in rote fashion and stress more abstract conceptual abilities. The assumption behind this trend is that it is more important for children to learn how to learn than it is for them to know specific facts. For example, it is better for children to be able to solve a problem like $2 + ? = 4$ than it is for them simply to memorize that $2 + 2 = 4$ in rote fashion. As a result, most elementary school teachers are spending less time requiring children to memorize multiplication tables and more time assuring that they know what multiplication is and that they understand the theory behind it. For the most part, this is a healthy trend, but it is important to keep in mind that this is emphasizing the kind of learning that retarded children and slow learners in general have the most difficulty with. There is a failure to capitalize on the specific strengths of these children. Jensen described a classroom of slow learners in which the teacher had been trying every day for some six months to teach them the alphabet, but with little success. Despite this, Jensen was able to demonstrate that these children could learn, on the average, 16 of 24 paired associates on one trial, completely on a par with children of the same age who were making normal progress. Observation of the teacher's behavior revealed that the teacher was spending little time on actual drill, and tended to reinforce the children's effort rather than their actual success. Because of this and because most of the things that the teacher was trying to teach were reflections of Level II (cognitive learning), these students were having few success experiences and were learning little.

Summary

Experimental research in learning and memory with the mentally retarded can be divided into two general types: research that compares retarded to nonretarded subjects and research that simply uses retarded subjects. The former type of research is usually oriented toward testing what could be called theories of mental retardation, explanations of why the behavior of retarded people differs from that of nonretarded people. One such theory is called the developmental theory and proposes that retarded people develop in the same fashion that nonretarded children do, going through the same cognitive stages, but their rate of development is slower and they do not reach the higher levels. To the extent that this theory is correct, when retarded children are compared to younger nonretarded children matched on MA, there ought to be no differences in cognitive functioning between the two groups. Another category of theories is called defect theories, and these propose that retarded people have specific defects in some processes but are relatively normal in others. Among the defect theories discussed in this chapter are the hypothesis that retarded people have a particular deficiency in the use of strategies such as rehearsal and generating mediators to aid memory, and the theory of Jensen that cultural-familial retarded children have a particular deficit in understanding complex relationships but have no deficit in simple rote learning.

There are a number of basic learning paradigms that have been quite heavily studied by experimental psychologists who are interested in the mentally retarded. The simplest of these is classical conditioning, which involves pairing a neutral stimulus such as a bell or tone (the conditioned stimulus) with a stimulus that normally elicits a response. The stimulus is called the unconditioned stimulus and the response is called the unconditioned response. After a number of such pairings, the conditioned stimulus also begins to elicit the response. Research on classical conditioning with the retarded indicates that as long as the learning is simple enough, there is no difference in performance between high IQ and low IQ subjects.

A second type of conditioning is called operant conditioning. This paradigm involves following a specific response with a reinforcement and thus, increasing the frequency or probability of the response. One type of operant conditioning that has been widely studied with the retarded is discrimination learning, training subjects to always select one stimulus and never the other when presented with two choices. Zeaman and House (1963) have shown that an important aspect of discrimination learning is getting the subject to pay attention to the relevant dimension, the characteristic that distinguishes the correct from the incorrect stimulus. Once they are doing this, there is little difference in learning rate between the retarded and nonretarded subjects, but it often takes retarded subjects a good deal longer to learn to attend to the relevant dimension.

Another type of learning is called paired associate learning, which involves teaching the subject to respond with a certain word when a stimulus word is presented. Research comparing retarded to nonretarded subjects on learning speed using paired associate learning has been mixed, some reporting that there is no difference between the two groups, others reporting that retarded subjects take longer to learn. One important way to facilitate learning in a paired associate task is to provide the subject with some sort of mediational link between the two words, some way to connect the two such as a sentence containing both words. When this is done, the speed of learning of retarded subjects improves dramatically.

A number of studies have shown that retarded subjects show impairments in short-term memory. However, research from a number of sources indicates that the main problem with retarded subjects is that they fail to rehearse, and this hurts their performance. Similarly, they are less likely to use other strategies to facilitate learning and memory, and this deficit rather than a deficit in learning rate per se, might be the important difference between retarded and normal subjects. In tasks where rehearsal or other strategies are not appropriate, as in long-term memory or in recognition memory, there seems to be little difference in performance between retarded and nonretarded subjects.

In a similar vein, Jensen has proposed that functionally retarded subjects are not impaired in associative or rote learning, but their deficit is limited to higher-level thinking. He proposed that the educational approach that is best for such children is one emphasizing facts and associative learning rather than conceptual learning, as is currently the case.

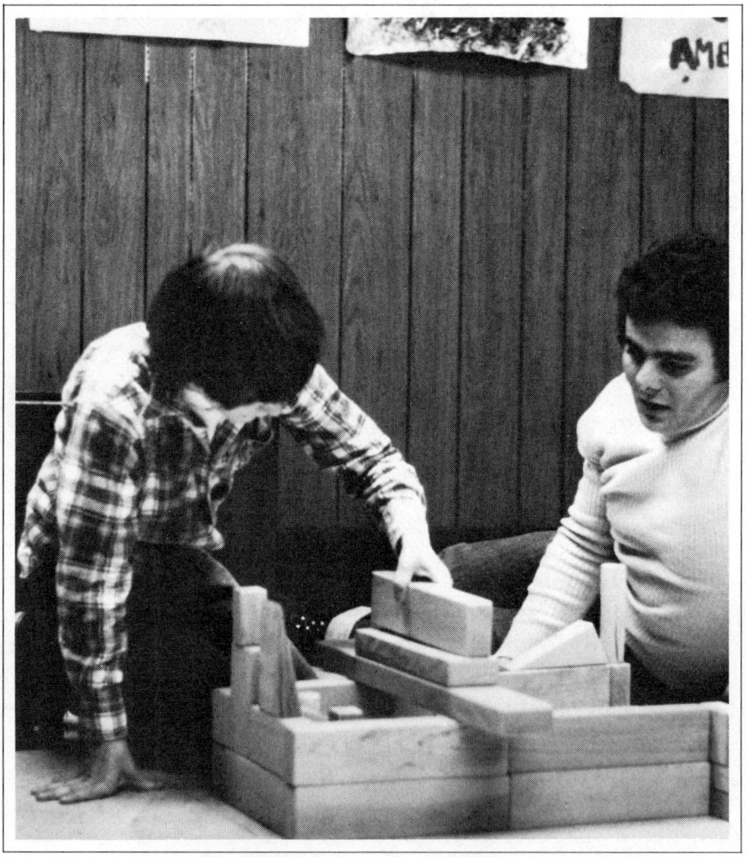

9
Language and Mental Retardation

Language and intelligence are so intimately related that some people have practically defined mental retardation in terms of a language deficit (Bereiter and Engelmann, 1966; Stamm, 1974). It is widely assumed that language is necessary for most higher-order thinking, and the vast majority of the items on most intelligence tests involve either a verbal stimulus, a verbal response, or both. A deficit in language skills is perhaps the single most important characteristic that distinguishes a retarded person from a nonretarded one. As a result, the subject of language in the retarded has received a good deal of attention both from a theoretical point of view and from the practical angle of trying to improve verbal skills in retarded children.

This chapter is divided into two sections. The first discusses the nature of language, emphasizing the mechanisms by which children become fluent in their native tongue. The second section considers the nature and prevalence of various speech and language disorders among the mentally retarded.

The Nature of Language and Language Acquisition

The process by which young children become fluent speakers of the language of their culture is a remarkable feat of learning. In a period of about three years, the typical child progresses from being an essentially nonverbal organism to having a vocabulary of thousands of words and being able to speak and understand complex sentences.

Let us consider exactly what the child has to learn. Language refers to a system of rules by which thoughts are translated into a series of sound waves in order to communicate information. The term language refers to the system itself, and thus it is distinguished from speech, which is a term referring to the actual behavior of an individual. Children must learn how to speak, of course, but, more importantly, they must learn a highly abstract system or code.

One of the most important characteristics of language, a characteristic common to all of the languages of the world, is the feature of openness or generativity. This means that all languages are infinite in capacity; there are an infinite number of acceptable sentences in any language. With the exception of a few ritualistic phrases, most of the sentences that people hear, they have never heard before, yet they understand them, and most of the sentences that they utter they have never heard before. This fact may be obvious, but it has important implications because it suggests that a child cannot learn a language simply by learning sentences. Children will seldom hear the same sentence more than once, and as soon as they begin to combine words, their own language is open since they speak sentences that they couldn't possibly have heard before. In other words, the child is learning abstract rules to construct sentences rather than sentences themselves.

This characteristic of openness is one feature that distinguishes human languages from the various forms of animal communication. Most species of animals have a set of signals by which one member of the species can communicate information to another. For example, various bird songs are used to communicate a message such as "Danger" or "This is my territory." All of these communication systems are finite in the sense that there are only a small number of total messages, and each always communicates the same thing.

If this were the case for human languages, it would be possible for children to learn language by association. They could simply learn which utterances go with which events similar to the way that Pavlov's dog learned that a tone meant that meat powder was coming. Very early in the language learning process, children might be doing just this. They learn by association that the utterance "cookie" stands for those little brown things that taste so good. However, very quickly children begin to say things that they have never heard before. They might use a phrase such as "Allgone jelly." The closest sentence that they could possibly have heard was a sentence such as "The jelly is all gone," and if they were imitating this, they would not say "Allgone jelly" but rather "Jelly allgone." Yet the statement "Allgone jelly" has meaning both to the children and to their listeners. There is no way that a simple process of association learning can account for this. Human language is more than a simple catalogue of sounds associated with meanings.

The component of language that makes this openness possible is syntax. Syntax, the linguists' term for what most people call grammar, is a system of rules by which the words of a language are combined together to make sentences. A sentence is more than just a string of words, however, because the specific reference of the various words in the sentence is affected by the syntax. The sentences "Bill hits Mary" and "Mary hits Bill" both have the same component words, but have entirely different meanings.

The rules of syntax are remarkably complex. Almost everyone has had several years of grammar in high school in which they learn that all complete sentences have a subject and a predicate, and they learn about prepositional phrases and indefinite modifiers and past participles and so forth. In order to speak English, it is necessary to use all of these various constructions correctly, and virtually all preschoolers learn how to use these rules by the time they are about five years old. Of course, small children cannot verbalize these rules, but by speaking sentences that correctly use these constructions, they demonstrate their competence.

Let us consider just one of the rules that the child has to learn, the rule for constructing passive sentences. Consider the sentence "Mary hits Bill." To make this into a passive sentence with the same meaning, the rule is as follows: Make the direct object (Bill) the subject of the sentence. Then add the appropriate form of the verb to be (in this case "is"). Follow this with the past participle of the verb and follow this with a prepositional phrase with the preposition "by," the object being the subject of the former sentence (Mary). The result is the sentence "Bill is hit by Mary." This seems like a horribly complicated rule, and it would be virtually impossible to teach such a rule to a five-year-old child, particularly when it involves an understanding of such concepts as subject, object, and past participle. However, although no five year old could verbalize this rule (in fact, most college students can't) most are able to use it correctly in the sense that they can construct and understand passive sentences.

The purpose of this rather elaborate example is to emphasize the point that language learning is a remarkable process. The child must learn hundreds and hundreds of rules like the one described above, yet all normal children accomplish this easily. This achievement is all the more remarkable considering the fact that children must learn the grammar of their language without the benefit of formal teaching. Since parents usually cannot verbalize the rules themselves, it would be impossible for them to teach their children. What teaching does occur is usually limited to a parent occasionally correcting a child's grammatical mistakes, and research suggests that this is probably ineffective for the most part (McNeill, 1966). Also, most learning occurs by repetition, but the process of language acquisition is hindered by the fact that the child seldom hears the same sentence more than once. If virtually every sentence that children hear is novel, it is difficult to understand how they can learn the underlying system. For example, at some time, the child must learn the concepts of subject and predicate since it is impossible to construct grammatically correct sentences without this knowledge. Yet the child must discover this merely by listening to other people speaking. Imagine yourself in a comparable situation of having to learn a language such as Chinese simply by listening to it.

The steps that children go through in acquiring language are remarkably similar regardless of what language the child is learning and how much or how little teaching and correction the child receives. During most of the first year after birth, the child can be considered nonverbal. For the first few months, the only sounds that the child makes are crying and cooing sounds that are not even prespeech. Sometime around four to six months, most infants begin to babble. Babbling refers to the combining of consonant and vowel sounds to form vaguely speechlike sounds such as "ba" and "goo." However, early babbling cannot be considered language development and probably does not even involve learning because all children babble in the same way at first, regardless of what language their parents speak. Even congenitally deaf children babble, although this behavior ceases after a while. In fact, although babbling seems to serve the purpose of letting the child practice forming speech sounds, apparently, it is not necessary for the later development of speech. Lenneberg (1966) describes a case of a boy who, as a result of an operation, had a tube inserted into his lungs through his trachea to facilitate breathing. The tube was put in when the boy was 8 months old and was removed when he was 14 months old. It effectively prevented him from making any speech sounds during this 6-month period. However, the day after the tube was removed, the boy began to produce babbling sounds typical of a 14 month old. Apparently, no previous practice or experience hearing his own voice was necessary.

Throughout language development, children's receptive language, their ability to understand what they hear, is generally several months more advanced than their expressive language competence, their ability to speak correctly. Sometime late in the first year of life, children begin to understand a little of what is said to them. Probably the first word that most children learn the meaning of is "No." A short while later, usually when children are about 12 months old, they will say their first meaningful word. For the next 6 to 9 months, children's expressive language develops relatively slowly. They may learn to speak two to four new words a month, but they will not combine them. However, receptive language skills during this time are more advanced.

Sometime between 18 and 24 months, children begin to combine words. Many psycholinguists consider this time the onset of true language (McNeill, 1966). At about the same time, children's expressive language vocabulary begins to grow very rapidly. The typical child has a speaking vocabulary of roughly 20 words when 18 months old, but 200 words by 21 months of age, and by the age of three years, the average child has a vocabulary of 1000 words or more (Lenneberg, 1966). This means that for a while, the child is learning two to three new words each day.

From the time that children first begin to combine words, they do not do so randomly, but appear to have a primitive grammar; that is, there are certain word combinations that are acceptable and certain combinations that are not, and the child only utters acceptable combinations. Children are obviously not directly imitating what they hear because they say things that they couldn't possibly have heard before.

Children's acquisition of grammar is also remarkably rapid. The best single measure of grammatical competence is mean sentence length. By the time children are three years old, they are speaking in sentences of five words or more and are able to use a large number of relatively complex grammatical rules such as grammatical agreement, the use of negatives and questions, inflections, and the proper use of pronouns.

Because of the fact that all children seem to learn so rapidly and so effortlessly at the same age, it is widely accepted that they can accomplish this task because they are biologically programmed to do so. In other words, the way that a child learns language is probably qualitatively different from the way a rat learns to press a bar in a Skinner box. The anatomy and physiology of the human nervous system are such that normal children will spontaneously acquire the language system of their culture when they reach a certain stage in development. In this sense, it is analogous to walking upright. Man's whole biology, brain, nerves, muscles, bones, and even sensory systems are designed so that man will walk in a certain fashion, and as a result, all children spontaneously walk upright when they reach a certain stage of development. They don't need to be reinforced for walking (children spend a good deal of time just walking around with no particular goal in mind), they don't need to see others walking (congenitally blind children walk at roughly the same age and go through the same stages as sighted children even though they have never seen anyone else walking), and specific training and practice seem to be largely irrelevant since Hopi Indian children who spend most of their first year strapped to a board walk at the same age as middle-class American children whose parents spend a good deal of time encouraging them to walk (Dennis and Dennis, 1940).

Language acquisition seems to be a similar process, with the obvious difference that children must be exposed to a natural language. All children all over the world learn their native tongue at roughly the same age, going through the same steps at roughly the same rate. Formal teaching is not necessary and probably not even helpful. Our biology has predisposed us to speak. Lenneberg (1967) has demonstrated that much of our vocal apparatus—our lungs, our larynx, and our mouths—seems to be designed specifically so that we would speak in a certain way. In fact, a number of people (e.g., McNeill, 1966; Chomsky, 1965) have suggested that the only way that children could master the complexity of grammar is by being born with a sort of innate knowledge of certain grammatical structures. For example, McNeill (1966) has suggested that knowledge of the subject-predicate relationship, the verb-object relationship, and the modifier-noun relationship might be prewired into the nervous system. Such knowledge could reduce language learning to a far more manageable task.

Lenneberg (1967) has extended this theory by suggesting that language learning can only occur at a certain time in development. Not only is it impossible to teach language to children before they are ready, but if they haven't acquired language skills before they reach puberty, they never will. Evidence for this assumption comes from two sources. First, if children suffer a certain type of brain damage, they can lose various language abilities, a condition known as aphasia. If this accident occurs before children have reached puberty, they will be very likely to start all over again learning language "from scratch." If the same accident occurs after puberty, language learning is a far more difficult process, requiring extensive therapy, and, all too often, the condition is permanent. The second type of evidence comes from observing children who are moved to a new culture where a different language is spoken. Young children seem to have little difficulty picking up the language of the new culture, while adolescents and adults learn the new language with difficulty, if at all, and will almost universally speak with an accent.

This theory is of little practical importance in dealing with most children, since virtually all normal children have mastered language by the time they start school. However, it has extremely important implications for language therapy with the more severely retarded because it implies that if individuals have not acquired adequate verbal skills by the time they reach puberty, they probably never will. A corollary of the theory is that language therapy will probably be considerably more effective with a young child than it will be with an adult.

Older theories of language acquisition tended to stress traditional learning processes such as reinforcement and imitation, while the more modern approach to language acquisition deemphasizes these processes. Before considering the role of reinforcement in language learning, a distinction must be made between language competence and language performance. Competence is the knowledge that people have about a language such as their knowledge about how to form grammatically correct sentences or their knowledge of how to express various relationships. Competence is purely a mentalistic concept, and an individual's level of competence can only be inferred from performance, what is actually said. A description of an unusual kind of language retardation might make this distinction clearer. Occasionally, otherwise normal children will remain largely mute until they are three or four years old, but when they start speaking, they will immediately speak at a level of grammatical and morphological complexity comparable to other children of their age who have been speaking for two years. These individuals' language performance was delayed, but their competence was not. Their knowledge about and understanding of language developed at the normal rate, but their performance, what they actually said, was deficient.

Most linguists would argue that reinforcement can have a considerable effect on performance, but only a small effect on competence. In other words, if certain children were heavily reinforced for speaking by their parents while other children of comparable mental abilities were not, after a period of time, the first group might well be speaking more than the second, but the grammatical complexity of the first group's sentences would be only slightly more advanced at best.

Modern linguistic theory also deemphasizes the role of imitation. Almost all children imitate what they hear, but imitation probably has little effect on competence. It is difficult to understand how imitation can play much of a role in the learning of grammatical rules because most of what children say they have never heard before, and imitation implies that children would be copying what they hear. Also, Lenneberg (1967) described a case of a child who was unable to speak at all, yet his competence developed normally in the sense that his receptive language skills, his ability to comprehend what he heard, developed at the normal rate.

Remember that children will grow up to speak whatever language they hear, and children who hear what is widely considered to be poor English (e.g., if their parents use "ain't", double negatives, and the like) will learn this language just as other children learn what is considered proper English. Children in the most culturally deprived homes seem to go through the same stages of language acquisition and at the same rate as middle-class children. However, they score poorly on tests of language skills because, of necessity, any language test must only test knowledge of one specific language, and culturally deprived children have learned a language different from the language on the test.

Implications for Language Training

Unfortunately the biological theory of language acquisition has little to say about what to do with children who have not acquired language spontaneously even though they have been exposed to an adequate sample of a natural language. Severe language deficiencies can rarely be attributed to inadequate teaching, and unless children have been reared in such a stifling environment that they have heard essentially no language at all, a very rare circumstance, a severe language deficiency must be attributed to a serious disturbance, either cognitive or emotional, within the child.

Most systematic programs to train language competence in children with essentially no language tend to emphasize the importance of traditional learning processes such as imitation and reinforcement, and they almost always break the language system down into its component parts and then teach each component individually. Children are first taught to form some of the sounds of the language, then they are taught to form a few simple words, then they are taught how to use these words appropriately, then they are taught how to form simple sentences, and so on. However, this entire procedure is directly contrary to the normal language learning process. All normal language learning is done on a whole task basis; the child hears only whole sentences and must learn the language without the benefit of sequential instruction (Cazden, 1972).

However, such component approaches are often successful in improving the language competence of children with very minimal language skills. For example, Guess, Sailor, Rutherford, and Baer (1968) taught a severely retarded girl to use plurals correctly with the following procedure: in step 1 the girl was shown an object and was asked "What do you see?" If she did not respond or responded incorrectly she was told the correct answer. This procedure was repeated until she gave the correct answer three times in a row. Then she was shown two of the same object, was asked the same question, and was expected to respond with the plural form. Again, if she did not respond correctly she was told the correct answer, and this procedure was repeated until she made the correct response three times in a row. The third step involved presenting the girl with either one or two of the object, and she had to respond with the correct answer in each case. After a number of such sessions, each with a different object, there was generalization to new situations. Similar procedures have been employed to teach the comparative and superlative forms of adjectives (Baer and Guess, 1971), verb inflections (Shumaker and Sherman, 1970), and other similar constructions. Snyder, Lovitt, and Smith (1975) reviewed some 23 such studies and concluded that most were successful in improving language competence, and in many cases there was generalization to new situations.

In other words the subjects were learning rules rather than simple responses.

However, it is possible that in cases where language skills are systematically taught, the learning process and perhaps even the language behavior of these children is quite different from the learning and language of children who acquire language in the normal fashion. Evidence for this assertion comes from the observation that children who are systematically taught language rather than acquiring it normally are unlikely to use speech spontaneously (Lovaas, 1968). Most normal children speak spontaneously a good deal even when they have little to say and no one is listening. However, children taught to speak in an organized program would only speak in the training sessions, and there was little carry-over outside the classroom.

A second piece of evidence supporting this contention is that the speech of children who are systematically trained often sounds very mechanical. The children speak in a monotone with little intonation similar to the way that robots speak in some science fiction movies. On the other hand, normal children imitate intonation patterns long before they can imitate actual words, and there is no stage of their language development when their speech lacks intonation (this observation was made by the author from watching a film by Lovaas, 1969).

However, the fact that there are differences between the language habits of children enrolled in such training programs and normal children is not a justification for changing these programs. In cases where normal processes have obviously failed, it is necessary to provide children with some sort of crutch, and while these children may never be completely fluent, their ability to adapt to their environment is certainly very much enhanced by their improved verbal abilities.

Speech Disorders Among the Mentally Retarded

A speech disorder can be distinguished from a language disorder in that it involves a difficulty in speaking, but does not necessarily imply any defect in the subject's knowledge of the language. The vast majority of speech disorders involve problems of articulation. This includes substitutions in which the individual substitutes one sound for another as in a lisp, and omissions, when an individual omits a sound entirely ('at for cat). Other types of speech disorders include disorders of rhythm, such as stuttering, stammering, and cluttering, and voice disorders, such as when an individual's voice is noticeably hoarse or else deviant in pitch or volume.

There is a large body of research documenting the fact that the prevalence of speech defects is far greater among the mentally retarded than it is in the general population. A survey by Martyn, Sheehan, and Slutz (1969) is typical. They administered speech examinations to 346 mentally retarded

Table 9-1 Speech Disorders in Relation to Level of Retardation

	Level of Retardation				
	Borderline IQ 84–70	Mildly MR IQ 69–55	Moderate IQ 54–40	Severe IQ 39–25	Profound IQ 24–0
Normal speech	3	29	20	20	2
No speech	0	1	5	16	36
Delayed speech	0	3	5	22	33
Articulation (severe)	3	7	12	26	18
Articulation (mild)	0	5	26	26	9
Stuttering	0	1	1	1	0
Other	0	3	6	4	3
Total	6	49	75	115	101

From M. M. Martyn, J. Sheehan & Slutz, K. Incidence of stuttering and other speech disorders among the retarded. *American Journal of Mental Deficiency,* 1969, **74,** 206–211. Copyright © 1969 by the American Association on Mental Deficiency. Reprinted by permission of the Association.

patients at Camarillo State Hospital in California. The results are shown in Table 9-1. Several interesting conclusions can be drawn from these data. First, only about 20 percent of this population had normal speech, the others had some kind of speech disorder. Second, the incidence of speech disorders increases with lower IQ. Among the mildly retarded, nearly 60 percent had normal speech, while less than 2 percent of the profoundly retarded did. More than a third of the profoundly retarded had no speech at all. Third, excluding the profoundly retarded, the most common disorders were disorders of articulation, and all groups had a higher prevalence of articulation disorders than is usually found in a nonretarded population. The prevalence of speech disorders among a normal school age population is estimated to be between 5 and 10 percent (Telford and Sawrey, 1972). However, the prevalence of stuttering was no greater among institutionalized retarded patients than it is in the general population.

Unfortunately, studies differ widely regarding the exact prevalence of various speech disorders. For example, Schlanger and Gottsleben (1957) found that 17 percent of a population of institutionalized retarded subjects were stutterers, a prevalence considerably larger than that noted by Martyn et al. The reason for such discrepancies is that the detection of speech disorders must be based to some extent on the subjective opinion of a speech therapist, and there is considerable room for disagreement. Everyone occasionally has disfluencies and blocks in their speech, and it is impossible to draw a precise line between such normal disfluencies and stuttering. Another problem is that it would be reasonable to expect quite discrepant results from different populations. For example, the Martyn et al. study was done on institutionalized retardates, and thus probably found a higher prevalence of speech disorders than would be found in a noninstitutionalized retarded population. However, prevalence figures differ widely even among noninstitutionalized retarded children. Wilson (1966) found that 53 percent of 777 children enrolled in EMR classes had speech deviations, while Donovan (1957) found a prevalence of only 8 percent among EMR children, not significantly different from the normal population.

Keane (1972) reviewed a large number of such studies and arrived at a number of conclusions.

1. The one undisputed fact that has been well documented is that there is a higher than normal prevalence of communication disorders found in the mentally retarded collectively.
2. A higher prevalence of speech and language disorders appears to be present in institutionalized retardates than in noninstitutionalized retardates.
3. The lower one proceeds on the IQ scale, the more one is likely to find not only more frequent, but more severe communication difficulties.
4. No unique configuration or pattern of speech and language problems has been demonstrated in the mentally retarded as a group or within any subcategory or syndrome under the aegis of mental retardation. The types of speech problems are generally the same as those found in the normal population, but they occur more frequently.
5. Articulation disorders are the most prevalent, with voice disorders in second place.
6. There is some agreement that a higher than normal prevalence of some form of disfluent speech behavior (stuttering) is present in Down's syndrome.

There are at least two reasons why speech disorders might be more prevalent among the retarded. Speech disorders are generally far more prevalent among younger children; all children have articulation problems up to the age of four or five and many of these problems persist until the child is seven or eight when they spontaneously clear up. Because retarded children have lower mental ages, it is reasonable to assume that they will behave similarly to normal children of the same mental age in many respects. Presumably, the majority of speech disorders can be attributed directly to low mental age. Second, various defects and anomalies of the vocal system are more prevalent among the retarded. For example, the prevalence of cleft palate is greater among the retarded than in the general population. Similarly, one of the distinguishing features of Down's syndrome is a large tongue that, of necessity, must interfere with articulation. This also accounts for a part of the increased frequency of speech disorders.

Language Disorders in the Mentally Retarded

A language disorder can be distinguished from a speech disorder in that it involves some sort of deficit in the individual's knowledge about the system of language. Examples would be an inability to use or understand complex syntax or a very limited vocabulary or an inability to use language appropriately. Because language competence is entirely a covert process, reliable assessment of language skills is even more difficult than is assessment of speech disorders, and it is difficult to classify language disorders into meaningful categories.

A most important consideration is whether the mentally retarded present unique kinds of language disorders or whether whatever language deficiencies they have are simply manifestations of their slower rate of development. This latter position is called the developmental theory of mental retardation and was discussed in the previous chapter. The best-known advocate of the developmental position of language acquisition in the mentally retarded is Lenneberg (Lenneberg, Nichols, and Rosenberger, 1964). In this study, 54 children with Down's syndrome were visited on various occasions over a three-year period to trace their language development. Although there was no normal control group, they concluded that each of these children was going through the same steps in the same order that all normal children go through, the only difference being that the rate of development was very much slowed down. They also found that the rate of language acquisition correlated quite well with other milestones of development such as gait and fine motor coordination. Consistent with Lenneberg's (1967) theory they found no progress in language development after the age of 14.

The developmental position could be questioned if it could be shown either that children of low IQ acquire language in a somewhat different manner than do children of normal IQ or if it could be shown that retarded children have a greater deficit in certain language skills than do nonretarded children of the same mental age.

Casual observation suggests that in general the developmental theory is an appropriate description of retarded language development. Since normal children have essentially mastered their native language by the time they are 5 or 6, it would be predicted that mildly retarded people, who achieve mental ages of 8 to 11 years at adulthood, should have adequate language competence, and in fact, this is the case. Although some mildly retarded children have articulation problems or have a limited vocabulary or speak in a ghetto dialect, very few have any difficulty in constructing normal sentences or in understanding complex syntax.

The majority of moderately retarded individuals also have a good deal of functional speech, although this group presents a great many more deviations from normal (Martyn et al., 1969). Even most severely retarded people have some functional language competence, and it is only among the profoundly retarded that one finds a high proportion of individuals with no functional language at all.

In order to measure language functioning more precisely, it is necessary to use some sort of standardized test. A number of general tests of language competence have been developed, but by far the most widely used is the Illinois Test of Psycholinguistic Abilities or ITPA (McCarthy and Kirk, 1961; Kirk, McCarthy, and Kirk, 1968). A number of the subtests do not measure language competence in the usual sense of the term, but it is still an extremely useful instrument because it provides a standardized measure of a number of important language functions. The earlier (1961) version had 9 subtests and the later edition has 12, but many of the subtests are similar in both versions. The following is a list of the 12 subtests of the more recent version:

1. Auditory receptive—a test that assesses the child's capacity to understand spoken language by asking questions that can be answered by "yes" or "no," for example, "Do boys play?", "Do chairs eat?"

2. Visual receptive—a nonlanguage test that measures the child's ability to understand what is seen. The child is shown a picture of something, such as a dog, and then is shown a series of choices from which he or she must select the one that was the same as the first one, in this case, a different kind of dog.

3. Visual sequential memory—a subtest that measures visual memory capacity by requiring the child to replicate a series of chips that have nonsense figures on them.

4. Auditory association—a series of verbal analogies such as "A daddy is big; a baby is __?__ ".

5. Auditory sequential memory—a test very similar to digit span on standard IQ tests in which the child is required to remember a series of digits.

6. Visual association—a nonverbal test in which the child is shown a picture, and then is shown a number of choices and must indicate which of the choices is associated with the original picture.

7. Visual closure—a nonverbal test in which the child is asked to find hidden figures in a picture.

8. Verbal expression—a test in which children are asked to tell as much as they know about several everyday objects, such as a ball.
9. Grammatical closure—a test that measures the child's ability to use inflections (grammatical endings) for example, "Here is a dog. Here are two __?__".
10. Manual expression—children are shown an everyday object and must show by gesture what is done with it. For example, if they are given a hammer, they must pound with it.
11. Auditory closure—the child hears words with a sound missing and must fill in missing sound, for example, airpla____.
12. Sound blending—the child hears sounds spoken at half second intervals and must combine them to make a word.

A number of researchers have looked at the patterns of subtest scores of mentally retarded children, and although there is far from universal agreement, there does seem to be a typical response pattern that characterizes retarded children. Mueller and Weaver (1964) administered the ITPA to a number of institutionalized and noninstitutionalized retarded children with an average IQ of 42. The first finding of their study was that the language age of the retarded children was more than a year below their mental age. This suggests that moderately retarded children have a particular deficit in verbal skills beyond their overall cognitive deficit. The two subtests on which the retarded children had the lowest scores were vocal encoding, a test that involves expressing ideas verbally, and auditory vocal automatic, a test that measures the child's knowledge of grammatical endings. The retarded children achieved higher scores on those subtests that did not involve language at all, in particular visual decoding and visual motor association.

Very similar findings are reported by Bateman and Wetherell (1965). They described a typical ITPA profile for retarded children based on some of the standardization research. As in the Mueller and Weaver study, the average language age of the retarded children was below their overall mental age, and they had a particular deficit on the auditory vocal automatic subtest. Other subtests on which the retarded children did particularly poorly were motor encoding, auditory vocal sequential, and visual motor sequential. As in the Mueller and Weaver study, the subtests on which the retarded children achieved the highest scores were visual motor association and visual decoding.

There are three general conclusions that can be drawn from the research on the ITPA with retarded children. First, retarded children tend to have lower language ages than they do mental ages. In other words, normal children of the same mental age have better verbal skills than do mentally retarded children. In contradiction to the developmental theory, retarded children have a particular deficit in language. Second, the subtest on which retarded children have the most difficulty relative to normal children is auditory vocal automatic, a test measuring knowledge of grammatical rules, inflections in particular. Third, the subtest on which retarded children achieve the highest scores relative to normal children is visual decoding, a subtest involving no verbal skills at all. There is a general tendency for retarded children to do better on nonverbal subtests; they have a particular deficit with the auditory vocal channel of communication.

Other researchers have investigated language skills in the retarded using techniques other than standardized tests. The hypothesis that retarded children have a particular deficit in the acquisition of the rules of grammatical inflection was tested by Newfield and Schlanger (1968) using a technique developed by Berko (1958). The subjects in the Newfield and Schlanger (1968) study were 30 institutionalized mentally retarded subjects with an average mental age of six years, two months and an average IQ of 60. These were compared to normal kindergarten, first-grade, and second-grade children. Knowledge of inflectional rules was tested by asking the children to fill in the blanks in sentences such as "Here is a wug, and here are two __?__." or "This dog knows how to zib. Here it is __?__." The correct answers are "wugs" and "zibbing." It is necessary to use nonsense words because if the children indicate that they know the plural of a real word, they may have simply memorized it, but if they indicate that they know the plural of a nonsense word that they have never heard before, they have certainly learned the rule.

Knowledge of inflectional rules of both real and nonsense words were tested. Even though the two groups were matched on mental age, there were striking differences in the performance of the two groups, with the normal children being consistently superior to the retarded children. Overall, the normal children made 90 percent correct responses to real words and 72 percent correct responses to the imaginary words, while the retarded children made 48 percent correct responses to the real words and only 29 percent correct responses to the imaginary words. However, the degree of difficulty for the various types of inflections was similar for both groups, suggesting that retarded and normal children learn grammatical rules in the same fashion.

A number of researchers have found that the language of the mentally retarded tends to be more concrete. For example, Papania (1954) compared the definitions given by retarded children to definitions given by nonretarded children of the same mental age on the vocabulary section of the Stanford-Binet. Because they were matched on mental age, there was no difference in performance between the two groups in acceptability of definitions, but the retarded subjects of all age levels tended to give less abstract definitions than did the nonretarded subjects. Similar findings are reported by Badt (1958). This is consistent with the research on learning in the retarded summarized in Chapter 8, which concluded that retarded children show more of a learning deficit on more complex, more abstract kinds of learning.

Lozar, Wepman, and Hass (1972) collected samples of the speech of retarded children and nonretarded children by asking them to describe and comment on a series of pictures. These samples were then analyzed according to the percentage of common words used and were broken down by parts of speech. It might be assumed that if the proportions of various parts of speech were different between normal and retarded children, then this would suggest differences in language usage and structure. There were no differences at all between any of the groups in the proportion of words used that could be classified as common (around 84 percent). However, 93 percent of the retarded children differed from the average of the nonretarded children on at least one part of speech found in their sample. That is, some retarded children used many more nouns than did the normal children, others used more adjectives or more pronouns. Very few of the nonretarded children showed such wide divergences from average. However, when the percentage of various parts of speech was averaged across the retarded subjects, there were no significant differences between retarded and normal.

This study illustrates an important consideration. Almost all of the individual retarded subjects deviated from the normal pattern in some fashion to a significant degree. Yet, it is impossible to make any general statements about language in the retarded beyond the observation that there is much more variation in retarded language usage than is found among the normal population. When averages are used, as is the case in virtually all research, certain important information might be lost, and it must be kept in mind that many individual retarded children (or normal children for that matter) will differ significantly from any average.

The studies described above are typical of the research on language in the retarded. Much of the other research is inadequate in some fashion either because there was no control group or because the results are inconclusive. Numerous good reviews have been written summarizing this research. The interested reader should consult McLean, Yoder, and Miller (1972), Schiefelbusch (1972), Schiefelbusch, Copeland, and Smith (1967) (in particular the article by Jordan in that volume), and Spreen (1965a, 1965b).

Summary

The acquisition of language in normal children is a remarkable process in a number of ways. First, children are able to learn whatever language is spoken around them incredibly rapidly, most normal children having mastered the fundamental rules of their language by the time they are four years old. Second, any language has an infinite number of correct sentences, and most of the sentences that children hear and speak, they have never heard before. This means that children cannot learn a language simply by copying what they hear; they must learn a highly abstract set of grammatical rules for combining words to make sentences. Children all over the world seem to go through the same steps in learning their language, regardless of what language they are learning or how much or how little they are deliberately taught or corrected by their parents. For this reason, it has been suggested that language acquisition, and, in fact, language itself, is part of people's biological nature.

There are several different levels of language, and thus, several kinds of disorders associated with the communications process. One level is a speech disorder, in which the individual has difficulty articulating the correct sounds. Examples of speech disorders include substituting one sound for another, omitting sounds entirely, and stuttering. There is a large body of research documenting the fact that the retarded have a considerably higher prevalence of speech disorders than do people of average mental abilities. As one goes lower on the IQ scale, the frequency and severity of speech disorders increases. However, the types of speech problems found among the retarded are exactly the same as those found among other groups.

More serious than speech disorders are language disorders, difficulties in the understanding and using of the vocabulary and the rules of syntax of language. Retarded people also have many language difficulties, although to some extent, these can be accounted for by their lower mental age. The most widely used test of language abilities is the Illinois Test of Psycholinguistic Abilities (ITPA), which is divided into a number of subtests measuring various components of language. Research with the ITPA and other research with the mentally retarded has generated the following conclusions:

1. Retarded children acquire language skills in essentially the same fashion as do normal children.

2. The rate at which they acquire language skills is slower than that of normal children. As a result, when retarded children are compared to normal children of similar chronological age, the retarded children show a distinct deficit.

3. Because language acquisition ceases sometime around puberty, many moderately retarded individuals and most severely and profoundly retarded individuals may not develop complete language skills.

4. On the average, retarded children are delayed in language development even when they are compared to nonretarded children of similar mental

age. In other words, retarded children have a particular deficit in language skills.

5. Retarded children have particular difficulty in acquiring the more complicated grammatical rules such as the rules of inflection.
6. The language of the mentally retarded is more concrete than is the language of nonretarded children.
7. The variance in language skills is greater among the retarded than in a normal population. At a given developmental level, one is likely to find a relatively wide range of verbal abilities.

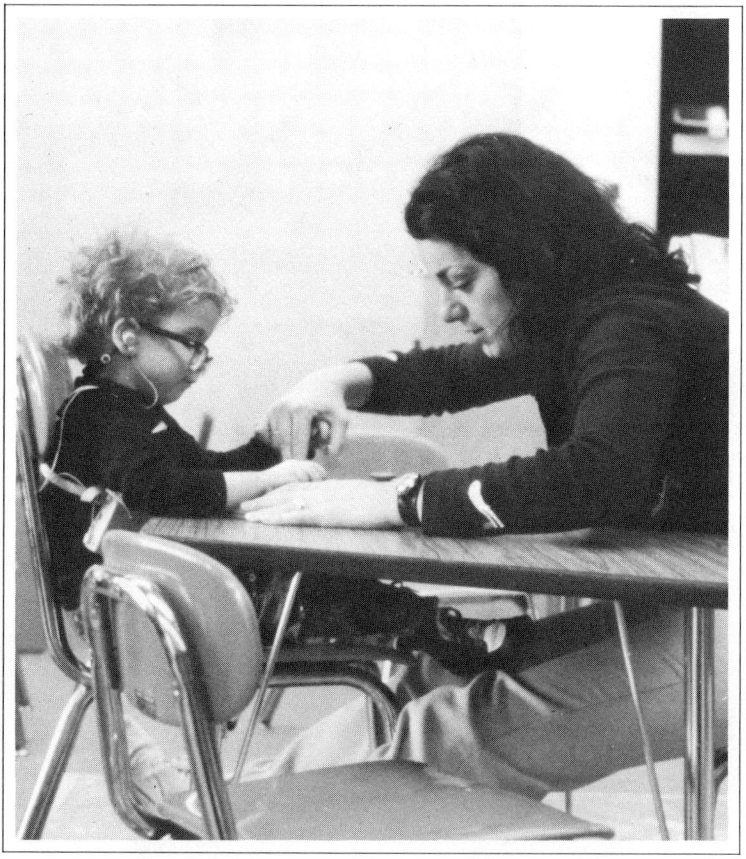

10

Cognitive Development in the Retarded: Piaget's Theory

Most of the research discussed in Chapter 8 did not have a strong developmental orientation; the researchers were not particularly concerned with how or even whether the various processes being studied developed and changed as the child got older. In fact, much of this research seems to assume that the basic processes of learning and memory were not qualitatively different between children of different age groups, and, as a result, the same research paradigms can be used for subjects at any stage of development. To many experimental psychologists the process of development is seen as quantitative rather than qualitative; children learn more skills and more knowledge and acquire more associations as they get older, but the basic underlying processes do not change. For this reason, attempts to determine specific deficits in the thinking of retarded children were more likely to compare them to CA-matched nonretarded children than to MA-matched subjects.

An alternative position, referred to as the developmental approach, tends to view mental functioning as being very different at different ages. In other words, the actual mental processes—learning, memory, mediation, perception, and the like—change qualitatively with age. An outstanding example of this developmental approach is the work of the Swiss philosopher Jean Piaget. His work, spanning more than 50 years, has created a revolution in the area of child study, and no discussion of cognitive development would be complete without considering his unique approach. This chapter first reviews the basics of Piaget's theory. This is followed by a review of research on applying Piagetian theory and research to mental retardation. The final section of the chapter is a general review of the developmental theory of mental retardation, incorporating not only the research discussed in this chapter, but also some of the research discussed in Chapters 8 and 9.

Piaget's Theory of Cognitive Development

It is assumed that most readers have had some exposure to Piaget's theory elsewhere, and thus, a thorough review of his theory will be unnecessary. The following is basically designed to be a refresher in Piagetian terminology and approach. The reader who would like more of a background than this chapter provides should consult one of the numerous excellent short reviews of Piaget's theory that have appeared in the last few years such as Ginsburg and Opper (1969) or Phillips (1975). Flavell (1963) provides a more thorough and complex review. The best summary of the theory by Piaget himself is probably *The Psychology of Intelligence* (1950).

Piaget's approach is considerably more mentalistic and philosophical than is true of most American psychologists. An important feature of his theory is that a child or adult actively constructs his world. The act of perception is considerably more than a passive response to stimuli; each individual has in his or her mind a cognitive structure, a model of reality that includes not only the specific facts but also the rules of logic by which reality operates, and all events are experienced in terms of this cognitive structure.

Most of Piaget's theorizing is concerned with how the child's cognitive structure, the model of reality, changes with age. He has proposed that there are four distinct stages of development that represent qualitative differences in cognitive functioning. The processes operating in the learning, thinking, and perception of the child differ in different stages, although each stage builds on the previous ones. It is easy to verify that the thinking processes of a child are very different from those of an adult by trying to explain something to a five year old using adult logic. Not only do adult rules of logic make no sense to the child, but it is difficult to avoid the impression that the child's whole world is quite different from that of an adult. This difference is a good deal more than the fact that the child has not learned as much as the adult; the child's whole cognitive style is very different.

The Stage Theory

Table 10-1 lists the four major stages in Piaget's theory with some of the substages and the more important characteristics of each level. There are a

Table 10-1 Piaget's Stages of Mental Development

1. Sensorimotor period. The child's thinking is limited to the here-and-now; the child's primary mode of perceiving and understanding his environment is by action rather than by symbolic representation. During this period the child gradually develops an object concept, the knowledge that objects exist independently of the child's experiences. Also during this time the child begins to develop an understanding of space, time, and cause-effect relationships.
   The sensorimotor period is divided into six substages.
   1. Exercising innate reflexes.
   2. Primary circular reactions.
   3. Secondary circular reactions.
   4. Coordination of secondary circular reactions.
   5. Tertiary circular reactions.
   6. Invention of new means through mental combination.
2. Preoperational period. The child is able to represent symbolically things and events that are not present. However, thinking during this period is still largely nonlogical. The child is perceptually bound; he takes all of his perceptions literally. The child is centered; he can only focus on one dimension of a stimulus at a time. The child is egocentric; he is not aware of the viewpoints of others. The child cannot understand the ideas of class or sets, and he gives immature answers in various conservation problems; he believes that the amount of liquid changes when it is poured from one container to another, that the number of objects can change when their configuration changes, and so on.
3. Concrete operational period. The child's thinking begins to manifest logical properties. He understands most kinds of conservation and can use classes in his thinking. The major limitation is that the child's thinking is limited to concrete rather than abstract objects and ideas, and thus it is impossible for him to outline a series of possibilities in his mind and test them systematically.
4. Formal operational period. The child begins to see reality as a subset of the possible. He can test a series of hypotheses systematically, he can understand second-order conservations such as conservation of volume, and he can perform operations on abstract ideas.

number of points that must be made about these stages. First, all children go through the same stages in the same order. No child ever skips a stage or inverts two stages. What distinguishes the gifted child from the average child or the mentally retarded child is not the stages that they go through, but the rate that they go through the stages. The one qualification to this statment is that people may differ in the highest stage that they attain. Not all adults reach the formal operational stage, and some mentally retarded children may not even fully achieve the concrete operational stage.

In at least one sense, the stage theory is misleading because it tends to suggest that these stages are discrete entities and that a child is entirely in one stage or another. In fact, most children manifest some features of several different stages of thinking simultaneously. Average children have begun to show some evidence of concrete operational thinking by the time

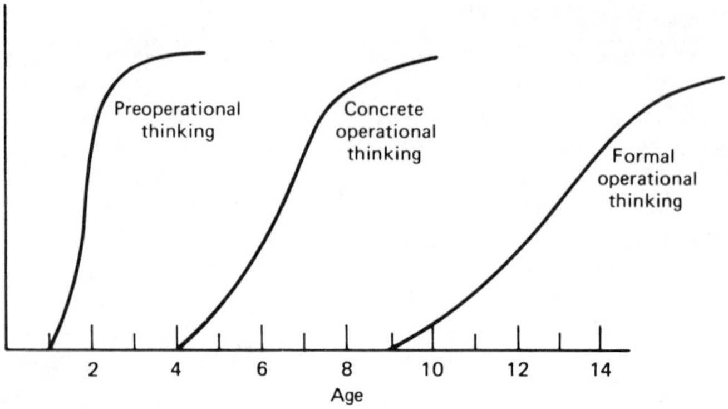

Figure 10-1 The development of Piaget's stages.

they are five or six years old but still retains some of the limitations of preoperational thinking when they are seven or eight years old. There is always a long transition period before the child fully attains a higher level of thinking, and by the time that they have attained one level, they have probably already begun the transition into the next period. Figure 10-1, adapted from Phillips (1975), is a more accurate representation of the relationship between age and stage than is the simple listing of age norms in Table 10-1.

The Sensorimotor Period

The first of the four stages is called the sensorimotor period and includes roughly the first two years of life (Piaget, 1952). As the name implies, this stage is characterized by the child's cognitive structures being predominantly sensorimotor in nature. The principal way which the child has of knowing about the environment is by acting on it, usually in response to specific stimuli. The major limitation of sensorimotor thinking is that children cannot symbolize; they cannot represent things or events or actions in their mind without the events being present. When the child's mother leaves the room, the child cannot form a mental image of the mother during most of this period. The child cannot think about things that are not present, and the only way that information in the environment can be assimilated is by the child acting on it, although the term action is defined rather broadly.

The sensorimotor period is divided into six substages. Substage 1 is characterized by children exercising their innate reflexes. Among these inborn behaviors are the sucking reflex, in which children will begin to suck on anything placed in their mouths, the rooting reflex, in which children will turn their head toward something that touches their cheeks, the grasp reflex, in which the children close their hand around something placed on their palms, and the various other reflexes that are discussed in most child psychology texts. Another type of innate behavior pattern is children focusing their eyes on stimuli that have a moderate amount of complexity. Research indicates that even very young children show definite preferences in what they focus their eyes on. For example, when they are shown a triangle, they focus almost entirely on the points (Salapatek and Kessen, 1966), and when given a choice between looking at a plain card and a bull's-eye pattern, they spend more time looking at the bull's-eye (Fantz, 1961). This research suggests that children are born with relatively elaborate schemes for looking, and that infants prefer to look at things from which they can extract the most information, although the information that they extract from what they are looking at is obviously very different from the information that an older child can extract from the same stimuli.

The second substage is characterized by primary circular reactions, and characterizes the child from one to four months old. A circular reaction is a motor scheme that repeats itself. Children at this age still have no concept of intention and they cannot "decide" to do something, but if they stumble across an activity that is pleasurable to them, they will tend to repeat it. The classic example of a primary circular reaction is children sucking their thumbs. Children accidentally put their hands into their mouths, which activates the sucking reflex. Because this is pleasurable, they try to repeat the activity. During this time, the child still does not have even primitive notions of the concept of objects or time or of cause and effect.

The third substage of the sensorimotor period is characterized by the development of secondary circular reactions, and the age range is roughly four to eight months in the normal child. A secondary circular reaction is similar to a primary circular reaction in that it is an action pattern that the child repeats, but it is called secondary because it involves objects other than the child's own body. For example, children with a rattle may bang it against the side of the crib. Because they enjoy the activity, they repeat it again and again. The most striking development during this period is that children are beginning to take an active interest in things other than their own bodies. Up through the beginning of this substage, children have no understanding that objects can exist independently of themselves. Children are totally egocentric in this respect, they cannot distinguish themselves from the events around them. When children are shaking rattles, they cannot distinguish the rattles as something separate from themselves. Piaget discusses the development of this object concept in detail. A mature object concept is achieved when children are aware that objects exist independently of themselves and maintain their existence even when they are not interacting with them. This is not possible until children have the capability of representing in their minds absent objects, a skill that they do not possess until late in the sensorimotor period. However, during the third substage, late in the first year of life, children show the first suggestion of being able to recognize things in their environment.

During the fourth substage, which normally goes from 8 to 12 months, children develop the ability to combine behavior patterns, and they begin to use one activity as a means to achieve another. For example, they may push the father's hand out of the way in order to get a desired toy. The object concept shows considerable development during this stage because children begin to actively look for disappeared objects. Their searching strategy may not be entirely appropriate in that they do not always look where the toy disappeared, but nevertheless, children's behavior indicates that they are beginning to be aware of the fact that there is an environment that continues to exist independent of themselves.

The fifth substage of the sensorimotor period is characterized by the development of tertiary circular reactions and runs from about 12 to 18 months. A tertiary circular reaction is like other types of circular reactions in that it involves repeating the same action over and over again, but now the child actively varies the pattern. For example, one of Piaget's children was playing with a soap dish and dropped it. The child picked it up and dropped it again, and then again. So far, this activity is a secondary circular reaction. Then the child began to vary how he dropped it, letting it go first on its end, then on a side, and so forth. Thus, the child is more actively exploring his capabilities. Rather than being content with simply repeating the same action over and over, the older child will actively seek out novelty for its own sake. Also during this stage, children develop a far more mature concept of space and objects. Their behavior indicates that they are quite aware that objects exist independently of themselves, and they will actively search for a missing object.

The sixth and last stage of the sensorimotor period is actually a transition into the next period because it is during this stage that the child develops the ability to symbolically represent objects and events. Now for the first time, the child can think about things that are not present. Piaget calls this stage the invention of new means through mental combination, which means that for the first time, the child can solve problems by thinking about performing certain actions.

Thus, in the first two years of normal children's lives, they make considerable progress in understanding their world. They progress from newborns who can do nothing but exercise their innate reflexes to children who have a good comprehension of space, time, objects, events, and actions, and are able to represent symbolically objects and events which are not present. Thus, in a very real sense, they have learned to think.

Preoperational Thinking

Probably the single most important feature that distinguishes preoperational thought from sensorimotor behavior is the ability to symbolize, to represent in one's mind objects and events that are not present. Piaget has devoted considerable thought to explaining the development of the ability to symbolize. He is firmly convinced that it does not arise from the child's use of language, which is developing at about the same time. This contradicts the ideas of many other psychologists who believe that thinking and symbolizing are intimately related to language, some even taking the extreme position that thinking is little more than internalized speech. Piaget, on the other hand, argues that symbols or mental representations arise not from language, but from internalized actions. Early in the sensorimotor period, the only way that children can understand something is by performing some action on it, and thus, it is natural that the first means that children have of actually thinking about things is by thinking about the actions that they perform on them. In this fashion, children gradually come to realize that objects can exist independently of their actions, and this knowledge is the beginning of a mature object concept.

The preoperational stage is perhaps the most interesting and certainly the most heavily studied of all Piaget's stages. The period of preoperational thought goes from about 2 to 7 years in the normal child, but it must be emphasized that there is a long transitional period between the preoperational period and the following stage, concrete operations. Most children show some evidence of concrete operational thinking as early as 5 or 6 and have not fully achieved it until they are between 8 and 10 years old.

Although the preoperational child is able to use symbols, thinking is still severely limited by adult standards. One of the beauties of Piaget's work is that he has pointed out the implicit logic that characterizes the thinking of adults. Most adults are totally unaware of this logic that characterizes their thought, and they are similarly unaware that the thinking of the preschool child does not manifest this logic. The best known example of this is a task that Piaget calls conservation of liquids. The child (or adult) is shown two glasses of the same size and shape and filled to the same level with a liquid. Even a preschooler will readily agree that the amount of liquid is the same in both glasses. However, if the contents of one glass are poured into a thinner glass before the child's eyes, the preoperational child will now insist that the thin glass has more liquid because it comes up higher in the glass. Mature adults, on the other hand, always assume that the amount of liquid remains the same even though the shape of its container may change. It is as difficult to convince most five year olds that the amount of liquid is the same even though it looks different as it is to convince an adult that the amount of water changed when it was poured into a different container. Yet most adults, unless they have read Piaget, have never thought about the fact that the amount of a liquid remains the same when it is poured into a different container, and they are equally oblivious to the fact that most five year olds don't know this.

This problem is called conservation of liquids (or of quantity) because the mature answer implies that the amount remains the same or is conserved, even though the shape or appearance changes. There are numerous different demonstrations of this concept of conservation, and in general, the preoperational child is unable to manifest conservation while the older, concrete operational child, is able to. For example, another type of conservation is called conservation of number, and involves the knowledge that the number of objects remains the same when their configuration is changed. If five year olds are shown the array in Figure 10-2 and are asked whether there are more forks or more spoons, they will reply that there are more forks because they are spread out. The children may answer in this way even though they are able to count. Most mothers have observed that children learn to count before they understand what counting and numbers mean. If the array were rearranged so that the spoons were more spread out than the forks, the child would now say that there are more spoons than forks. In other words, to the preoperational child, the number of objects may change when the configuration changes, just as the amount of liquid changed when it was poured into a different container. Other examples of conservation, or rather the lack of it in preoperational children, involve conservation of mass (or substance) and conservation of weight. These demonstrations are usually done with modeling clay. In conservation of substance, children are shown two balls of clay of the same size. After they agree that they have the same amount of clay, one is rolled into a sausage shape. Now the younger child will assert that the sausage has more clay than the ball (or the reverse). In conservation of weight, the procedure is the same except that children believe that one weighs more than the other. One important type of conservation, conservation of volume, does not manifest itself until the formal operational period. In this case, modeling clay is used as before, but children are asked to predict which will displace more water, the ball or the sausage. Not until children achieve formal operations will they know that the volume of the clay remains constant when its shape is altered, and thus, the amount of water displaced will not change.

All children acquire these various conservations in the same order. The first to be acquired is conservation of number, followed by quantity, weight, and volume in that order. When such conservation tasks are being used to test children's cognitive level, it is important not only to ask the children whether the amount has changed but also to ask them to explain their an-

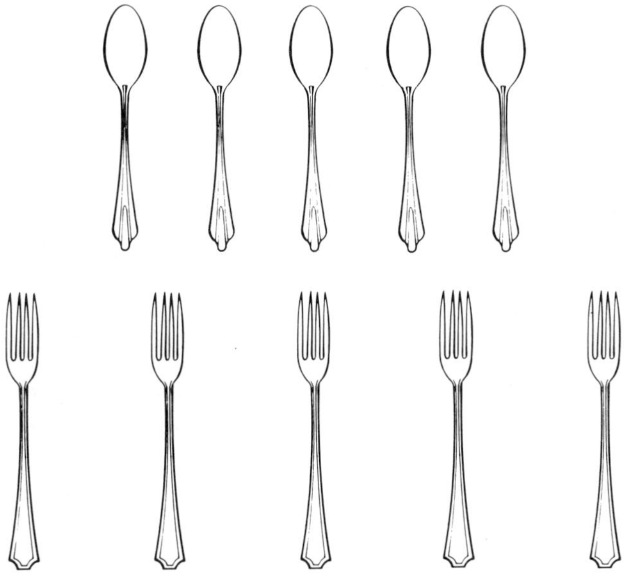

Figure 10-2 Conservation of number.

swer. It is fairly easy to teach children simply to give the correct answer but the important aspect of conservation research is whether children actually understand the concept or not, and this can best be determined by children's explanation of their answers.

Another example of the logic of mature thinking, which is lacking in the preoperational child, is the concept of classes and class inclusion, also known as sets. A class is a group of things that have something in common. For example, one class would be all of the red things in the room. Adults intuitively know a good deal about classes. For example, they readily understand that one class may include another (is a subset of another), and that if this is the case, the included class must be smaller than the more inclusive set. Similarly, adults can conceive of the intersection of two sets, for example, the set of blocks that are both red and round or all the teachers in a school who are women and have blond hair. Preoperational children do not have this intuitive knowledge about classes. If they are asked to group a large set of blocks of various shapes and colors into classes, they are unable to do it in a manner that makes sense to adults. They may start with a round red block, then follow it with a square red block, then select a green square block and so on. Similarly, they do not intuitively know that a subset must always have fewer than a more inclusive set. If they are shown a number of wooden beads, some of which are square and some of which are round, and they are asked whether there are more square beads or more wooden beads, they are likely to reply that there are more square beads.

There are a number of characteristics of preoperational thought that lead children to produce such apparently illogical answers. First, children's thinking is egocentric. The notion of egocentricity appears several times in Piaget's theory in different contexts. In this case, it refers to the fact that preoperational children are not aware that there are other viewpoints besides their own. One of Piaget's earliest observations is that much of the language of a preschooler is egocentric in the sense that it is not intended to communicate information. If children assume that everyone sees the world exactly as they do, there is no need to explain anything nor is there any real need to be logically consistent.

A second feature of preoperational thought that distinguishes it from more mature thinking is irreversibility. A mental action is reversible if children are aware that there is an opposite action that will return things to their prior state. Often, preoperational children seem to function as if they were not aware of this. One of the ways that concrete operational children are likely to use to justify their correct answer in a conservation problem is that the liquid could be poured back into its original container and it would come up to the same height.

A third characteristic of preoperational thinking is that children are perceptually bound: they take the superficial appearance of things to be the ultimate reality. The conservation of liquids problem demonstrates this principle. There appears to be more liquid in the thinner glass because it comes up higher. Adults know that even though there appears to be more liquid, in fact, there is not. However, the preoperational child, accepting the appearance of things unquestioningly, says that there is more liquid in the thinner glass. Because the liquid is higher, there must be more of it. Preoperational children are "centered," which means that they can only focus on one aspect of a stimulus at a time, such as the height. An older child is able to attend to both the height of the liquid and the width at the same time and knows that the extra height is compensated for by less width, while the preoperational child cannot think in this way.

Concrete and Formal Operational Thinking

The child overcomes these shortcomings in thinking only very gradually, eventually developing a stable system of mental *operations* and thus achieving the concrete operational stage. An operation, according to Piaget, is a mental action that can be fully compensated for and that is fully reversible. A child who has achieved a stable structure of operations with reference to a particular activity can now perform such mental activities and understand how they fit into a larger structure. For example, the child can fully compensate mentally for the action of pouring liquid from one glass into another, and this compensation results in a much more stable system. The concrete operational child is also fully able to understand the idea of classes and the interrelationship between them. For example, the child is able to comprehend the idea that all sparrows are birds but all birds are not sparrows, a relationship that was incomprehensible to the preoperational child. The concrete operational child has a far better understanding of the concepts of distance, time, and speed, and the relationships between them, ideas that the preoperational child can only vaguely comprehend. Concrete operational children are able to fully understand the concept of seriation, that is, they are able to put a group of things in order from longest to shortest, and, when given a set of eight dolls of different sizes and eight walking sticks of different sizes, can assign the proper walking stick to each doll, giving the shortest stick to the shortest doll, the next shortest stick to the next shortest doll, and so on. All of this was impossible for the preoperational child.

However, there are still some limitations to the thinking of the concrete operational child, and these limitations are not overcome until formal operational thinking is achieved. The most important difference between concrete operational thinking and formal operational thinking is that the former focuses on the real, while the latter focuses on the possible. The concrete operational child is primaily concerned with concrete reality, while to the formal operational child, reality is a subset of the possible. The older child is able to outline all of the possible relationships in a situation and then test each one systematically to determine which relationship is true. The classic experiment that demonstrates this involves giving the child a beaker containing a clear liquid and four test tubes that also contain clear liquid. The child is shown that when the liquid from the beaker is mixed with a certain combination of liquids from the test tubes, the resulting mixture turns yellow. The child's assignment is to determine which combination of liquids from the test tubes achieves this result. The concrete operational child may test 3 or 4 combinations randomly and may even stumble across the correct answer but is unable to imagine all of the 15 possible combinations of the liquids and try each one. The formal operational child, on the other hand, does exactly that, first testing A, then B, then C, then D, then A and B, A and C, A and D, B and C, and so on until eventually the child is certain to discover the correct answer.

A second difference between the concrete operational child and the formal operational child is that the latter is able to comprehend second-order conservations and relationships. One example of this is conservation of volume. Children do not seem to be aware that the amount of space taken up by a mass of modeling clay is the same regardless of what shape it assumes until they have reached the beginning of the formal operational period. An even more complex relationship that is not fully understood until the child is well into formal operations is the comprehension of specific density, which requires an understanding of the relationship between volume and weight. To test this, the child is given a bucket of water and a number of objects, some of which float and some of which do not. The child's task is to generate a rule to determine why some objects float and some do not. Concrete operational children are able to generate simple theories like large objects sink and small ones float or heavy objects sink while light ones float, but when they verify through experimentation that neither of these is adequate, they are stumped. The formal operational child, on the other hand, is able to conceive of a ratio of weight divided by volume, and can determine that when this ratio is small, the object will float, and when it is large, the object will sink. This is an example of a second-order operation, an operation on an operation, so to speak.

Causes of Cognitive Development

A question that is important from both a theoretical and a practical point of view is why children progress through these stages as they do. Piaget (1964) has stated that cognitive development depends on four things: maturation, physical experience, social experience, and equilibration.

The term maturation, as it is usually used by developmental psychologists, refers to development that results from organic or biological changes in the child, the unfolding of the genetic blueprint so to speak. As mentioned in Chapter 9, walking seems to be an example of a behavior that develops primarily as a result of the maturation of the nervous system. Many of the cognitive developments described above can be accounted for to some extent by this maturational process. Whenever children all over the world seem to go through the same stages of development in the same order at roughly the same rate, a maturational process must be suspected.

However, maturation by itself does not account for cognitive development. Little cognitive development would occur if the child were reared in a completely unstimulating environment. Children need lots of experiences with objects in order to develop mature concepts of number, amount, and the like. Evidence for this comes from the observation that children reared in some environments develop faster than in others. For example, middle-class children advance through the various stages faster than do children reared in presumably less stimulating low-income homes (Gaudia, 1972).

A third impetus to cognitive development is social interaction, not only with adults, but also with peers. Social interaction is not only a major source of factual information for the child, but it is also important as a developer of logic. When children play with each other and argue with each other and attempt to persuade other children to do something, they are forced to develop logical arguments to justify their position, and this makes them aware of their own and other people's thought processes.

The last and most important process that produces cognitive development is the uniquely Piagetian process of equilibration, the establishment of equilibrium between one's experiences and one's cognitive structure. Children experience disequilibrium when they become aware of a discrepancy between their cognitive structures and their experiences or, alternatively, when they can experience or perceive an event in two different and conflicting ways. For example, consider the case of children who believe that there are more forks than spoons in Figure 10-2 because they are spread out more. At first, the children are comfortable with their perceptions. They are not aware of any discrepancy. Later on, however, as they are beginning to develop a concept of number, they realize that there is something wrong with their belief that there are more forks than spoons, because when they count them both, they count the same number. Thus, they are in a state of disequilibrium, and this experience is an important motivator to achieve a higher level of functioning. Throughout development, and, indeed, throughout life, each of us is continually readjusting our cognitive structure to become more aligned with our experience, and the reason is that the experience of disequilibrium is a strong motivator for change.

Children will naturally seek out experiences from which they can learn, that is, experiences that are optimally discrepant from their cognitive structure, in order to produce a certain amount of disequilibrium. If an experience is too familiar, if it matches cognitive structure too closely, children will learn nothing and be bored. On the other hand, there are many experiences that are so discrepant from children's experiences that they cannot assimilate them at all or can experience them only in a way that is very different from the way that adults experience them. A five year old who watches the news on TV would be an example. Children do not spontaneously choose to do either type of activity. However, children may spend hours digging holes in the sand and filling them in. It can be assumed that the reason why they do this is because they are learning something from this activity.

Piaget's Theory and Mental Retardation

Piaget himself was not at all concerned with differences between children and why some children develop faster than others, and he did virtually no research with mentally retarded children. However, his most prominent disciple, Barbel Inhelder (1943, Translated 1968), did her doctoral dissertation on applying certain aspects of Piaget's theory to mental retardation. She performed a number of classic Piagetian experiments with retarded children at various levels, including conservation of amount, weight, and volume. Consistent with the theory, she found that the level of difficulty for the three types of conservation was the same as for normal children. In general, the responses of the retarded children were quite similar to those of normal children of younger ages, substantiating the developmental theory that retarded children progress through the same stages as normal children and in the same order, but their rate of development is slower. However, Inhelder also noted that some of the retarded children showed a good deal of oscillation between various stages. Apparently, not only was their rate of development retarded, but their development displayed what she called *viscosity,* meaning that even after they were sometimes capable of more advanced levels of thinking, they were likely to manifest less mature types of functioning. Inhelder suggested that the mildly retarded (morons) do not progress beyond the concrete operational stage of development, and that the moderately retarded (imbeciles) do not progress beyond the preoperational stage of development.

There has been a good deal of research in this country attempting to apply Piaget's theory to the behavior of retarded children. The primary goal of this research has been to show that his theory applies as well to retarded children as it does to children of normal mental abilities. Among the first studies of this type is that of Woodward (1959) who demonstrated that Piaget's six substages of sensorimotor development applied almost as well to the behavior of profoundly retarded adolescents as they did for normal children under two. She administered a number of tests to profoundly retarded children to assess which substage of the sensorimotor period they were functioning in. For example, children who were able to suck on their hands were placed at substage 2, children who manipulated objects were placed at substage 3, children who reached behind or removed a screen to get a toy or candy were placed at substage 4, and so on. Virtually all children who passed a test at a certain level were able to pass all tests below that level. She also developed various tests of circular reactions and tests of the child's knowledge of the object concept. These tests correlated quite well with the stage assignments made on the basis of other tests. She concluded that the behavior of the profoundly retarded could readily be classified into Piaget's six substages.

Most of the research on Piaget's theory both with normal and with retarded children has focused on the preoperational period and the transition into concrete operational thinking, and the bulk of this research has focused on the various kinds of conservation. Research by McManis (1969) is typical. His subjects were 90 mentally retarded children, 15 in each of six mental age groups between the ages of 5 and 10, and 90 nonretarded children matched to the retarded subjects on MA. Each child was tested for conservation of mass, weight, and volume. Three scores were obtained for each type of conservation for each child—a prediction score, a judgment score, and an explanations score. For example, to test for conservation of mass, children were shown two balls of clay the same size. Most children readily agreed that they had the same amount of clay. Then, the subject was asked if the amount of clay would still be the same if one of the balls were rolled into a hotdog shape. This was the prediction response. Then, one of the balls was rolled out and children were again asked if there was the same amount of clay in both. This was the judgment response. Then, the children were asked to explain their answers. Thus, the children could achieve a maximum score of three if all of their answers were acceptable. A similar procedure was adopted for conservation of weight and conservation of volume. Both were done with balls of clay.

Table 10-2 shows the percentage of each group that demonstrated conservation, defined as a score of three on a given task. We can see that the order of difficulty of the three tasks was as Piaget predicted for both groups, although there were a small number of subjects who showed inversions such as achieving a higher score on conservation of volume than on conservation of weight. Overall, the retarded subjects performed as well as the nonretarded subjects matched on MA, as would be predicted by the developmental theory. However, there were some differences on individual comparisons.

Other researchers have come to very similar conclusions. Brown (1973) compared retarded children to an MA-matched control group on conservation of number and of continuous quantity (liquid) and found no difference

Table 10-2 Percentages of Normals and Retardates at Six MA Levels Showing Conservation of Mass, Weight, and Volume

	Normal Subjects			Retarded Subjects		
MA	Mass	Weight	Volume	Mass	Weight	Volume
5	13	0	0	0	0	0
6	20	27	0	13	7	7
7	47	33	7	47	33	13
8	87	67	13	73	53	7
9	87	53	0	93	67	27
10–11	100	73	0	80	73	7

From D. L. McManis, Conservation of mass, weight, and volume by normal and retarded children, *American Journal of Mental Deficiency,* 1969, **73,** 762–767. Copyright © 1969 by the American Association on Mental Deficiency. Reprinted with the permission of the executive director of the association.

between the two groups, although another group of gifted children at the same MA level performed considerably worse. In a similar design, Gruen and Vore (1972) compared retarded children at three different MA levels to nonretarded children matched on MA on conservation of number, liquid, and weight and found no differences between the retarded and normal subjects.

Wilton and Boersma (1974) have reviewed the research on conservation with the retarded, and they came to the following conclusions: (1) Moderately retarded persons do not acquire conservation of substance, that is, they do not achieve concrete operations. (2) Mildly retarded children perform roughly as well as nonretarded children matched on MA on lower-order conservation tasks. (3) Mildly retarded persons do not usually acquire conservation of volume, that is, they do not achieve formal operations.

One research project in this area that deserves special mention is the longitudinal study of retarded and normal children done at Temple University by Stephens and her associates (Stephens, 1974; Stephens and McLaughlin, 1974). Most research that has been done testing Piaget's theory is cross sectional; that is, children of one age or stage are compared with different children of another age or stage. A preferable but more difficult experimental approach is a longitudinal design, in which the same children are tested at different ages or stages. This is precisely what Stephens has done. Subjects for this project were 75 mildly retarded children and 75 nonretarded children matched on CA. Twenty-five of each group were between the ages of 6 and 10 at the beginning of the project, 25 were between 10 and 14 at the beginning of the project, and 25 were between 14 and 18 at the beginning of the project. The findings discussed here were based on the development of these children over a two-year period, although the project is still going on. A total of 22 different cognitive tasks were used, including most of the standard measures of preoperational, concrete operational, and formal operational thinking such as conservation of substance, liquid, weight, volume and length, a number of class inclusion tests (e.g., the child is shown pictures of ducks, other birds, and animals and is asked "If hunters killed all the ducks, would any birds be left?"), tests of understanding of various relationships such as left and right, and the combination of chemicals test described in the section on formal operations.

Not surprisingly, on most of the tests the older subjects did better than the younger subjects, the nonretarded subjects did better than the retarded subjects, and there was general improvement in all groups over the two-year period. However, there were some interesting observations that refined our knowledge about cognitive development in both normal and retarded children. For example, substantial improvement was noted in the oldest group of normal children over the two year period of the study. This improvement indicates that cognition was still showing considerable development into the late teens. Despite the fact that Piaget suggested that children begin to manifest formal operational thinking at age 11, many of the normal subjects were unable to completely succeed at formal operational tasks at age 18. The retarded subjects also showed improvement over the two-year period in all age groups. However, the improvement in cognitive development for the oldest group of retarded subjects over the two-year period was slight, considerably less than the development of the normal subjects. This observation indicates that the cognitive development of retarded people begins to level off sooner than does the cognitive development of nonretarded subjects. This research also supported the conclusion of Inhelder (1968) that no retarded child showed evidence of formal thought. Even when they were compared to nonretarded children of similar MA, the retarded children showed deficiencies on certain tasks, particularly those tasks that involved the grouping, flexibility, and reversibility necessary for concrete operational thought.

Accelerating Cognitive Development with the Retarded

A question that often arises is the extent to which cognitive development can be accelerated through specific teaching. Piaget refers to the problem of accelerating cognitive development as "the American Question" because this seems to be the particular concern of American educators (1970). He himself is not concerned with how to accomplish this, or even whether it can be accomplished, and has stated that it is foolish and even dangerous to try to accelerate development. Children develop at their own natural rate, and any attempt to interfere with this natural rate will probably fail.

Nevertheless, a number of educators have attempted to develop programs to accelerate development, particularly to teach such concepts as conservation. Many of the early attempts in this area met with limited success and an early reviewer of this subject (Flavell, 1963) concluded that accelerating conservation was largely impossible. However, more recent attempts using a variety of different techniques have been more successful. It is still possible for skeptics to argue that while it is easy to teach children to give the correct answer in a conservation problem, it is quite possible that the child has not really developed an understanding of the problem, and thus, the learning is superficial. Brainerd and Allen (1971) provide a good review of attempts to teach conservation to normal children and some of the methodological and theoretical problems associated with this issue.

There have been a number of attempts to teach Piagetian skills to the mentally retarded. For example, Brison and Bereiter (1967) attempted to teach conservation of solid and liquid quantity to retarded, normal, and gifted children. The children were first given training in conservation with unequal quantities, then with equal quantities, and children who gave correct answers were encouraged to explain their response. There was no difference between the three groups in the number of children who acquired conservation, and less than half the subjects in each group were successful.

Lister (1969, 1970) attempted to teach conservation of weight and volume to retarded subjects, and reported a high degree of success in both cases, although her research has been criticized (Wilton and Boersma, 1974) because her techniques were poorly specified and many subjects apparently acquired conservation of volume before weight, a surprising result. Kahn (1975) replicated Lister's procedure and found a much smaller effect of training. Although a few retarded subjects showed evidence of formal thought in contradiction to Inhelder (1968), there was little evidence of transfer to other tasks, and there were no cases of inversion, subjects showing conservation of volume before weight.

Wilton and Boersma (1974), after reviewing this subject, concluded that while there is evidence of acceleration of understanding of conservation in retarded subjects, it is not at all clear what procedures work best or why they work. Similarly, it is difficult to determine whether cognitive structures actually changed significantly and children developed an understanding of conservation or whether these children were simply taught to say the correct answer with no real understanding.

In an effort to resolve this criterion problem, the issue of how to determine whether there has in fact been a change in cognitive structures, these same authors (Wilton and Boersma, 1974a) assessed conservation by observing eye movements and surprise reactions rather than the more customary verbal responses. After a period of training on conservation of liquids, they found that the trained group showed greater exploratory eye movements, while the control group tended to center their focus on the height. This pattern was consistent with natural conservers and provided strong support for the contention that such training programs do in fact train conservation rather than superficial responding.

Piaget's Contribution to Mental Testing

Psychologists of a Piagetian orientation have generally been critical of the traditional way that mental abilities have been assessed, viewing most of the widely used IQ tests as simply a hodgepodge of items selected with no real system or purpose behind them. A number of people have attempted to develop intelligence tests based on Piaget's theory. The advantage of such an approach is that unlike other intelligence tests that were developed with no particular theory in mind, these tests can be based on a rather clearly specified theory of intelligence and its development. As a result, many of the problems of validity that have plagued other intelligence tests can be avoided. There are at least two teams who are working on the development of standardized testing procedures for sensorimotor development, Corman and Escalona (1969) and Uzgiris and Hunt (1975). Both consist of a set of ordinal scales assessing object permanence, spatial relationships, and the like. Silverstein, Brownlee, Hubbell, and McLain (1975) have demonstrated the usefulness of both of these instruments with the profoundly retarded, although they found that the order of difficulty of test items was somewhat different for the retarded children than it was for normal children, a disconcerting finding.

Other people have attempted to produce standardized tests to assess cognitive development in older children. For example, Goldschmid and Bentler (1968) have developed a conservation assessment kit that assesses performance in a large number of different kinds of conservation. Undoubtedly, the most ambitious attempt of all to develop a standardized test of Piagetian concepts is that of Pinard and Laurendeau, who have developed a test battery made up of 62 subtests that has been standardized on some 700 Canadian children (Robinson and Robinson, 1976).

The Current Status of the Developmental Theory

One thread that has run through Chapters 7, 8, and 9 is the developmental theory, the theory that the behavior of the mentally retarded can be best explained by describing them as developing in the same fashion as normal children except more slowly. This theory is one way of accounting for the differences in learning, memory and language performances observed between retarded and nonretarded children, and it was the fundamental tenet of Piagetian interpretations of mental retardation. Because of its importance, this theory should be evaluated in some detail.

A developmental theory is only useful to the extent that there is a pattern to normal development, that is, that virtually all children proceed through roughly the same stages in the same order. As we have seen, this assumption is clearly valid for cognitive development as described by Piaget's theory, and it also seems to hold up fairly well in describing the development of language. There also seem to be developmental patterns in learning and memory of normal children, although these patterns have not been described in any detail here.

The next step in assessing the validity of the general developmental theory is to compare the performance of retarded children to younger nonretarded children who are at the same stage of mental development to determine the extent to which mental functioning is the same in the two groups. There are several difficulties here. The first is that it is difficult to arrive at an accurate assessment of stage of development both for retarded children and for nonretarded children. In practice, MA as measured by a standard intelligence test is generally used, although such tests are not based on any particular theory of mental development. Perhaps tests based on the Piagetian model will fill a real need here. A second difficulty is that there are likely to be clear motivational and personality differences between the retarded children and the nonretarded children, and, as a result, the performance of the two groups on a learning task might be quite different while actual learning competence for the two groups might be similar.

There is little question that the developmental theory is the single best description of mentally retarded children and adults. As a general theory, it is far superior in accounting for differences in performance between retarded and nonretarded people than any of the various defect theories that have been proposed. If one wishes to describe the functioning of a particular retarded child, the child's MA is almost always a reasonable estimate of his or her capabilities. A child with a mental age of five years is likely to be performing at roughly the five-year level in most areas of functioning, and if one were interested in which skills this child would be most apt to learn in the next year or so, an excellent guess would be those skills that the normal five and a half year old would be acquiring.

However, a close analysis of the research data indicates that there are simply too many differences between retarded and nonretarded children of similar MA to completely accept the developmental theory. The following are some generalizations that can be made about the performance of retarded children compared to the performance of normal children of similar MA.

1. Retarded children lag behind nonretarded children on normal language development, although they apparently acquire language in the same fashion that normal children do.

2. Retarded children show a particular deficiency in the use of certain grammatical constructions.

3. Retarded children are less apt to use verbal mediation, rehearsal strategies, and other control processes that facilitate learning and memory.

4. Retarded children have relatively more difficulty with learning and memory tasks that involve abstract and complex concepts and relatively less difficulty learning simple rote associations.

In other words, the developmental theory, while being a good rough approximation of retarded functioning, breaks down when it is examined in detail. The reader who is expecting an absolute answer such as "The developmental theory is right" or "The developmental theory is wrong" will be disappointed by this conclusion, but such ambiguity is very much the rule rather than the exception in the social sciences. The developmental theory will prove to be useful from time to time throughout the remainder of this book, but the reader must be cautioned not to take it too literally.

Summary

The theorizing of the Swiss philosopher Jean Piaget has dominated the study of cognitive development in children. He has postulated four different stages of cognitive development through which all children progress. The earliest of these stages is the sensorimotor period, which normally spans the first two years. During this time, children are unable to use symbols, and thus, their experiences are limited to the here-and-now. During the six substages of this period, children gradually acquire a relatively mature object concept, the knowledge that objects exist independently of themselves and maintain their existence even when they are not interacting with them. Children also develop knowledge about time, space, and causality.

The next stage is the preoperational period, which extends from two to about seven years old. During this time, children are able to use symbols, but lack many of the adult rules of logic. As a result, they fail many of the conservation tasks for which Piaget is so well known. Children are unaware that the number of objects remains the same when the configuration differs, they believe that the amount of liquid changes when it is poured from one container to another and that the weight of a ball of clay changes when it is rolled out into a sausage shape. Preoperational children are also unaware of the concept of classes, and are likely to believe that when they are shown a necklace of 10 wooden beads, 7 round and 3 square, there are more round beads than wooden beads.

The third stage is the concrete operational period, which normally extends from ages 7 to 11. During this period, children are able to think far more logically, and they do not make the sort of mistakes that characterized the preoperational child, but the object of their thinking is still the concrete world. Only in the last stage, formal operations, do children develop the ability to fully understand abstract ideas and to think of reality as a subset of the possible.

A number of research projects have demonstrated that this therory describes retarded development nearly as well as it does normal development. Profoundly retarded children seem to be functioning basically similarly to children in the sensorimotor period, and retarded children seem to acquire the various kinds of conservation in the same order that normal children do. In general, mildly retarded children will achieve the concrete operational level but not the formal operational level, while moderately retarded children will achieve the preoperational level but not the concrete operational level.

A number of people have attempted to accelerate cognitive development by explicitly teaching such concepts as conservation. Many of these projects have had some success, both with normal children and with retarded children, although there are numerous methodological problems and Piaget himself has questioned their value.

The Piagetian approach to mental retardation is the best example of the developmental theory of retardation, an idea that has appeared in chapters 7, 8, and 9. A general summary of research on the developmental theory is that it is an excellent rough approximation of a description of the functioning of retarded people, but there are a number of deviations from this theory. For example, retarded children show unusual deficits in language skills, the use of strategies in learning and memory, and in learning relatively abstract concepts, even when they are contrasted to MA-matched normal children.

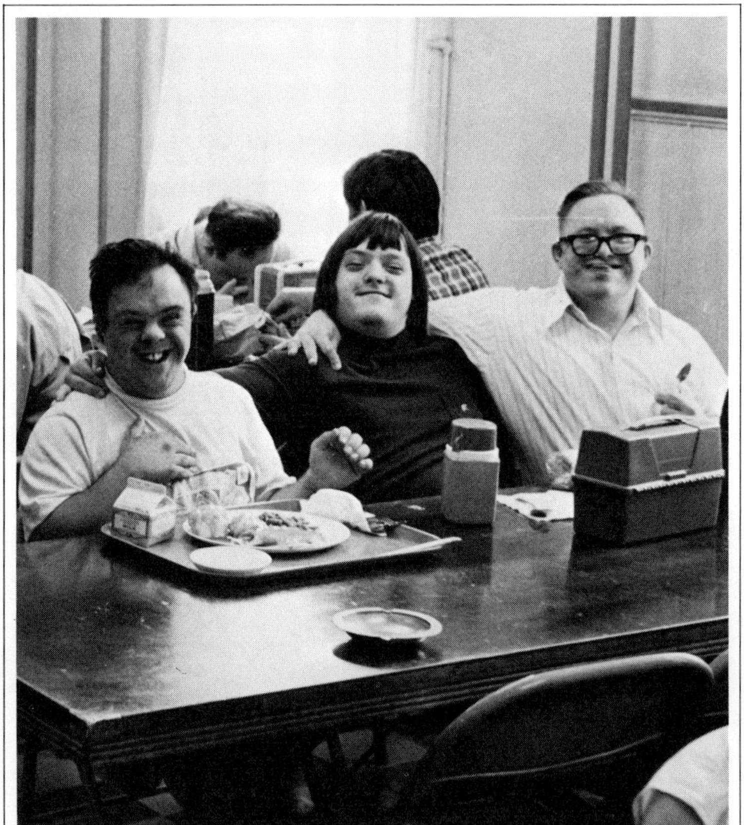

11

Personality and Social Psychology of Mental Retardation

A distinction is usually made between two basic kinds of psychological processes, the cognitive or intellectual processes such as thinking and memory, and the emotional, motivational, and personality processes such as anxiety and love. Mental retardation is primarily a cognitive disorder, and the vast majority of the experimental research in retardation has investigated cognitive processes. However, in many cases, the secondary effects on the retarded individual's personality and emotions are far more serious and present more of a barrier to effective adjustment than do the problems presented by deficient cognitive abilities, and there is a surprising lack of research into personality variables in the retarded. A number of writers who have reviewed this subject (e.g., Gardner, 1968; Heber, 1964) have commented on the dearth of research in this area, and this author's observation seems to be that the amount of personality research with the retarded is actually decreasing. Certainly, there have been few new theories or research techniques that have come out in recent years. One reason for this lack is the simple fact that retardation is usually considered to be a cognitive rather than a personality defect, but equally important is the fact that the entire study of personality is a very fragmented field. Techniques to measure such variables as self-concept or ego strength are relatively unrefined, and the most frequently used research techniques such as questionnaires, checklists, and projective techniques are often poorly suited to retarded subjects.

The chapter is organized into three sections. The first section outlines various reasons why there are personality differences between retarded and nonretarded individuals. A number of these differences are based on the fact that a retarded person is likely to have somewhat different social experiences than is a nonretarded person, and, thus, this section contains some discussion of the social psychology of mental retardation. The second section lists several specific personality characteristics that typify many retarded people. The last section reviews research on the prevalence of various kinds of emotional and behavioral disturbances among the mentally retarded.

Reasons Why the Personality of a Retarded Person Might Differ from That of a Nonretarded Person

Most people who work with the retarded have noted a higher degree of emotional disturbance as well as a number of other character disorders that seem to characterize many retarded people. There are a number of reasons why this might be the case. One's personality is shaped by numerous different forces and events, everything from organic factors such as a genetic predisposition or cerebral dysfunction to experiences in early childhood to the way we are treated by society in general. In many respects, the life histories of retarded people are just as diverse as those of any other group of people, but there seem to be certain experiences that are far more common among the mentally retarded in this society than among those of greater mental abilities, and these experiences can reasonably be expected to produce certain types of personality traits in the majority of retarded people.

Social Isolation and Rejection

There is a considerable body of evidence indicating that retarded children, regardless of whether they are in special classes or in regular classes, tend to be isolated by their peers. They have few friends and, for the most part, are outside the mainstream of social life in their schools. For example, Johnson (1950) asked schoolchildren to indicate who they liked best in their class and found that even though mentally retarded children were integrated into the regular classes, they were significantly less likely to be named as a friend by their classmates than were nonretarded children. This rejection was not due to the retardation label, but rather was attributed to the deviant behavior of many of the retarded children. Dentler and Mackler (1962), in a literature review, concluded that one consistent finding is a positive relationship between IQ and peer acceptance. In other words, the higher a child's IQ is, the more likely the child is to be accepted by and popular with peers.

The main cause of this rejection is the inability of the retarded child to learn many of the social skills that lead to acceptance and popularity. Popularity depends to a large extent on being able to make clever, interesting, and witty conversation and being able to understand the sometimes complex games that children play. These are the kinds of skills in which retarded children are most deficient and that are virtually impossible to teach. Unfortunately, social isolation tends to feed on itself. The more a child is rejected by peers, the more the child will develop inappropriate strategies to overcome this problem. A rejected child may bend over backward to be nice and to be accommodating to his or her classmates, giving them candy, running errands for them, and so forth, in order to win their friendship, but excessively accommodating children are seldom very popular. Other rejected children become aggressive in order to get attention, but this behavior is almost certain to lead to more rejection and isolation. Other isolated children may simply decide that they are worthless, and withdraw into themselves, making little attempt to change their situation. In other words, isolation is very likely to lead to deviant personality and adjustment patterns, and because retarded children are likely to be socially isolated, this tends to contribute to their unusual personality pattern.

Labeling and Stigma

The problem of social isolation and rejection is invariably made worse by the one experience that characterizes all retarded people, the experience of being labeled mentally retarded. Our culture puts considerable emphasis on being normal, and anything that signifies that an individual is somehow different is going to interfere with that person's acceptance by others. Such a sign of deviance is called a stigma. Almost any kind of handicap or deformity including such characteristics as having black skin or being an ex-convict can be a stigma, but they all have in common the fact that they tend to devalue the person and make the person seem less worthy than other people (Goffman, 1963). Many people feel distinctly uncomfortable in the presence of a blind person or an amputee or anyone else who has been labeled deviant in some way such as a mentally retarded person. Most normal (unstigmatized) people don't know whether to ignore the condition or whether they should somehow behave differently because of the individual's deviation. As a result, when they meet a stigmatized person, they tend to behave more formally and less spontaneously, producing an awkward and inhibited conversation. The all-too-frequent effect is that the unstigmatized person breaks off the conversation as quickly as possible. These reactions are even worse with children, who tend to tease mercilessly any child who happens to be different.

The stigmatizing effects of being labeled mentally retarded are further compounded by the fact that many people are quite ignorant about the nature of mental retardation. Old stereotypes that retarded people are violent or sexually promiscuous are still prevalent. As a result, some parents refuse to permit their sons and daughters to play with retarded children, giving the lame excuse that their children will pick up bad habits or will otherwise be harmed. Jaffee (1966) found that the label "mentally retarded" elicited more negative attitudes in high school students than did a description of a person who behaved like a retarded person.

As a result of the effects of labels, there is an active trend against the use of any kind of labels such as mentally retarded to describe children. Accompanying this is a tendency to place virtually all children in regular public school classes rather than establishing separate classes for various diagnostic categories. This practice, known as mainstreaming, is discussed in detail in Chapter 14 on education. However, some people feel that the detrimental effects of labeling have been exaggerated and that there is little solid evidence that labeling has harmful effects (MacMillan, Jones, and Aloia, 1974). Certainly, it is true that the social isolation of retarded children is due more to their immature social skills than it is to being labeled retarded, and research on whether integrating retarded children into regular classes improves their social acceptance is inconclusive. Some studies (e.g., Sheare, 1974) found that integration leads to more positive attitudes toward retarded children, while other research (e.g., Gottieb and Budoff, 1973) found that integrating retarded children did little to improve their social position.

Family Stress

One of the few things that virtually all social scientists can agree on is that the family is the single most important influence on the developing child. A child who is loved and accepted by his parents and receives the proper balance of discipline and independence is far more likely to develop into a well-adjusted adult than is the child from a rejecting family that is either overly permissive or too restrictive. Unfortunately, the presence of a retarded child in a family is likely to produce a good deal of tension and stress. Parents tend to receive the news that their child is retarded with either guilt or defense mechanisms or overprotectiveness or any one of a number of other behavior patterns that are likely to produce behavior problems and emotional problems in the child. The relationship of a retarded child to the family is so important that Chapter 13 is completely devoted to it, and it is sufficient to point out here that distorted family relationships are a major cause of adjustment and personality problems among the retarded.

Frustration and Failure

By the very nature of their impairment in adaptive behavior, retarded children are not able to accomplish many of those tasks that society demands of its members and that the retarded child's siblings and classmates are able to accomplish easily. This leads to many experiences of frustration and failure. The frustration experienced by a mildly retarded child who is unable to read after several years of intensive effort or that of the moderately retarded adolescent who is unable to fully deal with money will almost certainly have negative effects on the individual's personality development. In the first place, the stresses associated with repeated failure experiences are likely to result in anxiety reactions and defense mechanisms. In addition, retarded persons are likely to have lowered opinions of themselves and their abilities. Because they expect to fail at a task, they are likely to avoid undertaking new projects, and they have a general lack of confidence in their ability to effect change in their lives.

Cerebral Dysfunction

The role of cerebral dysfunction or brain damage in emotional and behavioral problems is unclear, to say the least, but there is a considerable amount of evidence that it is one contributing factor. For example, two of the characteristics frequently observed in children with brain damage are hyperactivity and emotional lability, the rapid movement from one emotional state to another with no apparent cause. In addition, brain damage has been implicated as a cause of more serious emotional disturbances such as autism (Bialer, 1970). Because brain damage is a direct cause of mental retardation in many cases, it would be predicted that accompanying emotional problems would also be prevalent among the retarded, particularly among the more severely retarded where brain damage is almost universal.

Lack of Insight

Personality processes and cognitive processes are often conceptualized as being independent of each other, but of course, they are not. Cognitive processes are intimately involved in the acquisition and change of personality patterns and even emotional reactions. Just thinking about one's behavior and becoming aware of the results of one's actions can occasionally bring about a significant personality change. As a result, it is reasonable to assume that people with less adequate mental abilities might be functioning at a less mature, more irrational, emotional level. For example, an important aspect of the development of personality is impulse control, the ability to restrain oneself from acting impulsively. Impulse control is related to cognitive development in the sense that as most children get older, they become better able to control impulses and delay gratification. This process requires a certain amount of foresight and insight into the effects of one's actions. As a result, it might be predicted that many retarded children, because they are lacking in cognitive skills, might be less able to control their impulses and delay gratification.

Cultural Deprivation

A final reason why there is a greater prevalence of personality and emotional difficulties among the retarded is that mentally retarded children are likely to be found among the lowest income groups and members of racial minorities. This means that their home environments tend to be characterized by a good deal of environmental stress and chaos that is conducive to adjustment difficulties. Retarded children are more likely to come from broken homes or homes where one parent is an alcoholic and are more likely to have experienced child abuse or other forms of relatively overt rejection. Research has shown that many forms of psychopathology are far more common among those of low socioeconomic status (Hollingshead and Redlich, 1958). This is a case where two characteristics, mental retardation and emotional disturbance, are correlated with each other, but neither one causes the other.

Personality Traits in the Mentally Retarded

There are a number of personality traits that are widely assumed to characterize most retarded people. This section lists some of these traits and describes some specific research and theorizing into the nature of retardate personality. The warning is repeated that the mentally retarded are a diverse group of people, and there will be numerous exceptions to any generalizations.

Expectancy of Failure

There are a number of general theories of personality, one of which is called social learning theory (Rotter, 1954). As the name suggests, social learning theory emphasizes the learned aspects of personality and social behavior. In the version of social learning theory developed by Rotter, constructs of particular importance are the significance of various goals to the individual and the individual's expectancy of achieving that goal. Both of these are determined by the individual's past experiences.

Social learning theory is unique among personality theories in that it has been systematically applied to the mentally retarded as well as to normal people, and this work has been reviewed by Cromwell (1963). Particular emphasis is placed on the assumption that most retarded individuals have experienced a good deal more failure than have nonretarded people. For this reason they are more likely to expect to fail in future undertakings. Early experiments (e.g., Ringelheim, 1960) found that retarded subjects did not differ from nonretarded subjects in verbalizing whether they expected to succeed at a task or not, so the theory had to be modified by postulating that many retarded people have more difficulty than nonretarded people in understanding whether they had failed or not. Also, it is possible that the verbalization of the retarded does not reflect their true attitudes, partially because of their lowered mental abilities, and partially because they might be more defensive about failure. However, the assumption of a higher expectancy of failure among the retarded receive some support in several recent studies by MacMillan (1969; MacMillan and Keough, 1971). In this research, subjects were asked to perform a cognitive task such as copying block patterns, and they were arbitrarily interrupted in the middle. Subjects were then asked why they were interrupted. Retarded subjects were more likely than were normal subjects to blame themselves, giving answers like "I was too slow" or "I couldn't do it."

If retarded persons expect to fail at most things that they try, this attitude is going to effect their behavior. In the first place, people who expect to fail are less likely to succeed. Zeaman and House (1962) found that after a long series of failure experiences, retarded subjects were unable to solve problems that they had previously been able to solve. In other words, diminished mental abilities tend to be magnified by a lowered expectancy of success. Another result is that retarded people are likely to be *failure avoidant* rather than *success striving.* Their behavior will be directed toward avoiding failure rather than trying to achieve success. For example, a mildly retarded girl who would like to be a cheerleader for her school may not try out because she expects that she will not make the cheerleading squad, and she is more concerned about avoiding this failure than she is about the possible success of being accepted. Experimental support for this postulate comes from research by Butterfield and Zigler (1961, cited in Cromwell, 1963) who found that nonretarded subjects learned better with a positive incentive than with a negative incentive (i.e., being correct to avoid being punished) while the retarded subjects learned better with a negative incentive.

An additional implication of the retarded person's expectancy of failure is his greater reliance on other people rather than on his own thought processes. Zigler (1973) has referred to this tendency as outer directedness. To demonstrate this tendency, he and his co-workers (Turnure and Zigler,

1964; Yando and Zigler, 1971) have done a series of experiments in which children were asked to perform some sort of task in the presence of another person doing the same thing. Retarded subjects were more likely than were nonretarded subjects to copy the behavior of the other person. Sometimes, imitating the behavior of others is a productive strategy, but retarded children persisted in it even when it was counterproductive, such as when the model was using a poor strategy and the retarded subject would have been better off not imitating the model.

External Locus of Control and Helplessness

Another postulate of social learning theory, also related to the many failure experiences of the retarded, is that retarded subjects are likely to have an external locus of control. Locus of control refers to individuals' perceptions of what determines what happens to them; individuals with an internal locus of control feel that what happens to them is determined largely by their own actions while individuals with an external locus of control feel that they have little control over their lives and that events are determined by chance or by the actions of other people. Bialer (1961) developed a questionnaire to measure locus of control in children and retarded people. Subjects had to either agree or disagree with statements such as "When people are mean to you, could it be because you did something to make them be mean?" (agreement suggests internal locus of control) or "When nice things happen to you, is it only good luck?" (agreement means external locus of control). His found that internal locus of control increases with mental age, and thus, retarded subjects had a more external locus of control at any given age than did nonretarded subjects.

An external locus of control tends to lead to a general feeling of helplessness. For example, a retarded person who hears that he or she must vacate his or her apartment may make no effort to look for a new one. Floor and Rosen (1975) developed some clever techniques to measure the phenomenon of helplessness in the retarded. For example, while the experimenter is showing subjects how to perform a simple task, a loud buzzer sounds. The experimenter turns it off, indicating that the buzzer turns on inadvertently. The subjects are then left alone, and after a while, the buzzer turns on again. The subjects are scored on whether they turn the buzzer off or not. In another case, the subjects are given a written test and are provided with a pen that doesn't work and several unsharpened pencils. The subjects are left alone and are scored on whether they use a nearby pencil sharpener to sharpen the pencils or not. The subjects were also asked a number of questions such as "What would you do if your wallet were stolen?" Retarded adults were more likely to get high scores on these various helplessness tests than were nonretarded adults. That is, they are more likely to just let the buzzer buzz, and they were less likely to sharpen the pencils by themselves. In other words, they were more helpless; they were less likely to take the initiative to improve their lives.

Increased Need for Social Interaction

There is little question that the work of Edward Zigler (1966, 1973) has had more of an impact on current thinking about personality in the retarded than any other individual. He is one of very few people to have conducted a long term, systematic research program into the nature of personality in the retarded. Zigler has been mentioned previously as an advocate of the developmental theory of retardation. He readily admits that many studies find differences in performance between normal and retarded children matched on MA, but he criticizes those people who attribute all such differences to differences in cognition. He suggests that a good deal of the poor performance of retarded subjects in learning tasks might be due to motivational factors. Specifically, he postulates that many retarded children and adults, particularly those in institutions, have experienced a good deal of social rejection, and as a result, they are more interested in pleasing adults and maintaining social contact with adults than are normal children, who are more motivated toward solving the problem. Thus, when it takes retarded children many more trials to solve a particular problem, this may not be because they have deficient mental capabilities; such a result could just as easily arise from their higher need to remain in the experimental situation as long as possible.

The first specific test of this theory was an experiment by Zigler, Hodgden, and Stevenson (1958). They asked retarded and nonretarded subjects matched on MA to perform several simple motor tasks such as placing pegs in a pegboard. Such an experiment is called a satiation task because the procedure is relatively boring, and the dependent variable is how long the subjects continue before they stop. Half the subjects in each group received a good deal of support and encouragement from the experimenter, while for the other subjects, the experimenter was nonsupportive and said nothing beyond telling the child what to do. The results supported Zigler's theory. Retarded subjects spent more time performing the tasks than did the nonretarded subjects, indicating their greater desire to please the experimenter. They also spent more time playing the game with the support condition than with nonsupport, but there was no difference between the support and nonsupport groups for the normal subjects. There was no difference in the number of errors made between the two groups, indicating that they were equivalent in cognitive ability.

In a further test of the theory, Zigler (1961) divided institutionalized retarded children into two groups, one who had experienced a great deal of social deprivation prior to being institutionalized and one who had experienced relatively little social deprivation prior to institutionalization. The procedure was again a satiation task, this time dropping marbles through a hole, and the results fully supported the theory. Those retarded subjects who had experienced more deprivation spent more time on the game than did the less deprived subjects. Similar results were obtained in an experiment by Green and Zigler (1962). They used three groups of subjects, institutionalized retarded, noninstitutionalized retarded, and nonretarded, all matched on mental age. The task was marble dropping. They found that the institutionalized retarded subjects spent more time on the task than did the noninstitutionalized retarded, who did not differ from the nonretarded subjects. An implication of this research is that many experiments comparing retarded to nonretarded children may have biased results because the experimenters used institutionalized retarded children and noninstitutionalized nonretarded subjects.

However, the generalization that retarded children, particularly socially deprived retarded children, are more willing to work to please adults and respond more positively to social support than are nonretarded children is complicated by an opposing tendency, the retarded child's reluctance and wariness to interact with strange adults. Zigler has called this a negative reaction tendency (1966, 1973). When retarded children enter an experimental situation with a strange adult, both their positive reaction tendencies—their need to be near and to please the adult—and their negative reaction tendency—their fear of the adult—are somewhat stronger than would be the case in nonretarded children. Evidence for this hypothesis comes from a frequent observation in work on satiation with the retarded (e.g., Zigler et al. 1958) that they frequently spend more time on the second of two boring tasks than they do on the first. This is almost never found with normal children. The explanation is that during the first task, the subject is somewhat wary of the experimenter, but during the second task, this fear has largely dissipated, leaving the positive reaction tendency much stronger than the negative.

Zigler has also postulated that there are differences in the reinforcement hierarchies of normal and retarded children. A reinforcement hierarchy is a rank ordering of things that are reinforcing to the child in the order of their strength as a reinforcer. Things that are strongly reinforcing to some children are only weakly reinforcing to others. Some children will work very hard for praise from the teacher, while praise has no effect for other children. Zigler has suggested that middle-class children of normal intelligence will work very hard simply for the reinforcement of being correct while lower-class children, the group from which most retarded children come, are not oriented toward being correct, but respond better with a tangible reinforcement. This hypothesis was tested in an experiment by Zigler and DeLabry (1962). They used three groups of subjects—institutionalized mentally retarded, lower-class nonretarded, and middle-class nonretarded. The children were required to learn a simple problem of concept switching. Some children received a tangible reinforcer for their performance, while others received the intangible reward of simply being told that they were correct. The retarded and the lower-class children learned faster with a tangible reward, while the middle-class children actually did slightly better with the nontangible reinforcement.

Defective Ego Functioning

While the psychoanalytic theory of Sigmund Freud is now somewhat dated, it would be difficult to overestimate its importance in the historical development of modern views of personality and psychopathology. As a result, no text on mental retardation can be complete without a consideration of how thinkers of a Freudian orientation view mental retardation. Unfortunately, as is the case with virtually all researchers in personality, few people have given mental retardation proper consideration, and there are only a handful of writers who have attempted to fit retardation into a psychoanalytic framework. Included here are Pearson (1942), Robinson and Robinson (1965), and Sternlicht and Deutsch (1972).

Freud divided the mind into three parts: the id, which is the seat of the innate impulses, instincts, and drives; the ego, which is concerned with testing reality and bringing the impulses of the id into harmony with the demands of this reality; and the superego, which is concerned with moral issues and is roughly synonymous with the term conscience. Mental retardation is primarily a defect of the ego. Normal ego functioning consists of learning about reality, understanding the results of one's actions, and learning to delay gratification and control impulses so that tensions can be released in a socially acceptable manner. A retarded individual is deficient in all of these processes. This means that retarded persons are less able to control their impulses and are thus more prone to outbursts of emotion or aggression.

As a result of these ego deficits, the superego, which develops out of the ego, also does not function in a normal fashion, and the conscience of a retarded person will be either overly harsh or overly permissive. An additional problem of the superego is to interpret actions in terms of moral absolutes instead of taking extenuating circumstances into account (Sternlicht and Deutsch, 1972). Thus, retarded children might overreact to school failure because their superegos have developed the value that failure is bad and they cannot easily modify this view to cope with specific circumstances (Robinson and Robinson, 1965).

The defective ego, which has difficulty in reducing tensions of the instincts in an acceptable fashion, is thus forced to depend excessively on the more primitive defense mechanisms to control this anxiety. A defense mechanism is a device adopted by the ego to defend against anxiety that usually involves some kind of distortion or denial of reality. The more primitive defense mechanisms such as repression (simply blotting a painful memory or thought out of consciousness) and denial (refusing to admit that a painful fact is indeed true) are often not as effective in reducing anxiety as are the more sophisticated defense mechanisms such as sublimation (channeling the tensions of the innate drives into socially acceptable endeavors such as art or music). As a result, the behavior of a retarded person is typified by irrational reactions and excessive anxiety. This problem is magnified by the fact that the retarded person must use an excessive amount of limited libidinal energy to perform everyday functions that for most people require little effort. The result is that even the primitive defense mechanisms don't work very well to reduce tension.

Because of retarded children's delayed development, their psychosexual development also tends to be deviant. Freud postulated a number of stages of sexual development that are characterized by different ways in which the child reduces sexual tension. During the first year or two of life, the child is in the oral stage and derives pleasure from sucking and chewing. During the anal stage, the primary erogenous zone is the anal area, and the child receives particular pleasure from defecation. This is the time when children are normally toilet trained. During the phallic, or Oedipal stage, the child is developing relationships with the parents and goes through the well-known Oedipal crisis, in which the male child falls in love with his mother and becomes very jealous of his father. Retarded children often cannot resolve these various crises in a satisfactory manner since they may not be ready to be toilet trained during the anal stage or ready for the processes of superego development or identification during the phallic stage. The result is that the retarded child becomes fixated to some extent in earlier stages and show manifestations of these various psychosexual crises throughout life.

Passing and Denial

One of the most fascinating and enlightening books on the nature of adjustment in the mentally retarded is *The Cloak of Competence* by Edgerton (1967). This book describes a study in which a number of retarded people who had been released from a public institution for the retarded in California were followed up to determine their adjustment to independent living. The title of the book comes from the observation that the central concern of all of these people was trying to pretend to be normal, competent, and "just like everyone else." This process of pretending not to be disabled is called passing and is typical of many handicapped people (Goffman, 1963). People who have a hearing loss may pretend to be asleep or feign inattention rather than admit to other people that they have difficulty hearing what was said. Occasionally, a person who is missing a hand will choose to wear a prosthesis that, although it is nonfunctional, looks very much like a normal hand rather than wearing a far more useful but less attractive hook. However, most people with a disability eventually stop pretending that they don't have a handicap and go on to live useful lives accepting their limitations. Apparently, it is far more difficult for a retarded person to do this since the label of retardation implies a far more fundamental defect than does a hearing loss or an amputation. Edgerton reported that all of his cases went to sometimes absurd extremes to prove to themselves and others that they were not mentally retarded. For example, not a single individual would admit that he or she had been institutionalized because of deficient mental abilities. Each one invented a more socially acceptable reason for institutionalization such as alcoholism, sexual promiscuity, being abandoned by their parents, or treatment of a physical illness. All felt that their institutionalization had been unjustified and that they were far more capable than the other people in the institution. This denial was not simply to impress others, but apparently it was equally important that these people convince themselves that they were not mentally retarded. Many of the people went to tragic extremes to convince other people that they were perfectly normal. For example, one woman bought a lot of snapshots of assorted strangers at a rummage sale and made a photo album, making up stories about each one to convince other people that she had friends and relatives just like everyone else. Although few of the ex-patients could read, a number of them had filled their apartments with old magazines and books because this was what other people did. "Normal" people get mail, and the ex-patients seldom did, so they would proudly display what little mail they did receive, even though it was usually addressed to Occupant. One woman even searched through other people's trash to find old letters that she could display on her desk. The ultimate possession was a car, something that few of these people could ever hope to afford, let alone drive. However, one man bought an old car that didn't run, parked it in front of his house, and never failed to stop to examine it whenever he was with someone that he wanted to impress.

Psychopathology and Mental Retardation

The terms psychopathology, psychiatric disturbance, mental illness, emotional disorder, and the like are generally used interchangeably to refer to disorders of personality, emotions, or behavior that significantly interfere with the individual's effective adjustment to his environment. There have been numerous attempts to classify such disturbances with category labels such as neurosis, schizophrenia, and psychosis among others, but most mental health workers agree that these labels are not used very reliably and precisely. In addition, the labeling process contributes little to our knowledge since the cause of most mental illness is unknown or uncertain.

There is general agreement that many kinds of psychopathology are far more common among the mentally retarded than they are in the general population, although there is some disagreement concerning the degree of overlap. At one extreme are psychiatrists like Phillips (1967) and Webster (1970) who comment on how rare it is to find a retarded child whose condition is not complicated by some sort of secondary psychiatric disorder. At the opposite extreme is Gorelick (1966) who reported that only 10 percent of a population of EMR high school students have emotional problems. Such large discrepancies can be attributed partially to the fact that different studies use different populations, but probably most of the differences can be attributed to the vagueness of the diagnosis of emotional disturbance.

A survey by Chess and Hassibi (1970) is particularly informative. They conducted psychiatric evaluations of 52 mildly retarded children who were living at home. Most came from middle-class families. Although only one child was considered psychotic and only one neurotic, nearly all of the children manifested some kind of disturbance in emotions or behavior beyond simply behaving more immaturely. Thirty children (58 percent) were considered restless or excessively active. Such hyperactivity seems to be frequently caused by some kind of cerebral dysfunction, and so finding a high prevalence of hyperactivity among retarded children is not surprising. More than half of the children engaged in some kind of repetitive, aimless motor activity. This included 8 cases of repetitive jumping, nine cases of arm flapping, 18 cases of excessive mouthing of fingers, and 12 cases of rocking. The authors attributed this to the children's lack of intellectual resources in inventing constructive activities for themselves. Four of the children (8 percent) showed explosive emotional activity. While engaged in some sort of play activity, they would suddenly stop and begin to shout, scream, throw things, or hit people for no apparent reason. Such outbursts would usually end as suddenly as they began. Emotional lability of this type is often reported to be a sign of brain damage (Strauss and Lehtinen, 1947). Fifteen children (29 percent) showed some kind of obsessional behavior. Examples include a child who, at his insistence, had been eating Rice-a-Roni every night for two years and a child who always insisted on carrying around pages of a telephone book. Fifteen of the children engaged in unusual seeking of sensory experiences such as pinching themselves or rubbing or hitting themselves. It must be concluded from this study that behavioral disturbances among the mentally retarded are clearly the norm rather than the exception.

The issue of how to classify emotional disturbances is most chaotic with regard to childhood psychoses. There are many children who display some combination of the following symptoms; extreme withdrawal, bizarre behavior, tantrums, aggressive outbursts, stubbornness, and generally delayed development, particularly in the area of language. A number of labels have been applied to such children, including childhood schizophrenia, autism, and central nervous system dysfunction, as well as mental retardation, but there is little consistency of usage. If the same child is seen by several different physicians, one might determine that the child is brain damaged, another may label the child autistic, and a third might make a diagnosis of retardation. Some writers (Kanner, 1946; Rimland, 1964) feel that autism represents a unique syndrome distinct from other disorders while other people (e.g., Menolascino, 1970) have questioned this assumption and use the term in a more general sense to describe withdrawn behavior.

An important consideration is whether such children should be considered mentally retarded. Many children with severe emotional problems are seen in clinics for the retarded, and most such children fit the definition since they have deficient mental abilities (at least they do poorly on intelligence tests), and they are certainly impaired in adaptive behavior. However, there is a certain reluctance to labeling these children as retarded. Rimland (1964) argues that autism is clearly distinct from mental retardation because autistic children do not look retarded and because they occasionally show indications of a superior memory. Similarly, Garfield and Witson (1960) argue that it is extremely dangerous for individuals suffering primarily from psychotic reactions and similar disturbances to be considered mentally retarded. Clearly an important diagnostic concern of many psychiatrists is determining whether a disturbed child is truly mentally retarded or only appears to be retarded because of emotional disturbance. The apparent assumption is that emotional disturbance can readily be alleviated by psychotherapy while mental retardation is hopeless. Neither of these assumptions is entirely correct.

This position has been criticized by many people (Bialer, 1970a; Cantor, 1960; Beier, 1964) on the grounds that the concept of pseudoretardation is being revived. A pseudoretarded child is one who appears to be mentally retarded but turns out not to be by functioning in the normal range at a later time. This is not generally considered to be a useful label, and the current definition of mental retardation (Grossman, 1973) has taken pains to escape this argument by avoiding any reference to the notion of incurability of retardation and defining it solely in terms of present functioning. Chess (1970) has accused psychiatrists of misdiagnosing many retarded children as emotionally disturbed. Such an error is extremely dangerous because not only does this require enormously expensive psychotherapy for both the child and the parents, but it also places the blame for the child's behavior squarely on the shoulders of the parents by assuming that it was their attitudes and relationship with the child that was responsible for the child's symptoms. Such an accusation is extremely difficult for almost any parent to bear.

Distinguishing between true mental retardation and the emotionally disturbed, pseudoretarded child would be an important issue if the treatment were different for the two different diagnoses, but this is not the case. If a child is both emotionally disturbed and mentally retarded, it does not really matter whether the child is retarded because of emotional disturbance or if the child is emotionally disturbed because of retardation. In both cases, the child can be given some form of psychotherapy for emotional disturbance and specific training in language, social skills, and any other skills in which there is a deficiency regardless of the diagnosis.

This question is still hotly debated, and readers who would like to pursue the various arguments further are referred to Balthazar and Stevens (1975) and the first six readings in *Psychiatric Approaches to Mental Retardation* by Menolascino (1970).

Stereotyped Behavior

One unusual category of behavior that is quite characteristic of more severely retarded children and adults is stereotyped behavior. Stereotyped behavior is any kind of repetitious behavior that has no apparent adaptive purpose. The most common example of stereotyped behavior is rocking, but the term also includes such behaviors as head rolling, twirling fingers in front of the eyes, jumping up and down, arm flapping, and picking at oneself as well as more dangerous self-destructive behaviors such as face slapping, banging one's head against the wall or the furniture, and even chewing on one's fingers. Stereotyped behavior is usually thought of as a problem of institutions. Some form of stereotyped behavior is found in about two-thirds of institutionalized retarded patients (Berkson and Davenport, 1962) but it is also observed in noninstitutionalized children (Chess and Hassibi, 1970). Usually, it is only a mild problem, but if individuals are extremely self-destructive, they may have to spend much of their lives in restraint or heavily medicated.

A number of different theories have been suggested to explain this peculiar behavior. Perhaps the most widely held is that stereotyped behavior serves the purpose of self-stimulation. Research suggests that organisms have a drive or need for a certain level of stimulation, and if their level of stimulation is insufficient, they will try to increase stimulation by whatever means is available. College students who volunteered to spend long periods of time in a minimally stimulating environment began to hallucinate. Subhuman primates who are kept in small cages are willing to work quite hard for the opportunity to look out a window. If retarded children or adults are in a situation where the level of stimulation is very low, such as an institution, or if they are unable to derive adequate stimulation from their surroundings because of their impaired mental abilities, they can increase their levels of stimulation by rocking or banging their heads against the floor. Evidence for this interpretation comes from several sources. First, stereotyped behavior almost exactly the same as that observed in retarded children can be produced in subhuman primates by rearing them in isolation. Chimps who have no opportunity to interact with other chimps almost always develop stereotyped behaviors such as rocking or head banging (Berkson and Mason, 1964). Second, when individuals are provided with increased stimulation, the frequency of stereotyped behavior decreases. Forehand and Baumeister (1970) placed severely retarded institutionalized subjects in a small cubicle and measured their rocking behavior. They found that when they showed slides to the subjects in the cubicle, rocking behavior decreased. Similarly, Davenport and Berkson (1963) found that giving retardates something to play with reduced stereotyped behavior.

A related theory is that organisms have a need for a certain amount of motor activity, and if they are deprived of an opportunity for adequate exercise, they will try to satisfy their need by stereotyped behaviors. Everyone has observed the compulsive pacing of lions and other big cats who are restrained in small cages in a zoo. Levy (1944) has observed that infants placed in small cribs in a hospital are apt to develop stereotyped behavior.

A third explanation of stereotypy is that it somehow reduces tension or anxiety. Evidence for this interpretation comes from a number of studies that suggest that the frequency of stereotyped behavior increases when the individual is frustrated or aroused. For example, Levitt and Kaufman (1965) and Hollis (1968) report that rocking increases when a loud noise is sounded on a ward. Food deprivation similarly increases the frequency of stereotyped behavior (Berkson and Mason, 1964), and Forehand and Baumeister (1970) noted a significant increase in rocking in institutionalized retarded subjects when food that they were eating was abruptly removed.

All of these explanations attempt to account for stereotyped behavior by postulating internal conditions within the organism. Another theory attributes stereotyped behavior to reinforcement contingencies within the environment. In other words, the child is somehow rewarded for such behavior. At first, it would seem that self-destructive behavior would be difficult to explain by reinforcement principles, since banging one's head against a chair is one of the least reinforcing behaviors imaginable. However, if children begin to bang their heads, one of the most certain reactions is that adults will rush over and start paying attention to them. In this way, the behavior is being reinforced. The author has observed a severely retarded girl who would bang her head against the floor several times, then look up to make sure other people were watching her. If they weren't, she would get their attention by calling their name, and as soon as they were looking, she would start to bang her head again. Further evidence for such an explanation comes from the fact that occasionally the frequency of self-destructive behavior can be decreased by extinction (removing reinforcement). Lovaas and Simmons (1969) isolated two self-destructive children for 90 minutes each day. The frequency of self-destructive behavior gradually decreased under these conditions in which no one was paying any attention to their behavior.

Probably all of these theories are partially correct since each has solid support in research, but none can account for all of the results. One observation that is difficult for any of the theories to explain is a finding by Green (1967) that head-banging behavior almost always originates in infancy. There are very few cases of children who start to be self-destructive for the first time after five or six. Such an observation makes it necessary to postulate some sort of critical period in development when certain stresses may lead to self-destructive behavior.

For a more complete review of research on stereotyped behavior, see Baumeister and Forehand (1973).

Summary

Although mental retardation is primarily a cognitive disorder, there are a number of reasons why one might expect that retarded people should differ from nonretarded people in noncognitive variables such as motivation, emotions, and personality. Among these reasons are the following:

1. Retarded people are likely to be socially isolated if not actively rejected by other people.
2. The fact that retarded people have been given such a stigmatizing label is likely to cause them to be self-conscious and is likely to cause other people to treat them differently.
3. The presence of a retarded child in a family is apt to cause family stress and tension, resulting in emotional disorders in the retarded child.

4. Retarded people experience a good deal more frustration and failure than do most other people.
5. Brain damage, which is found in many retarded people, is likely to result in emotional problems and disturbed behavior.
6. Retarded people have a lack of insight into their personality and motives and as a result are less likely to attempt to change themselves.
7. Many retarded people come from disadvantaged environments which are likely to produce emotional disturbances.

There are a number of personality characteristics that are generally found more often among the retarded than in the general population. Among these are the following:

1. Retarded people are likely to expect to fail. This expectancy means that they are likely to be failure avoidant rather than success striving; and they are likely to be outer directed, relying on other people rather than their own ideas to make decisions.
2. Retarded people are likely to develop a general feeling of helplessness, a feeling that they are not in charge of their own destiny.
3. As a result of social isolation, retarded people are apt to have an increased need for social interaction and to adopt unusual strategies to maintain contact with other people for as much time as possible.
4. The Freudian interpretation of mental retardation is that retarded persons have defective ego functioning. This means that they are more likely to rely on very primitive defense mechanisms such as repression or denial to reduce anxiety.
5. Retarded people are likely to go to great lengths to demonstrate to other people and to themselves that they are "normal," a process known as passing. Thus, they might park an old car in front of their house and show it off to other people even though they cannot drive because "normal" people have cars.

There is a general consensus that there is a much higher prevalence of emotional disturbance among the mentally retarded than in the general population. In fact, some experts claim that virtually all retarded people are characterized by significant emotional disturbance. Many professionals feel that it is important to distinguish those people whose retardation is secondary to emotional disturbance from those people who are primarily mentally retarded and also happen to have emotional problems. However, more common practice now is to regard this question as unimportant since the management is the same in both cases.

One common feature of mentally retarded people, particularly the institutionalized retarded, is stereotyped behavior, the compulsive repetition of a purposeless behavior that is often self-destructive. There are a number of theories that have been developed to account for this behavior, and each has some research data to support them. One such theory is that this behavior acts as self-stimulation for people living in basically unstimulating environments. Another theory is that it fills a need for motor activity. Still other people feel that stereotyped behavior reduces tension and anxiety, while still others feel that it is done because it is reinforced by other people through attention.

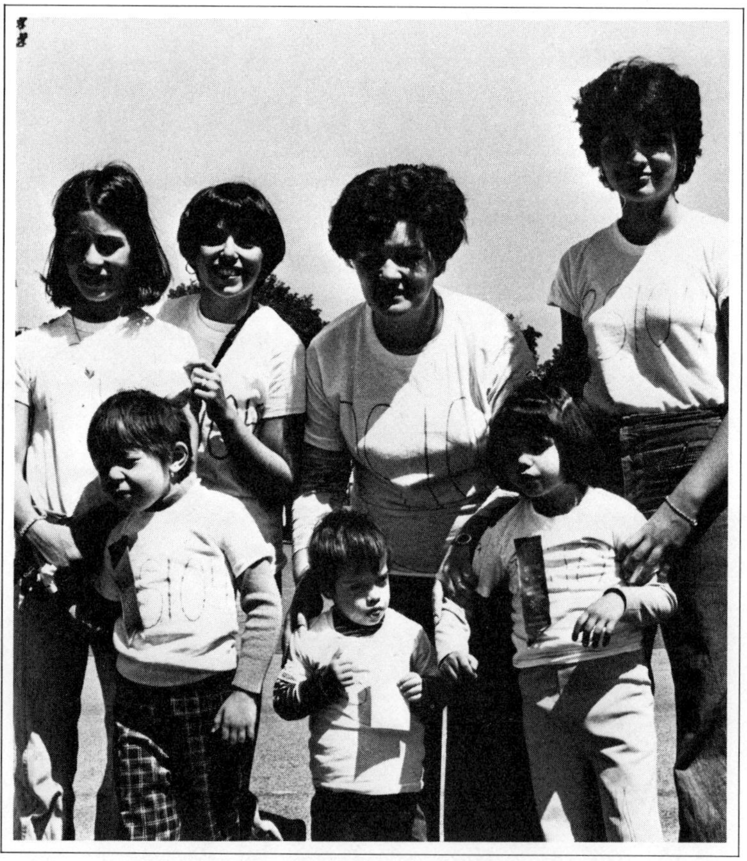

12

Treatment of Behavioral and Emotional Problems

The previous chapter discussed some of the reasons why there might be a high prevalence of emotional and behavioral disorders among the mentally retarded. This chapter reviews various approaches to treatment for such problems. Treatment of psychological problems can be divided into three broad categories. The first of these is psychotherapy, a term that includes a wide variety of techniques that have in common the fact that the client discusses feelings or otherwise communicates them to a sympathetic listener, and the assumption is that such an activity will be therapeutic. The second approach is behavior therapy, treatment based on the principles of operant and classical conditioning. The third approach is chemotherapy, the treatment of emotional and behavioral disorders with psychoactive drugs. None of these techniques is limited to use with the mentally retarded, and in fact all were developed for and are primarily used with people of normal mental capabilities. However, all have been used rather extensively with mentally retarded children and adults, and this chapter is limited to the use of these methods with the retarded.

Psychotherapy with the Retarded

The term psychotherapy originally referred predominantly to psychoanalysis, the technique developed by Freud that involved a patient meeting individually with a psychiatrist for the purpose of working out unconscious conflicts through free association, dream analysis, and an intense emotional relationship with the analyst called transference. However, classical psychoanalysis is seldom practiced any more, and it has been replaced by a bewildering variety of different techniques and methods with little in common beyond the fact that all have the goal of changing a person's behavior, feelings, or adjustment in a positive direction through communication with another individual. Psychotherapy is done either individually or in groups, it can be highly permissive and nondirective or it can be highly structured. It can be largely verbal or it can involve communication through nonverbal means. The clients range from severely disturbed psychotics to essentially normal people. It is virtually impossible to distinguish psychotherapy from a number of closely related techniques such as the supportive counseling of a social worker or rehabilitation counselor, various group activities such as sensitivity and encounter groups, or the advice and guidance provided by a clergyman. In fact, a good deal of what goes on in psychotherapy is similar to the support that two close friends or a husband and wife provide to one another. All of these methods are based on the assumption that a person's adjustment and emotional well being can be improved through talking with a supportive person about one's problems. In this section, the term psychotherapy will be used in a very broad sense to include not only traditional psychotherapeutic techniques such as those provided by a psychiatrist or clinical psychologist, but also the general process of support and guidance provided by a social worker, rehabilitation counselor, or other professional or paraprofessional who works with the mentally retarded.

Individual Verbal Psychotherapy

The traditional "talk" therapies carried out on a one-to-one basis with the therapist are not commonly used with the mentally retarded. There are at least two reasons for this. The first is that there is a lack of trained professionals to work with retarded people. The majority of clinical psychologists and psychiatrists have had little training in mental retardation and prefer not to work with them, and even if there were more professionals available, most facilities that provide services to the retarded would not have the money to hire them. It is far more efficient to provide such services on a group basis. A second reason is that many of the pioneers in psychotherapy specifically cautioned against using their technique with people of low intelligence and poor verbal skills. Freud felt that psychoanalysis would only be effective with those of above average intelligence because the retarded lacked insight into their own feelings and would have difficulty verbalizing them (Sternlicht, 1966). Carl Rogers (1951), the developer of client-centered therapy, gave the same warning, arguing that the retarded could not deal cognitively with acting out impulses and would be unable to view objectively the effects of their own behavior or the behavior of others. There is little question that low intelligence is a barrier to personality change and that many retarded people have difficulty verbalizing their feelings, but this certainly does not suggest that psychotherapy should never be attempted with the retarded. Individual psychotherapy is being undertaken with mentally retarded clients with increasing frequency, and there are a number of published reports of successful therapy with retarded clients (Thorne, 1948; Heiser, 1954).

It would be impossible to describe the process of psychotherapy with the retarded, and difficult even to make generalizations. Psychotherapy is a highly individualized process. What happens in a therapy session depends not only on the specific problems and circumstances of the client, but also on the unique personality and outlook of the therapist. Some therapists stick very closely to one system of therapy, such as psychoanalysis or client-centered therapy or transactional analysis, but most therapists are eclectic in their approach, which means that they do not use any one technique with all clients (Woody and Billy, 1966). Some therapists may focus on day-to-day adjustment problems of their client while others may attend more to feelings and conflicts. One therapist may make numerous suggestions of alternative behavior patterns while another may be almost completely nondirective.

Mentally retarded people seldom or never refer themselves for therapy but are referred by someone else, either a parent or a social worker or a teacher or an institutional staff member. This means that the presenting problem is usually some sort of antisocial behavior. For example, Thorne (1948) lists the causes of referral of 268 institutionalized retarded clients. Thirty-five percent were referred for insubordination, 21 percent for running away, 16 percent for fighting, 11 percent for sexual problems, 9 percent for severe tantrums, and 8 percent for stealing. Almost all of these complaints can be placed in the general category of impulse control, and thus, the single most important goal of most therapy with the retarded is getting the clients to better control their impulses. This can be done by getting the clients to discuss why they do what they do and increasing their awareness of the negative results that frequently follow such behavior. There are a number of other purposes of therapy that, while being important in their own right, also serve the purpose of helping the clients to control their emotions. One such purpose is making the clients more aware of their feelings. It is widely assumed that if individuals are more aware of their emotions, they will be better able to control them. A second purpose is increasing the clients' sense of self-worth. This is accomplished by the therapist accepting the clients for exactly what they are. Retarded people are accustomed to being rejected and ignored by most of society and a therapy or counseling session is one of the few situations, perhaps the only one, where the clients can find a person who is genuinely interested in them with all of their limitations. This experience by itself is often very beneficial to the client.

One possible goal of therapy with the retarded deserves special attention, and that is the goal of raising the client's intelligence, or "curing" the retardation. This is a reasonable possibility only in those cases where the individual's retardation is caused primarily by an emotional disturbance. In such a case, if the emotional block can be removed as a result of some sort of therapy, then there might be a corresponding increase in the person's mental functioning. However, although there are scattered reports of individuals whose measured intelligence rose into the normal range after therapy (e.g., Heiser, 1954), this is not a frequent occurrence.

Group Therapy and Counseling

Most therapy done with retarded individuals is done in a group setting rather than individually. There are several reasons for this, but the primary one is to maximize the effectiveness of what few counselors and therapists are available to work with the retarded. However, there are some advantages to group therapy beyond practical economics. In the first place, the clients have the opportunity to benefit from hearing about the problems of other retarded people. In this way, people can see that others have difficulties as bad or worse than their own, and they realize that they are not alone with their problems. Also, other people besides the therapist are able to provide encouragement and support. A third benefit of a group setting, perhaps the most important, is that it gives the retarded experiences in social skills and social situations. They can learn to be more sensitive to the feelings of other people, and a group counseling situation is one of the few opportunities available to many retarded people to get to know a number of other people on a fairly intimate level.

There are certain guidelines that most group leaders follow, although as with individual therapy there are a wide range of acceptable practices. The first is to encourage all of the members of the group to be as open as they can be. In other words, they should try to reveal their true feelings and not try to put up a front or try to impress the other members of the group. Nor should they be afraid to discuss some personal problem because they are ashamed of it or because they are afraid that others will criticize them or tease them. In order to encourage this process, it is important that any expressions of disapproval be minimized. This is called an atmosphere of psychological safety, a situation where the clients can say anything they want without fear because they know that the others accept them for what they are. After a period of time in such a situation, it is hoped that the members of the group will become less defensive; they will be able to discuss their problems and their fears openly and, in this way, they will be better able to understand themselves.

Group leaders must decide to what extent they should be directive and provide structure for the group by suggesting topics for discussion or whether they should let the pattern of the discussion be determined by the members. It seems to be the case that retarded clients require more direction and structure than do nonretarded clients (Sternlicht, 1966), and the most successful groups are those in which the leader is able to provide a good deal of structure.

A number of reports of group therapy with the retarded have been published. As is the case with most of the research on retardation, a disproportionate number of studies have been done with institutionalized patients. Many of these projects had the specific goal of preparing institutional residents for independent living. The report by Kaufman (1963) is typical. He conducted group therapy on a weekly basis for eight institutionalized mildly retarded patients who were about to be released. At first, the group sessions were rather chaotic. All of the remarks were directed toward the leader rather than to the group in general, and the members were concerned only with their own problems and tended to disregard what other people were saying. This led to a rapid shift from topic to topic. The leader then shifted from being relatively nondirective to providing a good deal more structure, and as time passed, a sense of group unity developed and they began to focus on common problems. One difficulty that most of the group had trouble with was controlling feelings, which resulted in frequent emotional outbursts and aggressive episodes. As the group progressed, the weekly meetings were supplemented by field trips to a nearby city where the members were given experiences in everyday activities that they would face on the outside, such as cashing a check, eating in a restaurant, or asking directions. These experiences provided additional topics for discussion, and the group members began to be concerned with specific problems that they would face after their release, such as what to do if they were lost. Kaufman describes four processes that developed during the therapy period. The first was catharsis, the release of emotional tension. The second was transference, a common experience in therapy in which unconscious emotions and feelings toward authority figures become manifest due to the relationship with the leader. The third development was a new motivation to learn. The experience of spending time alone in the city gave the members new impetus to learn social skills. The fourth was social pressure toward conformity. The author felt that the result of the group therapy was that the members had become more socialized, and as evidence, he mentioned that six of the eight received permanent discharges.

Another description of a group therapy program with retarded clients is described by Slivkin and Bernstein (1970). This one is instructive not only for its detailed description of group techniques, but also because it provides some interesting insights into various personality processes in the retarded from a psychoanalytic point of view. Group members were selected not because of their antisocial behavior as is frequently the case, but because of their ability to communicate. It was necessary for the therapist to assume a very active role in order to reduce disorderliness, and thus, the group was highly structured. At first, the group members mistrusted the therapist. They were afraid that he would report what happened to institutional authorities, and they teased him about being a "shrinker." The authors interpreted this as a defense against the need for significant relationships. The process of testing the limits was also evident and many of the clients were surprised to discover that they would not be punished for acting out, even when they engaged in violent activity such as throwing chairs or destroying property. Early in the session, a number of defenses were evident. Some patients adopted a blanket denial that they had problems. Others identified with the therapist by trying to become a deputy therapist. As the group members gradually learned to trust the therapist and began to develop a sense of group unity, these defenses fell and deeper problems became evident. For example, many of the members began to discuss their often unhappy relationships with their parents. Some of the girls transferred these feelings to the therapist, a common experience in psychoanalytically oriented therapy, and several of the girls physically assaulted him. One then spent the next session weeping copiously and begging for forgiveness. One boy told numerous stories about a father who loved him very much but was away in Vietnam. It turned out that the boy was illegitimate and had no father, but the therapist never tried to challenge such fantasies since they were so important to the clients.

The authors felt that despite the initial failure, such groups were highly successful in bringing out unconscious feelings and in helping the retarded group members to better control their emotions.

Play Therapy

Because so many retarded children and adults have problems with verbal communication, various kinds of nonverbal therapy have been developed, of which the most popular is play therapy (Axline, 1947). In play therapy, little emphasis is placed on communication of feelings verbally, but the clients, usually children, are encouraged to express themselves through the medium of play, which is children's natural mode of expression anyway. Play therapy is traditionally nondirective. Children are permitted to choose for themselves what toys to play with and how to play with them, with little or no intervention on the part of the therapist. There is usually a wide choice of toys available. Many of these are unstructured, which means that there is not one "correct" way to play with them, but they can be used in a number of different ways. Good toys for play therapy include a sandbox, clay, paints, puppets, and a dollhouse with a doll family. Only very minimum restrictions are set. For example, children cannot willfully destroy materials or physically attack the therapist, but beyond this, they are free to do whatever they feel like doing. As with other kinds of nondirective therapy, the assumption behind such an approach is that people have within themselves the ability to solve their own problems, but this ability is blocked by various restrictions placed on the child by society. At first, children are surprised to discover that the therapist is not going to punish or criticize them or tell them what to do. Once children discover that the therapist is not a threatening person, they can go on to do what they want to do without feeling the need to please other people. Meanwhile, the therapist is far from passive. The therapist's role is to develop a warm, friendly relationship with children in order to genuinely understand what the children are feeling and, in this way, reflect these feelings back to the children. The therapist must always accept children exactly as they are and maintain a respect for the children's abilities to solve their own problems. The discovery that there is a person who is sincerely interested in children as people is always beneficial to children, and this aids them in developing their sense of self-esteem and self-worth. Axline (1947, 1948, 1949) has described a number of cases in which a child's behavior improved rather dramatically after a number of sessions of her type of nondirective play therapy. Included are several cases who progressed from the retarded range into the normal range in intelligence tests.

Leland and Smith (1965) have written a book on applying various play therapy techniques to retarded children. They discuss four different types or levels of therapy depending on the capabilities of the specific child and the goals of the therapy. The crucial dimension is structure. Both the materials used in the therapy and the approach of the therapist can be either structured or unstructured. Unstructured materials have no particular function or use, such as water, clay, or sand, while structured materials are used in specific ways, such as toy trucks or dolls. An unstructured approach is one in which the therapist makes little attempt to direct the child in a certain direction, while a structured approach is one in which the therapist requests that the child do certain things. The most primitive type of therapy is an unstructured approach with unstructured materials. This is specifically directed toward very poorly functioning children who may not even be aware of themselves. Thus, an important goal of this approach is for children to learn to recognize themselves as people by learning that they can control materials and things. By interacting with these unstructured materials, they learn that they are responsible for what happens to them, and in this way, they discover that they have some control over their environment.

The next type of therapy is a structured approach with unstructured materials. This is the approach often used in various adjunct therapies such as art therapy, music therapy, or occupational therapy in which the client is asked to make or do a specific thing with relatively unstructured material. Examples range from having the client mold specific things in clay to having the client make a belt out of a piece of leather. Such therapy has the goals of improving self-concept, improving impulse control, and facilitating social interaction.

A third play therapy approach is using relatively structured materials, but with the therapist adopting an unstructured approach. The materials here would include many of the traditional childhood toys such as a dollhouse, a tea set, trucks, and a toy telephone. The therapist is not passive but makes few specific suggestions. This type of therapy is important for developing relationships with things and people and for dealing with social and cultural realities.

The last type of therapy, structured materials in a structured approach, begins to border on education because the therapist is asking children to use specific materials in specific ways. A major goal of this type of therapy is raising social maturity through improving cognitive functioning. The therapist is far more verbal in this type of approach and also encourages children to be more verbal. Children also learn how they fit into their environment and are aided in acquiring realistic levels of aspiration.

Creative Arts Therapy

Music, dance, and painting have been used for many years as a therapeutic technique with retarded children and adults. As in most play therapy, the approach is usually nondirective in the sense that patients are allowed to express themselves in what ever way they wish, and there is usually little criticism, the emphasis being on spontaneity and individuality.

The advantage of these techniques is that they can be applied to even the most profoundly handicapped people. For example, in music therapy, the more capable clients can be encouraged to sing along or even to learn to play a simple instrument, but even the most impaired can appreciate the rhythm of the music and maintain a beat with a tambourine. Many severely retarded people also enjoy dancing and can use this as a mode of expression. Painting is a particularly good way for nonverbal people to express their feelings, and even the most handicapped people can use and enjoy finger paints.

The goals of such therapy are necessarily nonspecific, and thus, it is difficult to evaluate the success of these programs. However, at the very least, such therapy provides an enjoyable activity for many people whose lives are often sterile and barren. In addition, music, dance, and painting can provide many nonverbal people with an opportunity to express their feelings. By actually creating something of their own that is admired by other people, severely retarded people learn that they can be productive, and this can enhance their self-esteem. Music and dance can also provide a socially acceptable way to release tensions, and this can result in fewer behavior problems.

A number of successful programs of music and art therapy have been described. The reader who would like to learn more about music and dance therapy is referred to Tyson (1957), Weigl (1959), and Alvin (1959), while Ludins-Katz (1972) gives some excellent ideas on the use of art with the retarded.

Evaluating the Effects of Therapy

The extent to which psychotherapy is effective in bringing about positive behavior change has been a controversial issue since the origins of psychoanalysis in the last century. While most people who actively do therapy insist that it is often a very effective treatment, there is remarkably little solid research substantiating this. A number of research projects (e.g., Eysenck, 1961) have concluded that the proportion of people who improve after therapy is about the same as the proportion who improve with no therapy, but there have been enough well-controlled studies done showing improvement as a result of various kinds of therapy (e.g., Bergin and Garfield, 1971) to suggest that psychotherapy is at least sometimes effective with some therapists. However, even the most avid defenders of psychotherapy agree that there are many cases where it is not successful and occasional cases in which it is damaging.

There are two problems related to research on the outcome of psychotherapy. The first is that psychotherapy is not at all a uniform process. Even therapists who claim to be using the same technique may differ widely in their style. Many readers may have been disappointed that the process of therapy was not described in more detail in the above sections, but the reason for this is that there is no one process of psychotherapy. Most reports of therapy are quite vague about what actually went on during a session, and, despite attempts by various medical and psychological organizations to describe it as a systematic technique, it is still much more of an art than a technology. However, the fact that therapy is a highly individualized art does not relieve the practitioners of the obligation to evaluate its effectiveness.

A more serious difficulty in evaluating the outcome of therapy is that the goals and purposes of therapy are usually quite vague. There is virtually no way to validly assess whether in fact a client has attained significant new insights or has improved self-concept or has achieved personal growth, and even if these things have occurred, has there been any improvement in the client's day-to-day adjustment. All too often, therapy programs are said to be a success based solely on the report of therapists, who say that they noted improvement in many of their clients. Such reports by themselves are not convincing. In the first place, a therapist is far from an unbiased judged. It is difficult for people to admit that a project to which they have devoted a great deal of time and energy has failed. More importantly, if improvement was noted in some of the clients, it is impossible to say that the improvement resulted from the therapy. Many emotional problems seem to clear up without therapy or treatment, a process known as spontaneous recovery. This is particularly true in the case of children, who often outgrow a behavior problem. If patients refer themselves for therapy when they are particularly disturbed or depressed, or if retarded children are referred when their behavior is particularly disruptive, and six months later, the clients are better, the improvement is as likely to be an example of spontaneous recovery as it is to be a result of the therapy. The only way that therapy can be proved to be effective is if there is a control group, a group of subjects matched on severity of symptoms and other demographic characteristics to the people receiving therapy but who receive no therapy themselves. Even if they are matched, subjects must be randomly assigned to therapy and control groups in order to demonstrate the therapy's effectiveness. Only a small proportion of therapy programs use adequate control groups, and without one, it is difficult to determine the value of therapy.

All of these problems are equally true with regard to therapy with the retarded. The most complete review of research in psychotherapy with the retarded is Sternlicht (1966). He concluded that while there are numerous studies describing therapy programs with the retarded, there are still no theoretical and empirical bases for this work, and there is little effective research dealing with the outcomes of therapeutic treatment. Browning and Keesey (1974) concluded that of 129 articles on counseling and therapy with the retarded, only one was properly controlled to draw conclusions about the outcome. Thus, it can be concluded that while psychotherapy is probably sometimes effective with some retarded people, there is currently little conclusive evidence that this is a viable technique, and there is no research at all indicating that one method is superior to another.

Behavior Modification

Another approach to treating disturbed behavior is called behavior modification, also called behavior therapy. This therapy is based on a very different conceptualization of disturbed behavior than is psychotherapy, and unlike psychotherapy, there is a considerable body of research demonstrating its effectiveness. As a result, the popularity of behaviorally oriented therapies has increased tremendously in recent years, particularly with the mentally retarded.

The Assumptions behind Behaviorism

Behavior therapy and behavior modification are derived from a school of psychology called behaviorism. Behaviorism was founded by John B. Watson (1914), but the name most associated with behaviorism today is B. F. Skinner (1974). Behaviorists make a number of assumptions, both implicit and explicit, about the nature of, the cause of, and the study of human behavior, and their viewpoint has been so influential, particularly with respect to the treatment of and the education of the mentally retarded, that it is important to review the assumptions underlying behaviorism in detail.

The defining assumption behind behaviorism is that only observable behavior can be fit material for scientific psychology. Behaviorists are not concerned with studying the mind or consciousness or thought or ideas or feelings or the ego or any of the other mentalistic constructs that are usually associated with psychology. If a process cannot be observed directly it cannot be studied scientifically, and, therefore, it is of no interest to behaviorists. They do not necessarily deny the existence of consciousness or feelings, but they argue that because such processes cannot be adequately defined or measured, they belong in the realm of philosophy or some other discipline where the methodology is armchair speculation rather than hard scientific observation. For the same reason, behaviorists deny the usefulness of the concept of intelligence, and thus they are little concerned with whether a child should be labeled mentally retarded or not. Behaviorists limit their diagnostic activity to describing observable behavior and its consequences rather than assigning labels.

A second assumption of behaviorism is that most behavior can be attributed to environmental causes. In order to understand why children are doing whatever they are doing, one should study their past and present environments rather than attempt to explain the behavior by postulating some hypothetical process within the children. Another way of stating the same assumption is that most human behavior is learned, and, because most behavior is learned, then it is possible to change almost any behavior by altering the individual's environment.

Among the most important aspects of anyone's environment are the reinforcement contingencies of various behaviors, in other words, what happens to children when they make a certain response. If they get a reward, more technically referred to as a positive reinforcement, for doing a particular thing, they are likely to do the same thing again in similar situations. For example, a child throws a temper tantrum, and his mother runs over, picks the child up, and gives the child lots of love, attention, and other kinds of positive reinforcements. As a result, the child is likely to have more tantrums in the future. In order to explain such behavior, it is not necessary to resort to such mentalistic concepts as feelings of frustration; the behavior is explained by the reinforcements in the child's environment.

This process of increasing the frequency or probability of a behavior as a result of reinforcement is called operant conditioning. A third assumption of behaviorism is that most learning can be best described through the relatively simple mechanisms of classical and operant conditioning. Even quite complex behaviors can be understood by breaking them down into their simple component parts and regarding each component as being learned through simple conditioning. A corollary of this assumption is that the process of learning is fundamentally the same in children at all developmental levels, and even in subhuman organisms. While this assumption may seem farfetched, much of what has been learned about classical and operant conditioning in rats and pigeons seems to apply to learning in college students as well.

Behaviorists have been among the most vocal critics of the use of traditional psychotherapy (Gardner, 1971; Stamm, 1974). A fundamental difference between behaviorists and more traditional psychotherapists is that the former view the specific behaviors of the child as the real problem, while most other psychologists regard the specific disruptive behaviors of the child as simply a symptom of an underlying conflict or problem. Hence, a behaviorally oriented psychologist is primarily concerned with changing the child's overt behavior, while many other psychologists and counselors tend to ignore the specific symptom and try to resolve the underlying personality problem.

A case described by Gardner (1971) can be used to contrast this difference. An institutionalized retarded girl who had also been given a number of other labels such as brain damaged was enrolled in a school program. After a few weeks in class, she began to vomit, and the frequency of this vomiting behavior increased rapidly and was accompanied by other disruptive behavior including screaming, tearing clothes, and destroying property. We can imagine how therapists of various persuasions might react to this problem. The girl might receive individual therapy in which she would discuss her problems for an hour or two a week with a therapist, or more likely, she would meet for several hours a week with a group of similar patients. If the therapist were psychoanalytically oriented, the girl might be asked to discuss her relationship with her parents and various events of her early childhood. If the therapist were nondirective, the client could talk about whatever she wanted to on the assumption that she could solve her own problems. She might receive some kind of play therapy, particularly if her verbal skills were poor. All of these methods have in common the fact that they attack the problem indirectly. The vomiting is seen as a symptom of a more serious problem, and it is necessary to treat the whole child, not just the specific symptom.

On the other hand, a behaviorist would observe the child in the classroom to determine what was reinforcing the behavior. In this case, it was observed that when the girl vomited, she was usually removed from the classroom and sent back to the dormitory. To change this behavior, the psychologist suggested to the teacher that the girl be kept in the classroom for the full period regardless of whether she vomited or not. At the same time, she was reinforced with tangible rewards and praise for desirable behavior. Within a month, the frequency of vomiting and accompanying disruptive behavior had reduced to zero.

Operant Conditioning

The underlying process behind most behavior modification is operant conditioning, although there is another type of behavior therapy that is based primarily on classical conditioning. As a result, the process and terminology of operant conditioning ought to be reviewed. Operant conditioning is little more than a new term for the observation that the frequency or the probability of a response will be increased if an organism receives a positive reinforcement immediately after making this response. A rat who receives a food pellet whenever he presses a bar begins to press the bar more and more often; a child throws a spitball at the teacher and everyone laughs (except the teacher), and the result is that the child will be more likely to throw spitballs in the future; a four year old works diligently at a puzzle and finally gets it all together, giving her a feeling of satisfaction and accomplishment, and in addition, the nursery school teacher praises her, and the result is that she will be more likely to work hard at future puzzles. The crucial factor in all of these examples is the concept of *reinforcement.* The food pellet, the laughter, and the feeling of satisfaction were all examples of positive reinforcement because they increased the frequency of the behavior that preceded it. Thus, a positive reinforcement is similar to a reward. However, people tend to define reward in mentalistic terms, as something that individuals like or something that makes them feel good, while reinforcement is usually defined in purely behavioral terms as anything that increases the probability of a preceding response being repeated. Different people are reinforced by different things. For some children, being hollered at by the teacher is aversive, that is, something they will work to avoid, but for others, being yelled at might actually be reinforcing since it is a form of attention. As a result, these children will do things that have the consequence of the teacher yelling at them.

Another type of reinforcement is negative reinforcement. Negative reinforcement differs from punishment in that it is something that the child will work to escape or avoid. Thus, negative reinforcement, like positive reinforcement, increases the frequency of behavior. If a child does homework to avoid being scolded by the teacher, this is negative reinforcement. Punishment, on the other hand, refers to any event that decreases the frequency of the preceding behavior. If a small child uses a word that is not supposed to be used, the mother may spank the child for this, and the frequency of the child's using that word will decrease (unless the attention value of the word is stronger than the spanking, in which case the frequency of the child's using the word will increase because of the reactions of everyone around the child).

An important variable in such learning is the time interval between the occurrence of the behavior and the reinforcement. If the reinforcement follows the behavior immediately, then it is more likely to be effective in increasing behavior than if there is a long interval between the response and the reinforcement. If there is a long delay between the time when the rat presses the bar in a Skinner box and the rat receiving a food pellet, the process of learning will be much slower. In fact, some behaviorists (Malott, 1972) feel that one of our biggest problems is that we respond to small immediate reinforcers rather than large, long-term reinforcers, and this explains why dieters are unable to stay away from chocolate cake and why textbooks under contract never get written. In the case of the dieter, the small immediate reinforcement associated with eating has more control over behavior than does the distant reinforcement of being healthier and more attractive. In the case of the book, there are not enough immediate reinforcements to maintain book-writing behavior, even though the long-term reinforcements of fame and fortune may be large.

If a behavior is not reinforced, the probability of that response being made again decreases. This process is called extinction. If a rat is busy pressing a bar in a Skinner box and the pellet dispenser jams, as they are prone to do, at first the rat may press the bar more than ever, but after a while, the frequency of bar pressing behavior decreases and eventually ceases completely. In similar fashion, if a child is throwing tantrums in order to get love and attention from mother, if the mother has been reading Skinner and decides to ignore the child whenever the child starts a tantrum, at first the tantrums may get worse, but if the mother can persist in ignoring her offspring, eventually, the frequency of tantrums will decrease.

With this background, it is easy to understand how behavior modifiers go about changing behavior in retarded subjects. They make little attempt to apply traditional diagnostic labels to their children. All behavior problems can be placed in two broad categories, those situations where children are doing something that they are not supposed to be doing, for example, banging their heads against a wall, and those situations where children are not doing something which they should be doing, for example, a six year old who is not yet talking. In the latter case, children can be taught the appropriate behavior by manipulating the child's environment so that the child will be reinforced for it. In the former case, the problem behavior can be eliminated either by removing the reinforcement for the undesirable behavior (almost all behavior has a reinforcement) or by reinforcing an incompatible response.

Steps to Increase the Frequency of a Behavior

Let us consider the prescription for each of these problems in detail. If the problem is that children are not doing something that they are supposed to be doing, the goal is to increase the frequency of the desired behavior. For example, consider the case of a special class teacher who is trying to get one of her students, Ronald, to do his arithmetic problems. She knows from past experience that if a child of his mental level spends enough time doing such problems, that he will master basic addition, and it is important for him to know how to add. However, doing arithmetic problems is not reinforcing for Ronald, and as a result, he spends very little time doing them. When he is given a specific assignment by the teacher, he may do it for a few moments, but soon he is staring around the room, and a while later, he is roaming around the room disrupting other pupils. There are six steps that a behavior modifier would follow to increase the frequency of arithmetic problem behavior in this child.

Step 1. *Specify the behavior to be increased.* In most cases this is an easy step since the diagnosis of the problem usually implies the solution. However, there are two precautions in connection with this. First, the behavior to be increased must be stated very explicitly and must be stated in behavioral terms. Deciding to increase "good student behavior" is not specific enough. The behavior ought to be somehow countable or otherwise measurable and stated in such a way that several different people observing the child's behavior would agree on the frequency of the behavior. In the case of Ronald, the behavior might be working 20 arithmetic problems and getting them correct each day. A second consideration is that the behavior must be within the capabilities of the subject. While behaviorists often appear to assume that anyone can be trained to do almost anything if the conditions are right, it is obvious in practice that this is not always the case. This is merely another way of saying "Set realistic goals." In the case of Ronald, the teacher has observed that the most problems that Ronald has ever worked in a single day is 20, and thus, the goal of 20 problems correct seems to be reasonable. However, it would be totally unreasonable to set a goal of 30 correct in a day, since this is probably beyond his immediate capabilities.

Step 2. *Determine an appropriate reinforcer.* This is the most important step. A reinforcer is anything that will increase the frequency of a preceding behavior, in other words, something that the subject will work for. Occasionally, small children will perform well with candy as a reinforcement, but for most older children and adults who are well fed, food is only a weak reinforcer and may not reliably increase the frequency of behavior. Another category of reinforcement that is commonly used is social reinforcement, such as praise, attention, and the like. Like most other reinforcers, this works very well for some children but not at all for others. A practice that is becoming increasingly common in schools is the use of privileges as reinforcement. Some children are willing to work very hard for the privilege of starting recess 10 minutes early or the privilege of looking through magazines or even being blackboard monitor. Table 12-1 shows a list of possible reinforcers that have been found to be effective with young and retarded children.

Each child is different, and what is highly reinforcing for one child may not be at all effective for some other child. Premack (1965) has developed a procedure that is often useful in finding a reinforcer for a given child. The Premack principle states that a more frequent behavior can be used as a reinforcement for a less frequent behavior. Thus, in order to find a good reinforcement for certain children, observe their behavior during free time and see what they spend a lot of time doing. If they spend most of their time talking with their friends, the privilege of talking with their friends can be used to reinforce a less frequent behavior such as doing their assignments.

In Ronald's case, the teacher observed that his favorite behavior was going out on the playground and shooting baskets, and thus, she decided to use this as a reinforcement for completing his arithmetic assignments.

It is frequently not convenient to dispense privileges as reinforcements

Table 12-1 Reinforcers Frequently Effective in a Classroom

Events	
Special lunch	Managing the token store
Cookout	Typing
Special field trip	Extra recess
Dancing	Playing with special games or toys
Class outdoors	Listening to stories
Baking	Seeing movies, slides
Leading class in singing	Using tape recorder
Jumping, tumbling	Being in class play
Serving lunch or tea to guests	Bringing in toys, books from home
Combing each other's hair	Talking to friend
Putting desks together	Being class leader, pledge leader, class monitor, messenger
Getting special desk in room	Passing out papers
Private time with teacher	Painting
Helping smaller children	
Cleaning boards, room	
Taking messages to office	
Dispensing or collecting tokens	
Tangibles	
Costume jewelry	Ball
Lipstick	Jump rope
Ribbons	Paint set
Candy, chewing gum	Snacks, beverages
Small toys	Photograph of self, friend, teacher
Coloring books, crayons	Baseball cards
Paper dolls	

From J. T. Neisworth & R. M. Smith, *Modifying retarded behavior.* Copyright © 1973 by Houghton Mifflin Co. Reprinted by permission of the publisher.

every time that a desired behavior occurs. However, it is important that some sort of reinforcer follow any desirable behavior immediately. A frequently used solution to this problem is to use tokens as reinforcers. A token is anything that can later be turned in for a reinforcement, such as a gold star, a check mark on a chart, or a poker chip. The advantage of using tokens is that each child in a class or on an institution ward can be reinforced immediately for any desired behavior when it would be a tremendous inconvenience for the aide or teacher to be dispensing privileges every time any child did anything that warranted reinforcing. It would certainly be disruptive for Ronald and his classmates to be running out to the playground every five minutes. Thus, each time that Ronald completes a certain number of problems correctly, the teacher could mark this on a card, and if he had accumulated enough check marks by the time that recess came around, he could go out to play. Otherwise, he would have to stay inside until he completed his assignment.

Another desirable feature of using tokens is that what is reinforcing for a child one day may not be reinforcing the next. If a whole class or ward is being reinforced with tokens, it is usually not necessary for the teacher to determine a reinforcer for each child; all she has to do is to develop a "reinforcement menu" that lists a large number of possible reinforcers, both privileges and toys, with a price in tokens for each one, and thus, at a certain time each day, each child can decide individually what reinforcement they want to turn their tokens in for.

Step 3. *Measure the baseline rate of the behavior.* The term baseline rate refers to the frequency of the behavior at the beginning of the project. This is the equivalent to a control group in an experimental design. Anyone establishing a behavior modification program will want to determine if, in fact, they are successful in modifying the behavior, and the best way to do this is to count the frequency of the behavior prior to beginning the program, and then to compare the frequency after the program has been in progress for a while.

Step 4. *Arrange the situation so as to maximize the probability of the desired response occurring.* Since the whole idea behind behavior modification is to wait for the desired behavior to occur and then reinforce it, it is important that the situation be arranged so that the desired response will occur as often as possible. If children never do what they are supposed to do, they will never be reinforced and no learning will occur. In dealing with children and adults who are only mildly retarded, this becomes a relatively trivial step, since one can simply tell the individual what the reinforcement contingencies are. One excellent way to expedite this is to draw up a contract with the subjects stating that if they do a certain behavior they will be entitled to a certain reinforcer, and that they agree not to ask for the privilege until they have performed the behavior. Thus, with Ronald, the contract would simply state that he would not be entitled to go out to the playground for recess unless he had completed 20 arithmetic problems, and both the teacher and Ronald would sign the contract.

In situations where one is trying to modify the behavior of a nonverbal child, it is often necessary to be a bit more clever in eliciting the desired behavior. One way that this can be accomplished is to get the child to imitate someone performing the response, a procedure known as modeling. Almost all children will imitate, and this is frequently an excellent method of getting children of very low mental age to do new things. For example, most programs which attempt to teach language behavior to retarded children usually teach the child to imitate the instructor as the first step.

Step 5. *Make the reinforcement contingent on the desired behavior.* Once these preliminary steps have been completed, the actual process of modifying the child's behavior can begin. This is done by observing the subjects' behavior closely and making sure that they get reinforced every time they perform the desired behavior. In the case of Ronald and his arithmetic problems, this is relatively simple since he will probably call attention to the fact that he has done the problems as soon as he finishes them.

Step 6. *Keep records.* Behaviorists are compulsive record keepers, but for good reason. It is very easy to determine how well a program is working if one has accurate records of the frequency of the desired behavior, and it is often quite difficult to assess how well the program is working if good records are not kept. It may seem like a waste of time to record on a graph or chart how many arithmetic problems Ronald works each day, but it certainly makes it a lot easier to determine whether there has been any improvement in his behavior. For one reason or another, many behavior modification programs do not work, and thus, it is necessary to change the program to improve performance.

Reducing the Frequency of Undesirable Behavior

The above procedure was appropriate for increasing the frequency of a desired behavior, but another common type of problem presented by most children at one time or another, particularly retarded children, is doing things that they should not be doing. Children engage in behavior that is dangerous to themselves or to others such as breaking windows or playing in the street. Many children also do things that are offensive or annoying to others. In working with retarded people, it is particularly important that such antisocial behavior be minimized since it will make it much more difficult for individuals to become a productive member of society if they have a number of annoying mannerisms. There are a number of different procedures that can be used to reduce the frequency of excessive behaviors.

1. *Extinction.* The easiest procedure, if it is possible, is simply to determine what is reinforcing the objectionable behavior and to remove this reinforcement. All too often, the reinforcer for objectionable behavior turns out to be attention from the child's parents, teacher, or other adults. Recall the example of the child who threw a temper tantrum and the mother reinforced the child's behavior so that the child began to have more and more tantrums. In this case, reducing the behavior is relatively simple, at least in

theory. If the child's mother can be instructed to ignore the child whenever a tantrum begins, the tantrums may actually become more severe for a while, but the child will soon learn that mother has caught on to the game and in the long run will throw fewer tantrums, just as the rat in the Skinner Box eventually stopped pressing the bar when the food dispenser jammed. In similar fashion, a child may be acting out in class in order to get attention from the teacher (being hollered at by an adult is reinforcing for some children). Thus, if the teacher is able to ignore the behavior, its frequency might decrease.

However, it is often the case that the trainer does not have control over the reinforcer of a particular behavior. Much of the misbehavior in classrooms is maintained not by the teacher's attention, but by the attention and laughter of the other students, and the teacher has little control over this. Other behaviors are simply self-reinforcing. Many children are excessively active simply because they enjoy running around, and they are not necessarily doing this to get attention. Other behavior may be maintained by attention from adults but is too severe to be ignored. If children bang their heads against a wall in order to get attention, ignoring it might eventually lead to extinction, but the children may have caused themselves tremendous harm in the meantime. In all of these cases, other procedures must be used.

2. *Train an incompatible response.* For example, a behavior that is incompatible with running around a classroom is sitting still in one's seat. If the teacher develops a program to increase the amount of time that children spend sitting in their seats, it follows logically that they will spend less time running around and disrupting others.

3. *Omission training.* Omission training is in some ways similar to training an incompatible response. In this case, the child is reinforced for *not* doing something. Suppose that an institutionalized child has the habit of rocking violently back and forth. While this behavior might be tolerated in an institutional setting, if this individual is ever released, such peculiar behavior could interfere with the individual's adjustment to the outside world. Extinction is not appropriate in eliminating most rocking behavior since it is self-reinforcing. However, suppose the individual enjoys smoking. Cigarettes can thus be used as an effective reinforcer to reduce rocking behavior if the individual is given a cigarette only after spending a certain amount of time during which the individual did not rock at all.

4. *Time out.* If children are in a situation that they enjoy such as a classroom (i.e., being there is reinforcing) if they are removed from this reinforcing situation when they are disruptive, the frequency of disruptive behavior

will decrease. For example, the teacher can send children to the coatroom or make them stand in the hall for a brief period. One danger of such a procedure is that for some children, the time out may act as a positive reinforcer, and in this case, the frequency of disruptive behavior will increase.

5. *Punishment.* A punisher is any event that reduces the frequency of the response that precedes it. The kinds of punishers usually used with retarded children are usually fairly mild ones such as a verbal reprimand, but occasionally, more severe punishers such as a slap or even mild electric shock or physical restraint have been used in behavior modification programs. The use of punishment has always been controversial, and most behavior modifiers use it sparingly. The occasional use of punishment has been responsible for a good deal of the bad reputation that behavior modification has in some quarters. Some people object to the use of punishment on ethical grounds. Others point out that punishment can be easily misused, especially by relatively untrained institutional staff. Still others argue that punishment should not be used because the results are unpredictable. Punishment may suppress all behavior or it may act as an example to produce aggressive behavior and it may produce unwanted emotional side effects.

However, many behavior modifiers argue that under certain circumstances, punishment can be an effective tool for bringing about desired behavior change, particularly in cases where a child has a behavior that is so disruptive that it precludes almost any other treatment or training. One of the most outspoken advocates of the use of punishment is Lovaas (1974). He described the case of a child who was so self-destructive that he had spent almost all of his life in restraint. Whenever he was untied, he would bang his face with his hands or bang his head against other things such as a bathtub. Lovaas untied him one day and he immediately started hitting himself, but this time, Lovaas gave him an electric shock. He hit himself a few more times, and each time Lovaas delivered another shock. Within a few minutes, the self-destructive behavior had entirely ceased. For the first time in many years, the boy fed himself and was given a bath and was allowed to roam around the room. Only after the self-destructive behavior was eliminated was it possible to begin a training program, and most people would agree that the benefit to the boy in the long run was greater than the temporary pain that he experienced from the shock.

The following is a list of guidelines that should govern the use of punishment in any kind of behavior modification program.

1. Punishment should only be used as a last resort when other methods such as extinction or reinforcing an incompatible behavior are inappropriate or have been shown to be ineffective.

2. The behavior that will be punished must be precisely defined.
3. Children must be aware of the circumstances for which they will be punished.
4. The punishment must be consistent. Every time that children perform the inappropriate behavior, they must be punished. Punishment should not be threatened but not carried out.
5. Children must have available alternative behaviors for which they will not be punished. A frequent abuse is punishing children for doing something over which they have little control, for example, spanking children for wetting their pants when they are not yet physiologically mature enough to control themselves.

Examples of Behavior Modification

Behavior modification in its various forms is now extremely widely used with the mentally retarded, and hundreds of reports of successful treatment using these techniques have been published. A classic example of the successful use of behavior modification to solve a severe behavior problem is described by Wolf, Risley, and Mees (1964). Their subject was a three and a half year old boy named Dicky. He presented a number of behavior problems including poorly developed social and verbal skills and severe tantrums. As is frequently the case with such children, Dicky had been seen by a number of different specialists and had been diagnosed as, among other things, mentally retarded, brain damaged, and psychotic. He had recently had an operation to remove cataracts from his eyes, and the physician told his parents that if he did not wear glasses regularly, he would become nearly blind. However, Dicky refused to wear his glasses and had broken several pairs.

The trainers tried the then relatively new technique of behavior modification to try to get Dicky to wear his glasses. Identifying a reinforcer was easy in this case, since they found that Dicky would respond readily to candy. Apparently wearing the glasses with full-strength lenses was particularly aversive, probably because it resulted in a drastic change in his visual preception, and as a result, they began by using frames without glass in them. At first, Dicky was reinforced simply for picking up and playing with the frames; then, by successive approximations, he was reinforced for bringing them closer to his eyes. However, Dicky balked at wearing even the empty frames correctly, and a number of weeks of training had failed to get him to wear his glasses correctly, even with the help of a special bar that went over his head and guided the ear pieces to their proper positions.

Since the candy reinforcement was no longer as effective, they started to use his regular meals as a reinforcement. For the first two meals of the day, he showed little interest, and thus, received little food. By midafternoon, he was particularly interested in ice cream, and this proved to be an excellent reinforcer. After a short while, Dicky was wearing his glasses for considerable periods of time, and he gradually became used to wearing them. Over the course of the next few weeks, he wore his glasses more and more until he could keep them on for most of the day, thus preventing further deterioration of his vision.

Repp and Dietz (1974) described the use of an omission training technique to reduce the frequency of severe aggressive and disruptive behavior in a number of mentally retarded children. For example, one of their cases was a profoundly retarded 12 year old who was consistently biting, hitting, scratching, and kicking other persons, and a training program was designed to reduce such behavior. After collecting baseline data in which it was clearly demonstrated that this behavior occurred at a high rate, the subject was reinforced with candy for periods of time in which he did not engage in such attack behavior. A timer was set to a prescribed number of minutes, and at the end of that time a bell sounded, and the boy was reinforced. If during that time he attacked someone, the timer was stopped and the boy was physically restrained for 30 seconds. Then the timer was reset. The time interval was originally very short, starting at 5 seconds, but was increased gradually so that by the twelfth session, the time interval was 15 minutes. Over the course of 17 sessions, the frequency of attack incidents dropped from the .19 incidents per minute observed during baseline to .01 incidents per minute. During the same period, an increase in the frequency of appropriate behavior was noted in this subject, although such behavior was not formally reinforced.

Neisworth and Smith (1973) described the case of a severely retarded woman who, when seated at a table with other people in a classroom, spent most of her time with her elbows together, her fists clenched over her ears, and her head bowed. If someone tried to force her to pay attention, she became violent and sometimes removed her clothes. A combination of extinction, time out, and positive reinforcement of appropriate social behavior was used to get her to increase the amount of time that she spent with her head up and attending. She was never given any attention for fussing or other undesirable behavior. Whenever she sat with her head down for more than 20 seconds, she was removed to a time-out room, and when she sat with her head up, paying attention, she was given praise and attention by the teacher. After 19 days of this treatment, she was paying attention for an average of 42 out of 45 minutes of a session, compared to an average of about 3 minutes prior to initiating the program.

Increasingly, behavior modifiers are focusing their attention on groups of subjects rather than on individual cases such as those described above. For example, a frequent problem with classes of trainable-level retarded children is their poor behavior in the school cafeteria. Neisworth and Smith (1973) described a program in which the cafeteria behavior of children was modified with the result that the general atmosphere of the cafeteria was improved. Three target behaviors were identified: (1) Children should use quiet, conversational voices when talking. (2) Children should stay seated until excused. (3) Children should line up quietly and wait for their teacher rather than running out of the cafeteria as they frequently did.

Before going to the cafeteria, each child was given three tokens in a plastic bag. The cafeteria was patrolled by volunteer parents who were instructed to take a token away from a child every time that child violated one of the three rules. As is customary with this type of program, children were not scolded or reminded of their infringement. A reinforcement menu was drawn up with the help of the children, and they could turn their tokens in either for privileges such as an opportunity to play on the monkey bars or for various toys. Each child kept a performance record on a chart in the classroom. The atmosphere of the cafeteria changed rapidly from one of chaos and noise to a quiet, pleasant place to eat lunch.

Abuses of Behavior Modification

Behavior modification methods such as those described above have been criticized on a number of grounds, and in fact, they have been declared to be illegal in some settings, primarily because some people feel that such methods interfere with the rights of the subjects to control their own behavior. Also, there have been a number of reports of abuses. May (1975) described some flagrant abuses of human rights which had been carried out in the name of behavior modification at a Florida institution for the mentally retarded. Adolescent boys had been forced to wear women's underwear, eat bars of soap, and masturbate in public as punishment for fighting and petty theft. In other cases, boys were beaten by attendants or locked in seclusion rooms for as long as four hours. One boy who had defecated in his pants had to hold his soiled underwear under his nose and rub his hands in it before washing the pants out. All of this had been done as a supposed behavior modification program.

Reports such as this one tend to give behavior modification a bad reputation, and, thus, any program using this technique must be extremely cautious that the clients' legal and moral rights are not being violated. One characteristic that seems to distinguish many of the most disreputable programs is the use of shame and public censure as a punishment. Such a practice only decreases the self esteem of the individual and often has little effect on the undesirable behavior. Aversive consequences should be used only rarely, and when they are used, it is far better to apply them quietly, with no hint of condemnation of the individual rather than to broadcast the punishment.

This section has provided only the sketchiest introduction to behavior modification. Subsequent chapters will describe some more specific ways that behavior modification has been used with the retarded to improve self-care, language, and academic skills. Readers who are interested in reading more about behavior modification have a tremendous number of books to choose from. Among the recent books that deal specifically with the mentally retarded are *Modifying Retarded Behavior* by Neisworth and Smith (1973), *Behavior Modification in Mental Retardation* by Gardner (1971), and a more recent book by the same author, *Children with Learning and Behavior Problems* (Gardner, 1974).

Drugs and the Mentally Retarded

In recent years, a large number of psychoactive drugs have been developed that have the effect of significantly reducing many of the most severe symptoms of psychosis and anxiety, and they have permitted large numbers of psychotic patients to be released from mental institutions to lead independent lives. While there are virtually no drugs that have been developed specifically for use with the retarded, an increasing number of retarded children and adults being placed on various psychoactive drugs in order to reduce the symptoms of emotional disturbance.

The best known of the psychoactive drugs are the tranquilizers. These are also known as antipsychotic drugs because they have the effect of reducing many of the symptoms of psychosis including extreme emotional reactions, anxiety, violent behavior, and hallucinations. However, they are also frequently used with patients who are not diagnosed as psychotic but who manifest various symptoms of emotional disturbance. The most widely used tranquilizer is chlorpromazine (Thorazine). Numerous studies have documented its effectiveness with severely disturbed patients, both retarded and nonretarded. For example, Bair and Herold (1955) administered the drug to some of the worst behavior and management problems in a state training school. Significant behavioral improvement was observed in some 90 percent of these subjects. Other frequently used drugs of the same type include trifluoperazine (Stelazine), which has been reported to bring out withdrawn patients as well as calming agitated patients, and thioridazine (Mellaril), which has been extensively studied with retarded children, all studies reporting positive results in reducing various symptoms (Freeman, 1970).

Another group of drugs is known as the minor tranquilizers because while they do not function as effective antipsychotic drugs, they have a calming effect and reduce anxiety. Included in this group are meprobamate, better known under its trade names as Miltown or Equanil, chlordiazepoxide (Librium), and diazepam (Valium).

There are also a number of psychoactive drugs other than tranquilizers that are frequently prescribed to retarded children and adults. Retarded people who are epileptic almost always receive some type of anticonvulsant drug such as Dilantin to control seizures. Hyperactive children frequently receive a stimulant such as Ritalin, which has the paradoxical effect of reducing activity in such children. The use of both of these drugs was discussed in Chapter 6.

There are several points that must be made regarding the use of psychoactive drugs with the retarded. The first is that drugs reduce the symptoms of behavioral disturbance, but they are not a cure. As soon as a person is taken off the drug, the symptoms are likely to reappear. A second consideration is that different people react quite differently to the same drug. A drug that is quite effective in reducing the symptoms of one individual may prove to be ineffective with another individual presenting similar problems. As a result, ideal dosages must be individually determined and continually monitored. Most psychoactive drugs are likely to produce a number of side effects in some people such as drowsiness, skin rash, blood disorders, jaundice, and tremors, and these further complicate the problem of determining an appropriate dosage. A third warning is that tranquilizers have not been shown to have any positive effect on mental abilities, despite the fact that many drug studies with the retarded have used IQ as one of the dependent variables (Sprague and Werry, 1971). For years, people have been searching for a drug that will have the effect of making people smarter. In the 1950s, considerable attention was focused on the drug glutamic acid that, it was claimed, had the specific effect of raising IQ. While some early research tended to confirm this, later, better controlled studies found it to be ineffective (Astin and Ross, 1960), and it is no longer used.

It is easy for drugs such as tranquilizers to be abused, and it is sometimes claimed that too many people, particularly institutionalized people, are on excessive dosages with the result that they are in a sort of chemical straitjacket, spending much of their lives in a semiconscious state in order to prevent them from causing trouble. Evidence for this comes from a survey by Lipman (1967) who reported that most public institutions for the retarded used large quantities of tranquilizers, particularly Thorazine and Mellaril, and that many residents had been on extraordinarily large doses for long periods of time.

Excellent reviews of the research on the use of drugs with the mentally retarded can be found in Freeman (1970) and Sprague and Werry (1971).

Summary

There are three basic ways of treating behavioral and emotional problems with the mentally retarded: psychotherapy, behavior modification, and chemotherapy.

Psychotherapy refers to any one of a variety of techniques and methods that have in common the fact that the client expresses feelings, emotions, and attitudes to a sympathetic listener or group of listeners. Psychotherapy is occasionally done with retarded people, although its value has never been clearly demonstrated, and many pioneers in psychotherapy, including Freud and Carl Rogers, have indicated that psychotherapy with the mentally retarded would be ineffective. Relative to most therapy, therapy with the retarded is likely to be more directive, with the therapist or group leader taking a more active role in the course of the session. It is also more likely to be done in groups rather than on an individual basis, and it is more likely to be oriented toward adjustment problems rather than toward the feelings of the client. Because many retarded people are not very verbal, such nonverbal therapy techniques as play therapy and creative arts therapy are particularly likely to be used with retarded people.

A second way of treating disturbed behavior is with behavior modification, also called behavior therapy, a method of treatment that has developed from basic learning principles. Advocates of this approach focus entirely on the observable behavior of the child, with little attempt to postulate inner motivations or other nonobservable, mentalistic concepts to explain the behavior. They assume the most human behavior can be explained by the rewards and punishments in the individual's environment. If individuals are rewarded (reinforced) for performing a behavior, they are likely to repeat it, and if they are not reinforced, he is less likely to repeat the behavior again. Therefore, in order to encourage retarded children to engage in more socially appropriate behavior, it is necessary to arrange their environment so that they will be reinforced for such behavior. If an individual is doing things that are disruptive, destructive, or annoying to other people, the frequency of such behavior can be reduced by extinguishing the behavior, that is, assuring that it is not reinforced, by reinforcing an incompatible response, by removing the child from the classroom—a procedure known as time out—or by punishing the behavior. Behavior modification has been quite successful in incorporating more socially appropriate behavior in mentally retarded children and adults and, as a result, is quite widely used.

Another effective way of treating emotional problems is with psychoactive drugs, particularly tranquilizers, that reduce the frequency and severity of psychotic symptoms, anxiety, and disturbed behavior. However, they are ineffective in raising intelligence, and the charge has been leveled that such drugs are overused with institutionalized retarded people.

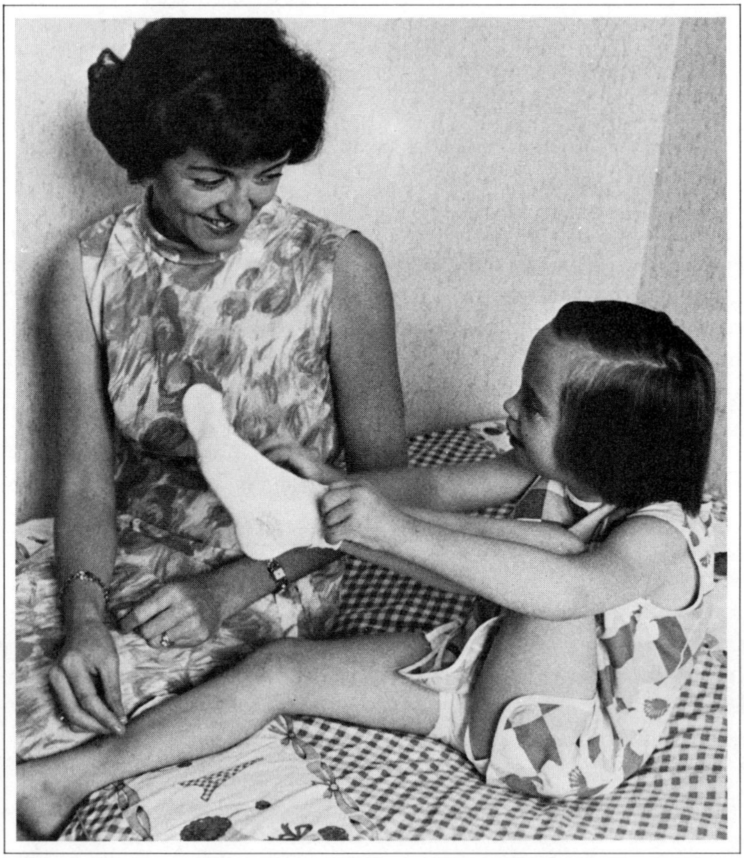

13

The Family of the Retarded Child

Much of the writing on mental retardation focuses entirely on the problems faced by the retarded individual and ignores the very different but just as serious problems faced by the parents and siblings of a retarded child. Anything that happens to the retarded child, any services that are provided or denied, will also effect the immediate family unit, and conversely, the dynamics of the child's family must be taken into account whenever a plan of treatment or management is considered. There is a growing trend in the mental health field to consider the client to be not just the retarded child alone, but the client's entire family, and there is an accompanying tendency to provide services on a family basis rather than simply to the one individual presenting problems.

This is a positive trend in many respects, but it also carries with it the negative side effect of treating the entire family as if there is something wrong with them. One of the complaints of many parents of retarded children is that psychologists, psychiatrists, physicians, and social workers often seem to assume that any parent of a retarded child has psychological reactions which need treatment. In a sense, it is automatically assumed that the family is sick and requires help, whether this help was sought or not (Wortis, 1972).

This tendency is magnified by most of the writing on the families of retarded children. Most of what has been written emphasizes the negative and pathological effects of the retarded child on the family. The parents are described as an anxious and guilt-ridden lot who are too engulfed in self-pity and defenses to adequately raise their child. The fact that much of the family dynamics are unaffected by the retarded child and that many families are able to effect a very positive adjustment is minimized.

Before reviewing this work, several notes of caution must be made. First, remember that the parents of retarded children are people, and people differ. Some parents are healthy, well-adjusted, and functioning at an effective level, while others may be poorly adjusted, neurotic, or psychotic even prior to the birth of their retarded child, and obviously, their reactions to their retarded child are going to be colored by their own personality and attitudes. Second, while a great deal has been written about parental reactions, most of it is based on casual observation of isolated cases and falls into the category of speculation rather than fact. There is very little good research to substantiate these speculations, and what research there is is as likely to contradict these speculations as it is to substantiate them. Third, almost everything that has been written about the parents of retarded children is based primarily on observations of middle-class mothers of more severely retarded children, particularly those who bring their children to outpatient clinics that provide services to retarded children and their families (Wolfensberger, 1967). This is far from a representative sample since the majority of retarded children come from lower-income groups and are only mildly retarded. It is probably the case that the reaction of a low-income parent of a mildly retarded child to the diagnosis of mental retardation is quite different from the reaction of a middle-income parent of a severely retarded child. In the first place, mildly retarded children tend to be diagnosed as retarded by the schools rather than by medical personnel, and many low-income parents have little understanding of the functioning of the educational system and a little faith in their local school system. These parents are less likely to take the diagnosis seriously since the discrepancy in behavior between the child labeled retarded and other children not so labeled is not very great. Thus, most of what is discussed below applies almost entirely to the families of more severely retarded children.

Impact on the Parents

Virtually all parents react with extreme shock and disappointment to the news that their child is mentally retarded. Menolascino (1967) and Wolfensberger (1967) have suggested that there are three kinds of crises that are precipitated by this news, in other words, three reasons why parents might react with such extreme emotions. The first of these is a novelty crisis. A novelty crisis is one that results from a major unanticipated change in one's life and one's conception of oneself. Thus, this is not a reaction to the retardation per se, but to the abrupt change in one's circumstances. The second type of crisis is a crisis of personal values. Most people have been reared with the idea that competence and achievement should be valued. Thus, when it suddenly becomes necessary for parents to love someone who has few of these desirable traits, the parent is put in a conflict situation and a good deal of stress can result. The third type of crisis is a reality crisis. This stems from the fact that there are a number of very concrete concerns that face the parents of a handicapped child, financial worries, limitations on their ability to take vacations, the extra time involved in caring for such a child, and so on.

These three crises, the novelty crisis, the value crisis, and the reality crisis will provide a basic outline for a discussion of parental reactions to their child's retardation.

The Initial Shock and the Novelty Crisis

The novelty crisis results from a sudden change in the parents' conception of themselves and their family and their future. Almost all parents have great plans and expectations for their children; they look forward to watching them taking their first steps, speaking their first words, getting all As in school, going to college, and being elected president. All parents seem to assume that their child will be the smartest, cutest, and best-behaved child in the neighborhood. With these expectations, it is not difficult to imagine the extreme shock and disappointment that almost all parents experience when they are told that not only will their child not grow up to be president, but may not even be able to be self-sufficient. In the words of one parent "It's like someone came to you and told you that your child was dead." (Waskowitz, 1959). All of the hopes and dreams of the parents are shattered, and the parents have to begin to rebuild their world in the light of this tragic news.

Naturally, the severity of the initial emotional reaction varies widely from one set of parents to another. Some parents are naturally calm and unemotional, and they accept the fact that their child is retarded with little outward expression of feeling. Other people who are naturally emotional may overreact in such a situation, irrationally blaming oneself or blaming others.

One important determinant of the reaction of the parents is the circumstances in which they learn that their child is retarded. The majority of the cases of Down's syndrome are diagnosed at birth or very shortly afterward, and thus, many of the most severe reactions occur at this time because the parents have had little prior warning that anything was wrong. In addition, the time of birth is generally an emotional period for the parents anyway. However, most other retardation is not diagnosed, or even suspected at birth, and the diagnosis is made at some later time, usually based on the child's slow motor development or the fact that the child did not learn to talk at the appropriate time. In many of these cases, the parents had begun to suspect that something was wrong prior to the diagnosis being confirmed. This process of gradual discovery could have the effect of reducing the emotional reaction, although often the thought of mental retardation does not occur to parents until it is suggested by the family doctor or pediatrician.

Obviously, how the doctor breaks the news to the parents is another important determinant of the extent of the novelty crisis. One complaint that a great many parents of handicapped children have is that they have been badly treated by professionals, and many of the complaints center around the callous manner in which they were first informed of their child's handicap. There are numerous reports of physicians determining that the child was retarded, but not telling the parents (Waskowitz, 1959; Zwerling, 1954). Other physicians have been very abrupt, or have seemed disinterested, or have emphasized the negative side of retardation, saying that the child will never be able to do anything and ought to be institutionalized. The following story is typical:

> *I first became worried about the child when at the age of 2½ he still did not talk. I was referred to the children's department of a London teaching hospital, where I saw a consultant physician, who in the space of not more than a few minutes, and in the presence of a group of students, informed me quite bluntly that the child was mentally defective. He added that it was pointless for me to be burdened with him and that he would arrange for his removal to an institution, although this would take some time because of the long waiting list. I picked up the child in my arms, and quite unable to utter a word, I left the hospital. To this day, I do not remember how I got home; the shock was so great that I had complete amnesia for about three hours (Tizard and Grad, 1961).*

The authors who related this account interviewed 80 mothers who had children with Down's syndrome to determine the circumstances under which they first learned of their child's condition. Only 7 parents were told when the physician first suspected mental retardation, and only 11 more were told when the diagnosis was confirmed. Twenty-eight of the doctors told the parents at some later time, and 29 physicians never told the parents at all, leaving them to find out for themselves that their child was retarded. Virtually all of the mothers interviewed agreed that the physician ought to tell a parent as soon as mental retardation was suspected rather than putting it off.

One reasons for this unfortunate situation is that many physicians feel uncomfortable about the subject of retardation. Most physicians have had little experience with retarded children and have no idea how to treat them.

Olshansky and his associates (Olshansky, Johnson, and Sternfield, 1964; Olshansky and Kettell, 1963), in a survey of physicians, found that many regarded a mongoloid child as totally unchanging and helpless. As recently as the 1960s, 40 percent of the general practitioners surveyed felt that immediate institutionalization was the appropriate recommendation for parents of retarded children, and only a small percentage felt that the decision to institutionalize the child was the responsibility of the parents rather than of the physician. Nearly half of the general practitioners had never heard of the local retardation clinic, and only a small percentage had accurate information about it. A great many physicians seem to hold the old stereotypes that a retarded child is hopeless.

In defense of the medical profession, however, it should be pointed out that much of the animosity that parents feel toward professionals is certainly due to the fact that they are the ones who have to inform the parents of the bad news, and messengers of bad news have often been scapegoats. Undoubtedly, many parents blame the doctor because the doctor is unable to help their child, and others blame the doctor irrationally as a result of their frustration and hostility toward the child.

The Crisis in Personal Values

The novelty crisis is short lived, but after the parents have overcome the initial shock, they begin to face other stresses. The value crisis comes about because the parents are in a situation of conflicting values. Virtually all parents have been socialized to the idea that they must love, cherish, and protect their child no matter how the child turns out. It is a rare mother who is able to admit, even to herself, that she sometimes dislikes her children and regrets having them. On the other hand, the child that they are obligated to love is often not very lovable, at least according to traditional values. Instead of being bright and alert and clever and amusing as most normal children are, their child, in addition to being very slow, may be physically unattractive and may be a major behavior problem as well. The whole concept of mental retardation is unacceptable to some people. Many parents are never able to fully accomplish this value shift, and as a result, they harbor ambivalent feelings toward their retarded child. On the one hand, they love the child because the child is theirs, but, on the other hand, they reject the child because of the retardation.

There are several characteristic responses to this ambivalence. Some of these reactions are indications of poor adjustment, such as excessive guilt or sorrow or the overuse of defense mechanisms such as denial or overprotectiveness. On the other hand, many parents are able to resolve their conflict and fully accept their child for what the child is.

Guilt. The parental reaction mentioned by the largest number of writers is guilt (Wolfensberger, 1967). Guilt, and the accompanying emotion of shame, is the feeling that one experiences when one has done something wrong. These feelings of guilt and shame are quite irrational in the case of giving birth to a retarded child. With rare exception, the retardation did not arise from anything that the parents did, and except in the case of Down's syndrome and a few other well-defined disorders, the cause of the child's retardation is unknown. Nevertheless, it seems to be a natural human tendency to attempt to provide explanations for purely random events, particularly events perceived as disasters such as the birth of a retarded child. Thus, the first question which many parents ask is "Why did this happen to me?" Even though there is usually no satisfactory answer to this, a surprising number of parents view their retarded child as some sort of punishment from God for past misdeeds (Kramm, 1963). Some parents believe that the child's retardation was caused by their past sexual misconduct or some other similar sin. This guilt reaction may be particularly strong if the retarded child was not wanted, or it can be magnified by the obsolete notion that most retardation results from genetic causes, implying that the birth of a retarded child is a sign of tainted stock.

Many parents feel guilty not about having a retarded child but about their own reactions toward their retarded child. A parent who is having difficulty working out this conflict in values and occasionally feels resentment toward or gets angry at the child may feel extremely guilty about experiencing such strong negative emotions toward a helpless individual. Actually, all parents probably dislike their children at one time or another, and it is probably better for all concerned if they can recognize that this is a normal reaction and not something to be ashamed of.

One of the overt symptoms of shame and guilt is that the parents seldom discuss their child's retardation either among themselves or with neighbors and relatives. Kramm (1963) in interviewing parents of children with Down's syndrome, found a number of families where the husband and wife never discussed the child because of the intense emotions involved. As an extreme example of such behavior, in earlier times, it was customary for families to institutionalize a retarded child and to tell other people that the child had died.

Denial. A second common reaction of parents to the discovery that their child is retarded is the defense mechanism of denial. This denial takes many forms. One relatively harmless version is referring to one's son or daughter as a slow learner, or even brain damaged or autistic rather than mentally retarded. Apparently, the label of mental retardation has more negative associations than do the other labels. A more serious type of denial is the refusal to admit that their child's condition is probably incurable and that the child will probably never be self-sufficient. A classic manifestation of this is going from one specialist to another trying to get a more precise diagnosis or searching for some kind of miracle cure. Krush (1964) described a case of parents who had contacted a total of 18 physicians, four teachers, a chiropractor, two hospitals, two clinics, and seven schools, all in search of a "magic key" that would restore their severely retarded boy to normalcy. While seeking a second opinion from another physician is a reasonable thing to do, bringing one's child to a large number of different doctors, hoping that one will make a more optimistic diagnosis or have access to some kind of miracle cure is clearly an irrational strategy and is a demonstration of the parents' inability to face reality. The extreme form of denial is simply not to admit that one's child is in any way different from normal children. Such parents persist in believing that their child will grow up to be a competent adult, able to go to college and become a professional or take over the family business.

Overprotectiveness. Another frequently described pattern of parental behavior is overprotectiveness (Maloney, 1958). Some parents, usually mothers, devote all of their time to their retarded child to the exclusion of their other children and their spouse. They consistently treat the child as if the child were less capable than he or she is. For example, such a mother may continue to dress the child after the child is able to dress himself or herself. Such parents never let their child out of their sight, and they give up all of their social life and all of their other interests to care for their poor retarded child. One interpretation of this behavior is that it is a type of reaction formation. Reaction formation is a defense mechanism in which one denies an unacceptable impulse by emphasizing its opposite. Thus, the mother appears to be saying "See how much I love my retarded child. I am sacrificing everything for him," but in fact the mother is trying to hide both from herself and from others the fact that she unconsciously dislikes and resents the child. Such an admission would be too painful and so she emphasizes the opposite.

Sorrow. Olshansky (1962) has speculated that almost all parents who have a retarded child suffer chronic sorrow throughout their lives. The extent of this sorrow may differ from one parent to another, but most will manifest this to some degree. He emphasized that this sorrow was in no way a neurotic reaction but is a perfectly natural and normal response, although many parents will try to hide their depression and sorrow in public. Other writers of a psychoanalytic orientation (e.g., Solnit and Stark, 1961) have postulated similar reactions, such as grief and mourning. They are suggesting that in a sense the reaction of a parent to the knowledge that their child is retarded is similar to the reaction of a parent who loses a child through death.

Acceptance. It is unfortunate that much of what has been written about parental reactions to having a handicapped child stresses the negative aspects of the coping process, the guilt, the developing of irrational defense mechanisms, and the like. While it is certainly the case that many parents do resort to various maladaptive behaviors at one time or another, the more positive processes of acceptance and adjustment tend to be deemphasized. Many parents are able to successfully resolve their crisis in values and accept their retarded child for what the child is. The word acceptance is often used to describe what is considered to be a healthy response to the fact that one's child is retarded. This process of acceptance involves a number of characteristics:

1. The accepting parent is able to accurately perceive the child's abilities and his potential, being fully aware of both his weaknesses and his strengths.
2. The accepting parent is able to view the child's retardation realistically, recognizing that it is sometimes an inconvenience for the family but not becoming so overwhelmed with self-pity or sorrow or guilt that the functioning of the family is impaired. Such parents should be able to discuss their retarded child freely, both among themselves and with neighbors and relatives without feelings of shame.
3. The accepting parent should attempt to provide the best possible medical, educational, and recreational services available within their means without neurotically searching for a miracle cure.
4. The accepting parent is able to provide the retarded child with as much love as is provided for other children, not rejecting the child, but not overloving the child either, not smothering the child with so much love that the child fails to develop independence. The accepting parent should not devote so much time and attention to the retarded child that the parent neglects the other children and spouse.

This concept of acceptance involves striking a balance between recognizing the child's disabilities and making compensation for them but not permitting the handicap to completely dominate family interactions. Obviously, judging whether a family has reached this level is entirely subjective, and thus, it is impossible to say what percentage of parents have accomplished this. However, there are certainly many families for whom having a retarded child is not viewed as the enormous tragedy that it is widely believed to be.

It is important to remember that such a value crisis is only an important source of stress for parents who place high value on success and achievement. In less competitive cultures where a place can be found for almost everyone regardless of competence, retardation is not considered to be the tragedy that it is among achievement-oriented middle-class Americans. For example, Eaton and Weil (1955) describe the Hutterite culture, a communal religious sect in the Midwest, where there is no emphasis on competition and achievement, and they report that among these people, retardation is not considered to be a tragedy at all.

The Reality Crisis

At the same time that parents of a handicapped child are forced to deal with these ambivalent feelings brought about by conflicting values, they must also face a number of more concrete concerns. The first of these is financial. Many retarded children have medical problems that require treatment, and unless these complications are covered under medical insurance, they can create a major financial drain. (Many medical insurance policies explicitly exclude coverage of congenital medical problems.) In addition to medical problems, it was the case until recently that many parents were obligated to find private training and education for their retarded child since many moderately and severely retarded children were excluded from the public schools. Other realistic concerns of parents include the way that relatives and neighbors will accept the child. Even though the parents themselves are often able to make a satisfactory adjustment to their child's retardation, the child's grandparents or other relatives may reject the child. There are many cases of grandparents refusing to come to visit a retarded child or not sending a present for the child's birthday as they do for other grandchildren. In addition, neighbors may shun the family. All of these attitudes stem from superstition and ignorance, but nonetheless persist even today, although probably to a lesser degree than was true in the past. Parents are also legitimately concerned about the effect of the retarded child on their own lifestyle. Will the child somehow restrict their ability to take vacations or go out socially? Many parents of retarded children report difficulty in finding a sitter, particularly if the child is a behavior problem as well as being retarded. Finally, there is concern about the long-term care of the child. What will happen to the child after the parents are no longer able to provide proper care. Most parents are familiar with the poor quality of the care provided in many of the traditional state institutions and legitimately fear that their child will have to be placed in such a location.

There have been several research projects investigating the impact of a retarded child on the day-to-day functioning of the family. Some of these studies emphasize the disruptive influence that a retarded child presents while others emphasize the more positive coping of the child's family. However, none of this research has actually compared the functioning of families of retarded children to comparable families without a handicapped child, and thus, the conclusions are only suggestive.

Holt (1958), in one of the most thorough research projects on the families of retarded children, painted a very negative picture. He interviewed 201 sets of parents in England to determine how the presence of a retarded child in the family affected them. Almost all of the parents stated that the retarded child required more care than did the nonretarded siblings, but some children were particularly troublesome. Fourteen of the children were so profoundly handicapped that they required total nursing care. These children were unable to walk or feed themselves and were not toilet trained, and thus, the mother had to provide continuous care, which was a tremendous strain. Another 63 of the 201 children were sufficiently destructive, aggressive, or hyperactive that they required constant supervision. In many cases, the mother could not even go to the bathroom without the risk that the child would do something dangerous or destructive. Thirty-one of the retarded children required attention at night, which meant that the parents, particularly the mothers, never got a full night's sleep. Many of the mothers never left their child. In 40 percent of the families, the husband and wife never went out together because of the problems associated with their child. Some mothers could not even go shopping because their child was too active; the child could neither be left at home nor brought to the store. In addition, many of the parents complained about the expenses associated with raising a retarded child.

A large number of the mothers showed signs of this tremendous strain. They were in poor health, continually exhausted, and showed other signs of stress. Several required hospitalization for these symptoms and two had threatened suicide. Many of the families were characterized by an unusual amount of quarreling as a reaction to the tension, and others complained of social isolation, in some cases because they had been rejected by their neighbors. The authors reported that not one of the families had made a full emotional adjustment to the problems.

Several other studies have found results basically similar to those of Holt (Tizard and Grad, 1961; Schonell and Watts, 1956) but a far more positive picture was described by Barsch (1968). He interviewed 177 parents of handicapped children in Milwaukee. Note that this research included all kinds of handicapped children, blind, deaf, and cerebral palsied as well as mongoloid and brain-damaged children, but he found few differences between the parents of retarded children and the parents of children with other kinds of handicaps. He interviewed the parents on a wide variety of attitudes and behaviors, and his general conclusion was that, with exceptions, having a handicapped child did not seem to produce major changes in outlook, attitudes, or child-rearing practices. He failed to substantiate some of the assumptions about these parents stated above. For example, while a few of the parents had gone to four or five different physicians in an attempt to obtain an accurate diagnosis, most had only gone to one or two. Of the Down's syndrome group, only 16 percent had gone to four or more different physicians. The one exception to this was the group diagnosed as brain damaged (not all of these children were mentally retarded). Because of the difficulty in diagnosis, these parents had a tendency to seek a wider variety of medical opinions.

Most of the parents reported that their child-rearing practices with the handicapped child were not very different from those used with their nonhandicapped children. They were not more lax with discipline or more overprotective, and they did not make more restrictions on these children than they had made on other children. Although this conclusion could be questioned because it is based on what the parent reported in an interview rather than on actually observing the parents' behavior, it is certainly necessary to reconsider the widely held belief that parents are more overprotective of handicapped children. Another widely held belief that parents of handicapped children are likely to become social isolates, seldom going out, not talking with neighbors, and so on, was also contradicted. Most of the parents reported that the handicapped child made few restrictions on their social life, and many of the parents were active members of various community organizations. Most of the mothers reported that they talked openly with neighbors about their handicapped child, and there was little indication of guilt or shame.

Because of the discrepancies between these studies, it is difficult to draw many firm conclusions beyond the fact that some parents are able to adapt to having a retarded child with few disruptions, while for other families, the presence of a retarded child is a major disruptive influence.

Having a retarded child is probably less traumatic now than it was in the past. There are several reasons for this. In the first place, the stigma of having a retarded child is gradually disappearing. People are less likely to see a retarded child as an indication of "tainted stock" or as a punishment from God. Second, each year more and better services are being made available to these families. Complete diagnostic services are now available in many communities and counseling is usually a possibility for most parents who desire it. Many communities are providing day care or nursery school services as well as a regular school program for even the most severely handicapped, and as a result, few parents are forced to put up with an extremely disruptive child for 24 hours a day every day. In some cases, homemaker services are available to help harried mothers. Various government agencies are taking care of an increasing proportion of the financial burden, thus taking a major strain off many families. If all of these trends continue, much of what has been written about the strains imposed on a family by a retarded child might be obsolete in a few years.

Determinants of Parental Reactions

Parents differ widely in their reactions and their attitudes toward their retarded child, and it is worthwhile to consider why some parents react well and others badly.

One variable that seems to be important is the socioeconomic status of the parents. It is reasonable to assume that middle-class parents might tend to react somewhat differently to a retarded child than would a low-income family. Farber (1972) has proposed that there are two kinds of crises that can be precipitated by a retarded child in the family, and that one is more typical of low-income families while the other tends to characterize middle-class families. A *tragic crisis* is one in which the aims, aspirations, and the anticipation of a happy family life are frustrated. This is similar to the value crisis described above because the parents' expectations for themselves and their child are blocked. A tragic crisis is more typical of middle-class, achievement-oriented families who tend to have high aspirations for their children. The second type of crisis is the *role organization crisis.* In this case, the parents are more concerned with the day-to-day problems imposed by the retarded child. This crisis is more typical of low-income groups. Such parents are too overwhelmed by daily events and crises to be very concerned with the long-term development of their children. This is roughly similar to the reality crisis proposed by Wolfensberger (1967) because the parents are very wrapped up in the financial problems of the retarded child, obtaining proper medical and educational services and the like. In other words, the difference between the lower-income family's response and the response of the middle-income family is that the former is more concerned with the present, the here-and-now problems, while the latter, being more able to cope with the daily problems, becomes concerned about the future. A major research project by Farber and his associates has tended to substantiate this hypothesis.

One characteristic that is clearly related to the parents' acceptance of their retarded child is their understanding of the nature of mental retardation (Stone, 1967). Parents who have an accurate comprehension of what causes retardation, particularly the cause of the retardation in their own child, are far less likely to manifest feelings of guilt and shame and are less likely to use defenses such as denial. It follows from this that an important principle of counseling these parents is to provide them with as much information about mental retardation as they can readily absorb.

Perhaps the single most important determinant of parental reaction toward their retarded child is the parents' own level of adjustment. Parents who prior to the birth of the retarded child are functioning at an effective level, who are relatively free of defenses, and whose marriage is stable will tend to have few problems with acceptance. On the other hand, parents who were having difficulty coping with their lives and who had tendencies toward pathological symptoms prior to the birth of the child will probably continue to have difficulties with coping and are likely to use irrational defenses such as denial. It has been suggested (Hastings, 1948) that the presence of a retarded child does not generate new problems in family integration but only magnifies already existing problems.

Brothers and Sisters of Retarded Children

One of the concerns of many parents is that their other children, the brothers and sisters of the retarded child, will be harmed in some way by the presence of the retarded child in the home, and this is occasionally given as an excuse to institutionalize the child. Fortunately, there is little evidence to substantiate these concerns. Most siblings of retarded children claim that there are few adverse effects (Graliker, Fishler, and Koch, 1962), and there also does not seem to be a greater prevalence of adjustment problems among the siblings of retarded children than would be expected in any group of comparable children (Schipper, 1959).

Naturally, there are occasional practical problems. A sibling, usually a sister, may be called on to help care for the retarded child, and this can interfere with her social life. Occasionally, children are so ashamed of the retarded brother or sister that they refuse to bring friends home. However, such a reaction of shame is almost always learned from the parents. The siblings, unless they are much older than the retarded child, have no opportunity to experience a novelty crisis or a value crisis; as far as they are concerned, having a retarded brother or sister is not at all unusual. However, even small children pick up the attitudes of the parents, and if the parents seldom talk about the retarded child and seem to be ashamed, then the normal siblings are likely to acquire the same attitudes.

One study of the siblings of retarded children deserves special attention. Grossman (1972) extensively interviewed a large number of college students who had a retarded brother or sister in order to determine their reactions, and there were a number of interesting findings. Consistent with other research, the ability of the normal sibling to adapt to having a retarded child in the family seemed to be closely related to how well the parents accepted the problem as well as how openly the parents discussed the retarded child. However, although there were a wide variety of different reactions reported, there was no significant difference in the overall level of adjustment to college between the siblings of retarded children and a control group of college students who had no handicapped people in the family.

A number of the students expressed a frank dislike of their retarded brother or sister, but a comparable number expressed strong positive feelings. One of the most impressive findings was that 45 percent of those interviewed felt that they had benefited from having a retarded child in the family. They felt that they had a greater understanding of people and were more tolerant of them, that they had more compassion and were more sensitive to prejudice, and that they had a greater appreciation of their own good health and intelligence. Some also felt that the experience had drawn the family closer together.

However, an equal number felt that they had been harmed by the experience. They expressed feelings of guilt and shame, in particular, a sense of guilt for being in good health. They also felt guilty about harboring negative feelings toward their retarded sibling, and several resented the fact that their parents had had to devote so much attention to the retarded child that they felt that the normal children had been slighted.

One of the concerns expressed by many of the group was the fact that they felt that they had to avoid identifying with their retarded brother or sister. That is, they had to emphasize the fact that they were not like the retarded sibling. Related to this, there seemed to be much more embarrassment and shame if the retarded child was the same sex as the college student than if it were of the opposite sex. They also reported more difficulties with adjustment when the retarded sibling was older than when the sibling was younger.

Counseling Parents of the Retarded

With all of the various types of problems facing parents of mentally retarded children, it is not surprising that many of them seek some sort of counseling with their problems, both practical and emotional. As a result, counseling with the parents of retarded children is a rapidly growing service. However, the term counseling refers to so many different kinds of services that it has lost whatever meaning it once had. On the one hand, it can refer to a single session with a family doctor in which the doctor explains the results and prognosis of a diagnostic study and tries to calm their worst fears. On the other hand, it can refer to a long series of sessions with a psychiatrist, psychologist, counselor, social worker, or psychiatric nurse in which the parents discuss their deepest feelings toward themselves and toward their retarded child. Group counseling overlaps with other activities of parent groups such as parent seminars and educational groups.

Wolfensberger (1967), in reviewing the research on parental counseling, noted a trend away from single interview, "one shot" counseling with the parents at the time that they first hear that their child is retarded. It is now recognized that the impact of a retarded child on the family unit is an ongoing thing. Certainly, parents may need counseling at the time when the diagnosis of retardation is first confirmed, but many parents are too distraught at that time to absorb much information or effectively face their feelings. As a result, a number of sessions, perhaps spread out over a considerable length of time, may be required in order to assist parents in working out their feelings and recognizing the ramifications of their child's problems. In addition, as the child develops, new types of crises are continually presenting themselves. When the retarded child first goes to school, the family is faced with a host of new problems (as well as releasing the mother from old problems). The child may be teased by the other children or the parents may not feel that the program in which the child is placed is appropriate for him or there may not be an appropriate program available at all. Any other family crisis is likely to be magnified by the presence of a retarded child, and crises faced by all families, such as the breadwinner being laid off or a member of the family becoming very sick or the family moving to a new community can be made much worse if there is also a retarded child who requires special attention. Similarly, when retarded children leave school, a whole new set of problems present themselves; where can they get a job, or if they can't get a job immediately, what should they do with their time? Is it best for the child to continue living with the parents or should some other kind of placement be sought? In all of these situations, the parents are likely to want to seek guidance and advice, and as a result, whoever does the initial counseling with the family should encourage the parents to seek help whenever they feel that they need it, and they should be informed that such help is always available.

Counseling endeavors can be distinguished on the extent to which they are primarily educational in function versus the extent to which they are concerned with the client's attitudes and feelings. Counseling at the latter end of this continuum resembles psychotherapy, in that discussion of day-to-day reality problems is discouraged in favor of considering the parents' deeper feelings, not only toward their retarded child, but also toward themselves and their marriages and their lives. (e.g., Cummings and Stock, 1962). The goal in such counseling is to make the parent more aware of his or her defenses and anxieties. At the opposite extreme is counseling whose primary function is to increase the parent's knowledge about mental retardation, of the causes and probable prognosis of the retardation in their own child, and of specific management techniques. Such counseling borders on education. Obviously, most counseling is not at one extreme or the other, but addresses itself to some extent to both practical and emotional problems.

Wolfensberger (1967) has noted a distinct conflict between parents and professionals regarding the aim of counseling, parents being more interested in the solution to practical, everyday problems such as what is the best way to toilet train my child or what day care facilities are available or am I disciplining my child enough. Professionals, on the other hand, are more interested in focusing in on the parents' feelings. This difference in outlook is one source of parental dissatisfaction with professionals, and is often a barrier to effective counseling.

Most of the principles of counseling parents of the retarded are the same as they are for any other type of counseling. Roos (1963) has listed a number of guidelines for counselors. The most important of these is that the parents be treated with acceptance and respect. By doing this, the counselor is able to help them to overcome their feelings of shame and the loss of self-worth which are common among these people. The parent must be led to realize that having a retarded child is nothing to be ashamed of and that the child in no way reflects poorly on them. Second, the counselor must also permit total freedom in the expression of emotions. In ordinary social interactions, people are expected to save face and not allow their feelings to show themselves, and many parents need a place where they can express their feelings to a sympathetic listener. By expressing these feelings, not only does the parent feel better, but he or she can learn to realize that these feelings are perfectly normal and are not to be condemned, even though they are not usually permitted to express them in public.

A third principle is to let the parents make decisions for themselves. They are the ones who will have to live with the child, and they are the ones who ought to make the decisions regarding the child's welfare. An important function of the counselor is to outline the various options that are available to the parents with the advantages and disadvantages of each, but the final decision should be left to the parents. Related principles are that the counselor should not assume an authoritarian role and must let the parent determine the direction of the interview. The parents know what is bothering them, and any preconceived notions that the counselor may have about the parents of the retarded are likely to be wrong. If this means that most of the discussion is centered on practical questions rather than on feelings, the counselor should accept this.

A fourth principle of counseling is that the counselor must be honest. The counselor should not attempt to mislead or encourage the parents by presenting an overly optimistic picture of the child's potential because such a strategy can only lead to frustration later on. Similarly, the counselor should not pretend to be more knowledgeable than he or she is. If the counselor is not able to answer a question, he or she should say that he or she doesn't know rather than try to fake an answer.

Group Counseling

Parents who seek professional support for their problems are far more likely to find themselves in a group setting rather than meeting individually with the counselor. The reasons for this are not only economic—the counselor's time is used more efficiently, but also the parents are able to benefit from the experiences of other parents. They see that there are other families with problems as difficult or worse than their own, and this frequently gives them a new perspective on their own problems.

There is no single best approach to group counseling; it is probably safer to say that there are as many different techniques as there are people doing counseling. Ramsey (1967), in reviewing a number of published studies, found that the number of members in a group ranged from 3 to 36, although most had around 10. The purposes ranged from strictly educational, where the parents were primarily listeners rather than discussants, to the informal and unstructured groups where the emphasis was almost entirely on feelings rather than on practical problems. The number of sessions ranged from 3 to 63, and the group leaders came from a wide variety of different professional backgrounds. Although all of the reports enthusiastically praised the benefits of group approaches with these people, little attempt was made to systematically demonstrate that in fact the group sessions were resulting in positive changes in the clients.

Wolfensberger (1967) has criticized most of the group work that has been done with parents of the retarded because of its lack of direction. Publications on the subject are characterized by "contradiction, speculation, subjectivism, and conceptual and terminological confusion," and as a result, any real summary of this work is impossible. He feels that many clinics and parents groups simply decide that it would be a nice thing to do to organize a parents group, but little thought is given to specifying goals or integrating the group sessions into a systematic program.

Nevertheless, many parents are undoubtedly able to benefit from a well-organized discussion group made up of people with problems similar to their own. In the first place, simply being aware that other people with retarded children have similar problems is often comforting. In addition, almost everyone welcomes an opportunity to talk about their problems with a group of sympathetic listeners. Any feelings of shame that the parents may have are very much mitigated by the fact that everyone else in the room also has a retarded child in the family. This process leads to the breaking down of defenses such as denial, and this enables the group members to make more realistic decisions about their children. Another obvious benefit is that parents are often able to help each other with everyday management problems and with information about the availability of community services. A final benefit is the support and encouragement provided by group members in times of unusual difficulty.

Parent Education

Probably the single most important factor that contributes to parental acceptance of a retarded child is the parent's knowledge about mental retardation. For this reason, an important function of many parent organizations is the dissemination of information. Many parental guidance groups serve primarily an educational function by having speakers, films, and the like. Parents frequently join a counseling group not so much to work out their feelings, but to obtain practical knowledge in the management of their child, and many programs that are defined as group counseling actually resemble a course on mental retardation and its management. Wolfensberger (1967) lists a large number of topics that ought to be covered in such a course.

1. Causes of retardation, including certain genetic aspects.
2. The diagnostic process.
3. Treatments, both preventive and secondary.
4. The effects of a retarded child on the family.
5. Home management, with emphasis on habit training, behavior and discipline, sexual behavior, and so on.
6. Speech and language.
7. Seizures.
8. Normal child development and its relevance to retardation.
9. The retarded child's feelings and needs.
10. Interpretation of retardation to relatives, friends, and neighbors.
11. A review of retardation facilities in the area, perhaps with visits.
12. A review of relevant national and state laws, from taxation to sterilization.
13. A review and display of appropriate reading materials.
14. Legacy planning.

15. Historical trends in retardation, both of the past and the present, with a discussion of the President's Panel Report.
16. Research trends in mental retardation (Wolfensberger, 1967, p. 367).

Genetic Counseling

A particular concern of many parents is whether subsequent children will be mentally retarded and whether their normal children might have retarded offspring. Answering these questions is the special function of a relatively new type of professional, the genetic counselor. As information accumulates about the inheritance patterns of various forms of retardation, genetic counseling has assumed an important role in the overall management of the parents. Genetic counselors obtain as much information as they can, both about the probable cause of the child's retardation and the pedigree of the parents. The counselors are then able to determine the chances of any subsequent child being mentally retarded or having other disorders. In some cases, this is relatively simple. For example, if the retarded child has a disorder transmitted by a single recessive gene such as PKU or Tay-Sachs disease, it is known that the chances are one in four that another child will also be afflicted. This is usually considered to be too great a risk, but most genetic counselors stress that the final decision is always up to the parents. If the child has Down's syndrome, the situation is more complicated because this disorder has several different causes. Usually, Down's syndrome results from nondisjunction, and if this is the case, the probability of another child also being retarded is quite small. However, sometimes Down's syndrome is also caused by translocation, in which case, the probability of another child also having the disorder is very much greater. As a result, if parents of a child with Down's syndrome wish to have another child, it is wise for them to have a chromosome examination first.

Many parents need more information than the simple probabilities of having another retarded child. If the retardation is caused by a genetic problem, this can not only be a severe blow to self-esteem, but the parents may require practical information about various forms of birth control and sterilization procedures. Some parents may seek information about adopting more children. If the parents have religious or moral convictions against artificial forms of birth control, then additional problems are presented. As a result, genetic counselors need to be more than just a geneticist; they must be able to provide support and comfort to parents to whom they have communicated bad news, and they need to be knowledgeable about other kinds of medical and social services.

Parents as Teachers

There is universal agreement that child-rearing methods have an important impact on the mental development of the child, and there has been a major thrust in recent years toward training parents, particularly low-income parents, to provide a more stimulating and enriched environment for their children with the hope that mental retardation can be prevented. There have been a number of well-publicized programs with this aim. Parent involvement is frequently an important component of various compensatory education programs for preschoolers, the assumption being that parents will be able to carry on the work of the school in their own home, thus providing a good deal more training for the child than can possibly be provided to a child who attends the program for a few hours each day. These are not technically mental retardation programs since the children involved have not usually been formally diagnosed as retarded, but their aim is to prevent retardation among children of families where retardation is likely. The usual procedure is for a social worker, teacher, or paraprofessional to visit the child's home about once a week and show the child's mother one or two specific exercises that she can do with her child. These exercises range from training in self-care skills to language stimulation to specific training in cognitive skills to generally encouraging the mother to interact with her child more often. A number of these programs report success in raising the IQs of disadvantaged preschoolers. Caldwell, Bradley, and Elardo (1975) provide a good review and evaluation of a number of these parent education programs.

Parents as Behavior Modifiers

The problems of central concern to most parents revolve around day-to-day home management; they worry about how to control a hyperactive child or how to toilet train a severely retarded child or how to teach their child to dress himself or herself. One solution to this type of problem is to train parents in behavior modification techniques. There are two advantages to such a procedure. The first is the economic issue; there are not enough trained professionals to provide proper service to all of the children who need it. In a school situation, one teacher must deal with a number of children at the same time, but in the home, most retarded children have one and perhaps two parents who are willing to devote a considerable amount of time to that one child. A second advantage is that the problem of generalizing from the school or clinic to the home does not exist. It is often the case that a conscientious teacher will be able to teach a retarded child a number of new skills that the child performs adequately in school but does not do at home. If the parents themselves teach these skills to the child in the child's own home, this problem cannot exist (although there can be the opposite problem of a child performing well at home but not in school).

The principles of behavior modification are sufficiently simple that most parents have little difficulty acquiring the basic concepts. Even if they do not fully understand the theory, all but the most limited parents are able to carry out a simple behavior modification program designed by someone else. Salzinger, Feldman, and Portnoy (1970) describe a typical program of this type. They taught 15 sets of parents, each with a brain-damaged child (no further diagnostic information was given, but from the descriptions, many could be considered mentally retarded), the basic principles of behavior modification. The first step was to train them to accurately observe their child's behavior, for example, to record "cried and stamped his foot" rather than "got angry." The parents were also given several tests of reading comprehension. Each parent, with the assistance of the trainers, developed their own programs. Each program was highly individualized since each child presented somewhat different problems. For example, one child habitually went into his parents' room and woke them up at about two in the morning. Apparently, this behavior was being reinforced by the child's mother who would converse or argue with the boy and sometimes permit him to spend the night in their room. In order to reduce the frequency of this behavior, the boy was given points toward a reward for every night in which he did not get out of bed. If he did get up, he was immediately sent back to bed with a minimum of conversation, and if he did not go into someone else's room, he was ignored altogether. The frequency of this behavior dropped from almost seven nights per week to nearly zero after four weeks of this regimen.

The authors reported that the program was a success in every case in which the parents, in their judgment, conscientiously carried out the program. Unfortunately, this was only true in 4 out of the 15 families. The rest of the families either failed to keep accurate records or were inconsistent in their contingency management. However, limited success was observed in another four cases. Interestingly, almost all of the parents were far more concerned with reducing the frequency of negative behavior than they were with increasing positive behaviors. Among the behaviors successfully reduced were hyperactivity, tantrums, sniffing people, disrupting meals, and continually changing TV channels. The more successful parents tended to be the ones with more formal education and better verbal skills.

Books for Parents

Since the most important function of parent counseling is probably the dissemination of information about mental retardation, many counselors recommend that parents read one or more of the many books that have been written about retardation specifically for parents. Some of these deserve special note. For example, *Mentally Retarded Children: What Parents and Others Should Know* by Blodgett (1971), *The Retarded Child: Answers to Questions Parents Ask* by Atwell and Clabby (1971), and *Developmental Handicaps in Babies and Young Children—A Guide for Parents* by Brown (1972) all answer general questions about retardation, and in the latter case, other handicaps as well. Other books have a more specific purpose. For example, *The Child with Down's Syndrome* by Smith and Wilson (1973) and *To Give an Edge: A Guide for New Parents of Down's Syndrome (Mongoloid) Children* by Horrobin and Rynders (1975) are both directed toward the parents of Down's syndrome children as their titles imply. Books such as *Ice Cream, Poker Chips and Very Goods: A Behavior Modification Manual for Parents* by Williams and Jaffa (1971), and *Isn't It Time He Grew Out of This: A Training Program for Parents of Retarded Children* by Baldwin (1973) are typical of a number of books that attempt to teach behavior modification principles to parents. The Planned Parenthood Association has published a little book for parents called *Love, Sex, and Birth Control for the Mentally Retarded: A Guide for Parents,* (Kempton, Bass, and Gordon, 1973) which answers parents questions in this sensitive area.

Summary

The birth of a retarded child or the discovery that a child is retarded almost always has a severe emotional impact on the parents. It has been suggested that these parents experience three kinds of crises, a novelty crisis, which is a reaction to the sudden impact of a major change in one's life; a value crisis, brought about by the fact that it is necessary to alter one's values to accept a child with few desirable characteristics; and a reality crisis, a reaction to the concrete kinds of problems presented by having such a child in the family.

The novelty crisis is short lived, and is a response to the news of a sudden change. The severity of the novelty crisis is determined to some extent by the way that the news is broken to the parents. Parents often complain that professionals treat them rather callously and delay telling them about their child's retardation, often even after the diagnosis is confirmed.

The value crisis is somewhat more serious. It results from the fact that parents must deal with conflicting values. They have been taught to love and cherish their child no matter what happens, but they have also been taught to value competence and achievement, and, as a result, they may experience feelings of rejection toward their child. There are a number of characteristic reactions to this conflict. One is guilt, both from having a retarded child in the first place and from feeling negatively towards their child. Another reaction is denial that the child is retarded or that the condition is incurable. A third reaction is overprotectiveness, perhaps arising from unconscious feelings of ambivalence. Another response is chronic sorrow, similar to the feeling which a parent would have if a child died. While most of what has been written about parents of retarded children stresses the negative side, many parents are able to resolve this conflict in values and fully accept their child, recognizing his limitations, but not overprotecting the child or feeling guilt or shame.

The third type of crisis is the reality crisis, a response to the concrete problems presented by raising a retarded child. Some retarded children can require a good deal of medical care or other kinds of costly treatment. Also, the family may be rejected by relative or friends who have old ideas about retardation. Some children can make severe demands on the parents' lifestyle, preventing them from going out or taking vacations. Most parents also worry about what will happen to their child when they are no longer able to take care of the child.

There have been several major studies about the effects of a handicapped child on the family, but the results are inconclusive. Some children, particularly the more severely handicapped and the severe behavior problems, can cause considerable stress and tension, but apparently, many families are able to adjust to the presence of a handicapped child with few disruptions.

Many parents are concerned about the impact of the handicapped child on the normal brothers and sisters. Fortunately, there is no evidence of a higher prevalence of adjustment problems among the siblings of retarded children than would be expected in a comparable group without a handicapped child in the family. Some siblings report a frank dislike of their retarded brother or sister, but just as many feel that they have benefited from the experience by having a greater understanding and tolerance of people.

Many parents seek some sort of counseling for their problems. The term counseling covers a variety of different procedures, everything from a single session with the family doctor to a much longer series of sessions with a psychiatrist or psychologist. Counseling endeavors can also be distinguished on the extent to which they are primarily educational in function versus the extent to which they are concerned with the client's attitudes and feelings. There seems to be a conflict between parents and professional counselors in this area, parents being interested in solutions of practical, everyday problems while professionals would rather that the counseling focus on the parents' feelings and emotions. Most counseling with parents is done in groups rather than individually, because not only is this arrangement more economical, but parents are able to see that there are many other families with problems as bad or worse than their own, and there is less shame about talking about one's retarded child in such a group.

Probably the most important function of any kind of parent counseling is education about mental retardation. Parents are interested in learning about how to discipline their child, what kinds of services are available, what their legal rights are, and so on. A particularly important type of education for some parents is genetic counseling, discovering whether their child's retardation had a genetic cause and whether they should risk having more children. Another rapidly growing area of parent education is training parents to use behavior modification techniques with their children.

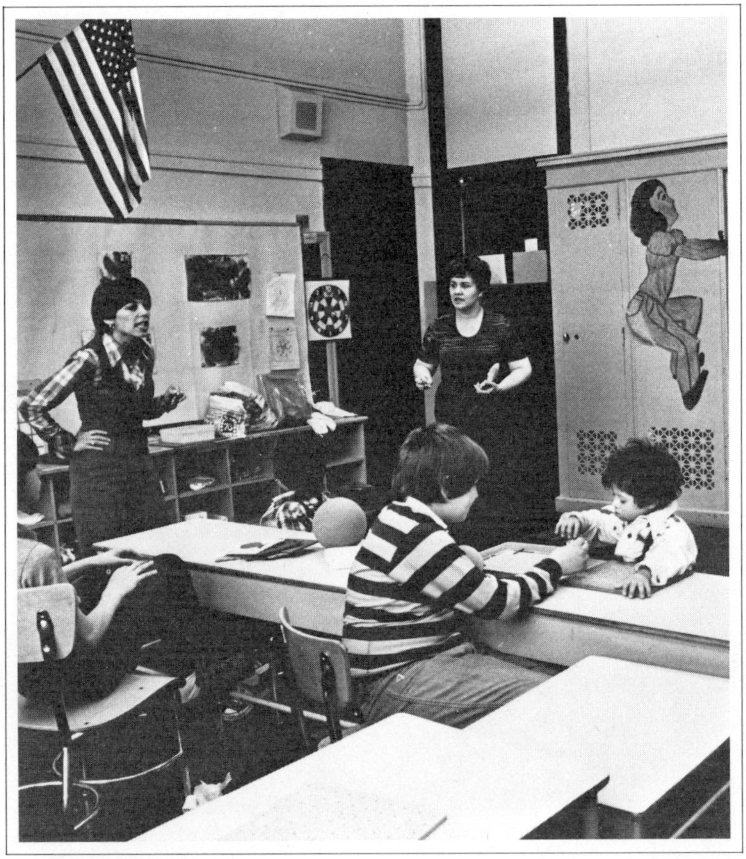

14

Education of the Mildly Retarded Child

The American educational system is in a period of rapid change. Responding to pressures both from within the system and from outside it, more innovations are probably being introduced now than at any time in the past. Almost every school district can boast of several experimental programs, ranging from open classrooms to engineered classrooms to special programs for the gifted to resource rooms for children with learning disabilities. Special education for the mentally retarded is in the forefront of this wave of innovation, and the past decade has seen major shifts in almost every aspect of special education, how retarded children are taught, what they are taught, where they should be taught, even in the very definition of who is eligible for special services. This chapter discusses some of the current issues involved in teaching mildly retarded children. After a brief review of the characteristics of mildly retarded students, the currently hotly debated issue of the extent to which these children should be taught in special classes or in regular classes will be discussed. The next section reviews a number of traditional approaches to teaching retarded children, with special emphasis on a more recent approach called clinical teaching. The final sections consider some selected topics in the education of the mildly retarded child, such as reading and the retarded child, and high school and vocational education.

Characteristics of the Mildly Retarded Child

It is important to keep in mind that many children labeled mildly retarded do not differ in important ways from their nonretarded peers. Most of them have no serious physical problems, and their poor school performance can rarely be attributed to a specific organic cause. Frequently, the social skills of these children are not nearly as retarded as their academic skills, and they are considered mentally retarded solely on the basis of the results of an IQ test and poor school performance. They often come from an ethnic minority and speak a dialect of English rather than standard English. Some even have a foreign language such as Spanish as their native tongue. While many mildly retarded children have emotional or behavioral problems, this is certainly not a universal problem.

Mildly retarded children are usually referred to by the school system as educable mentally retarded (EMR), and these terms are used interchangeably in this chapter. This label refers to those children who are able to learn basic academic skills. Most people who are labeled EMR can be expected to live independently and obtain competitive employment after they leave school. Thus, the goals of education for EMR students differ only slightly from the educational goals of nonretarded children. They must be taught the basic tool subjects to as high a level as their potential allows, and they must be taught enough basic adjustment skills so that they can lead independent and productive lives. The primary difference in curriculum goals between EMR students and nonretarded students is that the former are likely to receive less stress on the traditional academic subjects, particularly at the high school level, and more emphasis on very practical applied skills such as how to get and keep a job.

Organizational Considerations: Special Classrooms or Special Programs in the Regular Classroom

Prior to the late 1960s, if a child was having difficulty in mastering the basic tool subjects, the most common practice was to refer the child to a psychologist, who would administer an intelligence test such as the Stanford-Binet or the WISC, and if the child achieved a tested IQ of less than 70 (or 75 or even 80 in some cases), the child would be likely to be assigned to a self-contained special class for the mentally retarded. The self-contained special class was rarely challenged as being the best way to provide education for the slow learning child until the late 1960s when rather abruptly it became the target of a good deal of criticism. Now, in the late 1970s, placing EMR children in a special class for the entire day has far fewer defenders, and the majority of experts in special education are advocates of a policy called mainstreaming, integrating retarded children (and other handicapped children) into the mainstream of the educational process for as much of the day as possible, and giving them special attention in an integrated rather than a segregated setting.

Advantages of Self-contained Special Classes

Where a retarded child is placed is an important educational decision, and it is wise to consider both sides of this complex argument. Although some type of mainstreaming is favored by most special education experts at the present time, the self-contained special class still has its defenders (e.g., Kolstoe, 1972), and it is important to realize that there are a number of clear advantages to such an arrangement. Perhaps the most compelling argument in favor of self-contained special classes is that if a slow-learning child remains in a regular classroom, each year the child will fall farther behind and would soon reach a point where most of what happened in the classroom would be incomprehensible. If the child were only reading at the second-grade level, a fifth- or sixth-grade reader or a social studies book written at that level would be completely incomprehensible, and it would be inconvenient and difficult for the teacher to make special provisions. Until recently, the only nonspecial education option available for such children was keeping them back several grades, and this was unsatisfactory because of the social problems associated with assigning a ten-year-old child to a class of seven year olds. In the special class, on the other hand, the child could be exposed to reading and other materials at his or her own level, but at the same time would be in a classroom with other children of approximately the same age.

A second justification for placing a child in a self-contained special class is that the child can be exposed to teaching methods and materials specially designed for slow-learning children. Many special educators insist that slow-learning children require teaching methods somewhat different from those used in regular classes. They feel that the teaching needs to be more structured with less emphasis on incidental learning, that the material needs to be simplified, and that slow-learning children require more individual attention than do normal children in order to learn. Ideally, in a special class, the teacher would be specially trained in special education methods, and thus, the children ought to learn more and progress faster in a special class than in a regular classroom.

A third argument in favor of special classes is that the quality of education in the regular classes can be improved if the slow learning children are removed. One or two retarded children in a regular class may require a disproportionate amount of the teacher's time. The teacher may have to develop a special curriculum just for them, and this will detract from the overall quality of the teaching that the other children receive. In addition, mentally retarded children are likely to be behavior problems, and they may be disrupting the classroom activities almost continually, particularly if much of what goes on in the class is beyond their understanding.

Another argument concerns the relationship of the retarded child with peers. Research has shown that retarded children tend to be socially isolated whether they are in a special class or not (see Chapter 11). For the most part, they are ignored if not actually teased by their normal peers, and as a result, there is little social damage done by placing these children in a special class because they are not apt to benefit very much by being with nonretarded children anyway. In addition, it is possible that retarded children will suffer damage to their already low self-esteem if they are required to compete with children of normal intelligence. A retarded child will certainly not have very many success experiences if compared to children of normal intelligence. On the other hand, if all of the retarded children are placed in a special class, they will be compared to each other and will have a much greater chance to experience winning and success.

Arguments Against Self-contained Special Classes

In the later 1960s, a number of trends began to converge to bring about a shift in the attitudes of educators toward self-contained special classes, and beginning with an article by Dunn (1968), an increasing number of people began to question some of the assumptions behind special classes, arguing that the majority of slow-learning students might be better served by placing them back in regular classes.

One of these trends was an increased emphasis on individualization in education. For years, one of the major criticisms of the whole educational process has been the lock-step way in which children have been taught. All of the six year olds are in the first grade, learning the same thing at the same time, all of the seven year olds are in the next grade, all reading second grade readers, and so on. It has always been recognized that children differ widely in abilities. Some first graders are not quite ready for first-grade work, while others are ready for third-grade work, but in the past, it was difficult for the educational system to make provision for these individual differences, and so they didn't. It has only been in recent years that education has made a real effort to provide for a more individualized educational program, and most of the current innovations in education are aimed at providing a more individualized education for children. Such innovations as teaching machines, programmed learning, and open classrooms have just this purpose in mind. As long as education was carried out in a group, lock-step fashion, little provision could be made for unusually slow learning children, and assigning them to special classes was probably the best strategy. However, now that many teachers are making an effort to individualize the instructional process, regular classes are more able to accommodate slow-learning children, and the need for special classes is decreased.

The renewed emphasis on individualization has also had another impact on special classes. Assigning all of the children in a given IQ range to one class makes sense only if all of these children learn in about the same way. However, teachers have come to realize that the label of mentally retarded implies very little in the way of specialized teaching methods. There are lots of different reasons why a child may be having trouble learning in school. Some children may have perceptual problems, others may have language problems, still others may have motivational problems or emotional difficulties. There might be almost as many different kinds of learning problems in a class of children labeled EMR as there were children in the class.

At the same time, people began to be more aware of the stigmatizing effects of labeling a child as mentally retarded. It is usually impossible to place children in a special class without labeling them, and this label could have an important impact, not only on their self-esteem, but also on their ability to get a job and become a functional member of society after they leave school. Although research has not fully substantiated the fears that many educators have about the stigmatizing effects of labeling (MacMillan et al., 1974), there is general agreement now that labeling still ought to be avoided unless the label implies a definite type of treatment, and the label mental retardation certainly does not.

Another criticism of special classes is the self-fulfilling prophecy phenomenon discussed in Chapter 7. If a teacher knows that certain pupils are mentally retarded, the teacher will not expect very much of them, and, as result, they will not achieve very much. It is often felt that the curriculum of a special class is nothing more than a watered-down version of the regular class curriculum; the same material is taught, but at a more superficial and less challenging level. Some special educators feel that the major criticism of special education is that it underestimates the learning abilities of the students and that it fails to provide sufficient challenge (Greene, 1972). This is far less likely to happen if the retarded child is retained in the regular class, particularly if the child is not labeled mentally retarded.

A fourth criticism of special classes is that they become dumping grounds for all kinds of problem students. If teachers have a difficult student in class, one who has trouble learning or one who presents unusual behavior problems, it is easier for the teachers to arrange to have the child moved out than it is for them to confront the problem directly and give the child the special programming necessary. A related argument is that special classes represent a form of racial segregation since a grossly disproportionate number of children who are assigned to special classes are either black or Mexican-American. A study by the California Department of Education reported that while blacks and Mexican-Americans comprised, respectively, 8 percent and 13 percent of the pupils in the California school system, they made up, respectively, 26 percent and 26 percent of the pupils in special classes for the mildly retarded (Jones, 1972). In other words, there were more than three times as many black children and twice as many Mexican-American children as there should have been if these groups were proportionately represented. Notice also that these two ethnic minorities made up more than half of all the students in EMR special classes. Similar situations exist in other parts of the country. Studies of children in special classes reveal that there is usually a considerable amount of overlap in abilities between children assigned to special classes and the slower-learning students in regular classes (Garrison and Hammill, 1971). Students are assigned to special classes only partially on the basis of low IQ and poor school performance. If children are doing poorly but are otherwise not creating any problems, they are not likely to be referred to a special class, particularly if they are from a white, middle-class background, but if children are disruptive or from a low SES family, their chances of being placed in a special class are greatly increased (Rubin, Krus, and Balow, 1973).

Recent court decisions have had an impact on this situation and on the whole issue of self-contained classes for the mentally retarded. In a California case, *Diana* v. *Board of Education* (1971), nine families of Mexican-American children who had been placed in special classes argued that the placement had been unfair because the intelligence test used in the placement process had been based on English rather than the child's native language. The court ruled that children whose primary language was other than English must be tested in their native tongue as well as in English and that school districts must submit plans to reintegrate most children of Mexican-American and Chinese descent who were in special classes back into regular classes.

Another court decision on the same issue was even more far reaching in its implications. In *Hobson* v. *Hansen* (1967), the court ruled that the entire tracking system in the Washington, D.C. school system was illegal because the use of IQ tests to make class assignments resulted in a form of *de facto* segregation, with black children being overrepresented in the lowest track and white children overrepresented in the higher tracks. Although the judge explicitly excluded special classes for the retarded from his ruling, nevertheless, the whole practice of placing children in classes based on test scores suffered a serious setback.

A fifth argument against the segregated special class is that children in regular classes are seldom exposed to children with handicaps of various types, and as a result, they develop misconceptions, stereotypes, and unrealistic fears about handicapped people. Our society has a long history of segregating people with disabilities, placing them in institutions far away from their home communities where they are unable to participate in the mainstream of life. This tends to stress that handicapped people are very different from the rest of us and do not really deserve full human rights. The best way to overcome these misconceptions is to integrate handicapped people of all types into society as much as possible rather than deliberately segregating them. If normal children are routinely exposed to retarded children and to children who are blind or have cerebral palsy as they are growing up, they will learn that the handicapped are people just like everyone else and discrimination against them will gradually disappear.

Perhaps the strongest indictment of special classes for the retarded is the result of outcome studies on their effectiveness. When retarded children are removed from regular classes and placed in special classes, there ought to be a dramatic improvement in their academic performance because they are being placed in a smaller class where they can receive individual instruction and be taught by a teacher who has had special training in teaching slow-learning children. Because not all retarded children are placed in special classes, it is possible to determine whether in fact this is true by comparing the academic performance of retarded children in special classes to comparable retarded children who remain in regular classes.

In reality, this is difficult research to do because very few school districts will permit their retarded children to be assigned randomly to either a special class or a regular class, as good research practice requires. The best designed study of this type was done by Goldstein, Moss, and Jordan (1965). They screened all of the entering first graders in three communities for children with tested IQs of less than 85. These children were then assigned randomly to either special classes or to regular classes; and after four years, they were tested on academic achievement and social knowledge. There were no significant differences between the two groups on either test. There was no evidence that the children assigned to special classes learned any more or any better than did the children who remained in regular classes. However, children in both groups gained significantly in IQ. At the beginning of the study, the average IQ of the children was 75, but a year later, it had risen to 82, and many of the children in both groups had IQs well above 85. When the performance of those children who had final IQs of less than 80 was considered, the children who had been assigned to special classes performed somewhat better than those children assigned to regular classes.

A number of other studies have also compared the academic performance of retarded children assigned to special classes to supposedly equivalent retarded children in regular classes, and although in many cases, the two groups cannot be assumed to be equivalent, none has found any advantage for special classes. Either there was no difference between the two groups, or more likely, the children in the regular classes actually outperformed those children placed in special classes. Excellent reviews of this research can be found in Cegelka and Tyler (1970) and in Wiegerink and Simeonsson (1975).

Another piece of evidence suggesting that special classes are not more effective than regular classes in educating retarded children is their disappointing record in returning children to regular classes. Gallagher (1972) reported that less than 10 percent of children in special classes ever improved enough to be reassigned to a regular class on a full time basis. In other words, once children are assigned to a special education program, they will almost certainly remain in special programs for the remainder of their school career.

This is a very serious indictment of special classes and of the whole concept of special education. For years, educators have argued that retarded children need special types of instruction, special materials, specially trained teachers, and the like, yet there is little evidence that any of these special methods are in any way more effective than simply placing retarded children in regular classes. While it is often argued that the reason why special classes have failed to show substantial improvement in their pupils is that the teachers do not in fact use the special methods and materials advocated by special education experts, it is clear that this research has contributed substantially to the mainstreaming movement.

Alternatives to Special Classes

As a result of court decisions, outcome studies, and concerns about labeling, the defenders of self-contained special classes are clearly on the defensive. However, this does not mean that school districts all over the country are rushing to integrate their retarded children. There are a number of influences that tend to slow down the mainstreaming movement. In the first place, many teachers, both regular classroom and special class teachers, are opposed to it. Regular class teachers are afraid that if retarded children and children with other types of learning and behavior problems are reintroduced into their classes, this will result in more problems for them. This is a legitimate concern because many teachers have had little training or experience in teaching retarded children. Special class teachers fear that their jobs will be threatened. Many administrators, perhaps reflecting the attitudes of their teachers, similarly oppose mainstreaming. A survey by Payne and Murray (1974) revealed that about 40 percent of suburban school principals and 54 percent of urban school principals did not accept the idea of integrating educable retarded children into regular classes.

An additional barrier is the need to develop adequate programming within the regular classes for these slow learning children. There is almost universal agreement that retarded children and other pupils with specialized learning problems should not be returned to regular classes without some sort of special programming. The idea behind mainstreaming is that most of this special programming should be provided in the regular classroom rather than in a self-contained special class. Thus, it becomes necessary to alter the organization of the regular class to some extent to accommodate handicapped pupils.

There are a number of different administrative arrangements by which this might be accomplished. The most conservative arrangement is to assign retarded children to a special class for a part of the day, where they receive instruction in the basic tool subjects such as reading and arithmetic, but to assign them to a regular class for instruction in the less academic areas such as art, music, and physical education in which retarded children are at less of a disadvantage. In this way, they are able to benefit from being with their nonretarded peers for at least a part of the day, but much of the special class stigma still remains.

A more popular arrangement is to assign retarded children to a regular class, but to provide them with supplementary instruction on a part-time basis in a resource room. There are many different kinds of resource rooms. Some only provide services to a single disability category such as the EMR, but increasingly, resource rooms are noncategorical, providing services to any child with special needs, regardless of diagnostic label. A resource room can be staffed by a single highly trained teacher or by a number of different educational specialists such as a speech correctionist, a remedial reading teacher, a learning disabilities expert, and a mental retardation specialist. Students could be pulled out of their regular classes for special attention either individually or in small groups several times a week. Such an arrangement has several advantages. First, handicapped children would be in regular classes on almost a full-time basis and thus would be able to benefit from interacting with their normal peers. Second, there would be less stigma attached to going to the resource room because retarded children would not be the only ones going. Children with other special needs, such as a child with a speech defect or a child with a specific learning disability, would also be using it. A third advantage is that the valuable time of special education experts can be used more efficiently because they can devote their full time to their specialty without spending time on activities that could just as easily be done in a regular classroom. In this way, the resource room can provide services to more students than can a special class. One of the best resources currently available on the theory behind and the implementation of a resource room is Hammill and Wiederholt (1972).

The widespread use of resource rooms is a relatively new innovation in special education for the handicapped, and there is as yet little research into its effectiveness. However, what little research there is has been more positive than the efficacy research with special classes, indicating that at least in some cases, children learn more in resource rooms than they do in traditional special classes (Weigerink and Simeonsson, 1975).

One problem with the resource room concept is that it requires close coordination between the resource room teacher and the regular classroom teacher. Each must know what the other is doing, and in many cases, the resource room teacher may want the regular classroom teacher to give the child special exercises. Thus, it is necessary that the two meet with some regularity.

This problem can be overcome with a different type of administrative arrangement in which the regular classroom teacher does all of the teaching, including whatever special programming is required for the children with learning problems in the class. However, each teacher would be visited by one or more consultants on a regular basis who would assist the teacher by providing special exercises and individual prescriptions for any exceptional children in the class. In this arrangement, the mental retardation specialist or the learning disabilities expert would do little or no actual teaching but would devote all of his or her time to consulting with regular classroom teachers.

Ideally, each school district ought to be able to provide services to exceptional children on a number of different levels. Deno (1970) has described seven different levels of special educational services arranged in a hierarchy from the most integrated to the most segregated. These levels are shown in Figure 14-1. Although a given district should provide services on a number of different levels, an important aim of the educational system ought to be to keep each child at as high a level as possible, that is, in the most integrated setting possible, and there ought to be progressively fewer exceptional children at each lower level. A child should only be moved from a higher to a lower level if there is compelling evidence that such a move would be beneficial. A related consideration, too often lacking in special education programs, is that there should be a continuous reevaluation of each child who is at less than the highest level in order that children will be able to be moved back into the educational mainstream as quickly as possible. In the past, special education has usually represented a one-way street in that once a student was assigned to a special class, the student had little hope of ever returning to a regular class. Gallagher (1972) has gone so far as to propose that children be assigned to special class programs for two-year periods only, and, at the end of this time, they would be automatically returned to

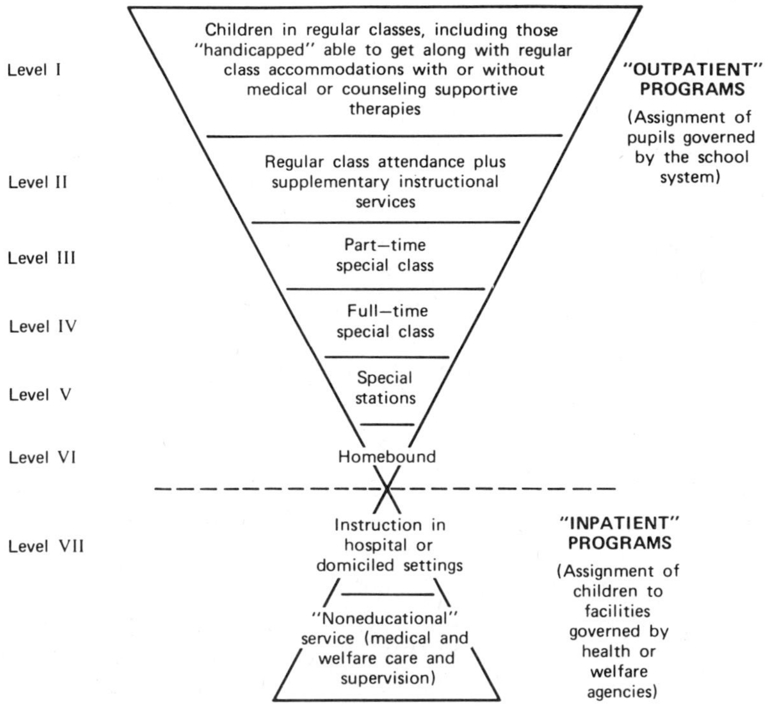

Figure 14-1 Seven levels of special education. From E. Deno. Special education as developmental capital. *Exceptional Children,* 1970, **37,** 229–237. Copyright © 1970 by the Council for Exceptional Children. Reprinted with permission of the Council and the author.

the regular class unless there was good reason not to. Such a proposal makes sense for several reasons. If the special education program is doing its job properly, then children assigned to special programs ought to be advancing more rapidly than they did in the regular class, and thus, should nearly have caught up. On the other hand, if children assigned to special programs are not advancing any faster than they did in regular programs, they ought to be placed back in a regular program anyway where at least they can avoid the stigmatizing effects of special placement.

Special Education Methods

The field of education has always been characterized by a tremendous diversity of approaches, methods, and theories. The education section of any college library contains shelf after shelf of books on teaching methods, and educators often disagree on even the most basic issues underlying the teaching process. Most educational research is unable to show that one teaching approach is superior to another (Stephens, 1966), and it is important to keep in mind that there is probably no one best way to teach children (or if there is, no one has found it yet).

This same situation exists in the field of education for the mentally retarded. Experts in special education have proposed a number of different systems and approaches to teaching, and while each has had an impact, no one approach is dominant. Theories of special education are too numerous to review in detail, and so this section will provide only a brief coverage of some of the more traditional approaches to teaching the retarded. However, the more current approaches will be covered in some detail.

Seguin's Physiological Method

Edouard Seguin (1846, 1866) was the first to publish a book on the education of mentally retarded children. His method was called the physiological approach because the sequence of instruction was organized to parallel what was then thought to be the general pattern of physiological development. The first step was education of the muscle system, a procedure that is now called motor training. He emphasized physical activity, particularly encouraging those activities that satisfied the child's own needs and desires. Particular stress was placed on the training of the hands because of their importance in effective adjustment. Perhaps his most important contribution were his ideas on the training of the senses. He felt that one of the major problems with a mentally retarded child was that many sense impressions failed to reach the nervous system, and that this lack could be overcome through systematic exercises. He proposed that children be required to discriminate between different weights, textures, sizes, shapes, and so on. Auditory training was done through the use of music. Consistent with his idea of training the muscles first, Seguin proposed that reading be taught by first teaching the child to write. The emphasis in all of his work is on learning by doing, an approach that has a strikingly modern tone.

Montessori's Autoeducational Method

Unlike Seguin, who is now only of historical interest, Maria Montessori (1912) is still widely read by teachers today. While at the present time, her approach to education is usually associated with the preschool instruction of normal children, Montessori developed most of her teaching methods with children who would now probably be labeled mentally retarded. Her method is an autoeducational approach because the child is largely self-taught. Montessori emphasized the fact that teachers and schools cannot directly teach, but they can only provide an environment that is conducive for the child to learn. Her approach is based on the assumption that children want to learn and have a natural drive to improve their own competency. In this sense, her method is similar to the modern open classroom in which each child is engaged in activities of his or her own choosing, and the teacher plays a supporting role rather than a directing role.

Like Seguin, Montessori placed a good deal of emphasis on the training of the senses. She developed many instructional materials that are still widely used today, such as a stack of blocks of progressively smaller size to teach size concepts, surfaces of different textures to train the sense of touch, and buttoning and zipping boards to teach self-care and fine motor coordination. All of these materials had in common the fact that they were inherently interesting to small children, and they each taught a specific skill.

Some of Montessori's ideas have been incorporated into modern educational practices while others have been rejected. For example, her assumption that each child should work at his or her own pace on materials of his or her own choosing was considered a somewhat radical idea at the turn of the century but is now almost universally accepted. Similarly, her idea that education is only effective if it is enjoyable and should be based on the child's own interests has wide popular support. At the time of her initial work, most education was based on the assumption that the mind needed to be trained like a muscle, and therefore, education should not be too pleasant. However, her emphasis on the training of the senses is no longer popular because research has shown that the senses do not need training and probably cannot be trained in the way that she proposed.

Piaget's Contribution To Education

In a number of ways, Piaget is a direct intellectual descendant of Maria Montessori. Both stressed the natural curiosity of the child and minimized the role of direct teaching, emphasizing that children had to discover relationships for themselves and that material that was directly taught was often learned only superficially. Piaget was a philosopher, not an educator, and he has said very little about the best way to educate children, but a number of educators have enthusiastically adopted his approach and attempted to generate some principles from his theory that could be applied to the classroom. (Elkind, 1970; Ginsburg and Opper, 1969; Schwebel and Raph, 1973). These principles presumably apply as much to the education of retarded children as they do for the education of children of normal abilities.

The first principle of education which derives from Piaget's theory is that children learn through action. Children learn about numbers and quantity and space and time by playing with objects and with each other, not by listening to a teacher. To the extent that this is true, much of traditional education has been ill-conceived. In the traditional classroom, children are encouraged to sit still, be quiet, and listen to the teacher, and it is difficult to imagine an atmosphere less conducive to learning.

A second principle is that children are naturally curious and are attracted to experiences and objects from which they can learn. Thus, the ideal classroom is a relatively unstructured and permissive one in which children are permitted to choose for themselves what to do from a wide variety of different materials, with the teacher taking a relatively passive role.

A related implication is that individual differences should be encouraged and accepted. Some children naturally develop faster than others, and teachers should not arbitrarily decide that at a certain time the whole class will be doing a certain lesson.

Another principle is that children must learn primarily by discovering things for themselves. Knowledge that is explicitly taught is likely to be superficially learned and quickly forgotten. This is particularly true of the various logical rules on which Piaget has placed so much emphasis. Simply telling children that the amount of water remains the same when it is poured from one container to another is futile; it is necessary for children to discover this for themselves by pouring water back and forth.

A final principle is that teachers should not assume that children think in the same way that adults do. Virtually every parent and teacher has at one time or another tried to explain something to a child using adult logic, and the explanation was completely beyond the child. Such occurrences are difficult to avoid entirely; it is nearly as hard for an adult to think like a six year old as it is for a child to think like an adult. However, if teachers are made aware of the nature of children's thinking, the frequency of such problems in communication can be minimized.

The Unit Method

During the 1920s and 1930s, the philosophy of education began to shift away from instruction in formal disciplines and toward training practical skills and more applied knowledge. One manifestation of this movement that was particularly popular in special education was the method of teaching through units or projects. Instead of dividing the instructional time up into the various subject areas, so much time for reading, so much time for arithmetic, and so on, much longer blocks of time would be devoted to a unit of experience, a problem area selected from real life such as health, family life, or leisure time. Students would collect information on the unit, go on field trips, listen to outside speakers, make scrapbooks or notebooks, and so on, all in connection with the unit topic. The emphasis is on firsthand experience and applied practical knowledge, and the assumption behind it is that students will learn practical skills such as how to plan a project, how to manage time, where to get information, and how to go about solving problems. The basic tool subjects can be taught in connection with the units rather than independently in order to maintain interest.

The best known advocate of the unit approach to special education was Christine Ingram (1935), who described a number of possible units for retarded children of different levels. Among the suggestions which she made are the following:

1. The units should evolve from the real life experiences of the children and should be based on their interests.
2. The choice of the unit should depend on the children's level of mental, physical, and social development.
3. The unit should develop both individual abilities and interests and group activity and cooperation.
4. The units should offer opportunity for the development of basic habits and attitudes.
5. The unit should develop interests in out of school activities. It should go beyond the classroom into the home and community.
6. The unit should include activities that utilize the tool subjects.

The unit method, or at least variations on it, is still in wide use today, although few teachers use this method entirely. Meyen (1972) provides some up-to-date guidelines on how to develop units for exceptional children.

The Modified Traditional Curriculum

It has only been in the past few years that most teachers of the mentally retarded have received much special training in special educational methods. Most teachers of special classes were trained in and had experience in regular classroom teaching, and thus, tended to use basically the same approach that was used to teach nonretarded children. The difference between the special class and the regular class was not so much in what was taught or how it was taught, but in the rate at which material was covered. The special class teacher would spend more time on any given topic and would in general progress more slowly. Thus, less material was covered and the teacher would go into less depth on what was covered. This approach is often referred to as a watered-down curriculum. Although few textbooks advocate this approach, it is probably the best description of general special education practice. In other words, most of what goes on in most special education classes on a day-to-day basis is not very different from what is occurring in regular classes down the hall. The teacher may provide somewhat more individual attention because the class is smaller, but the general approach to what is taught and how it is taught is basically the same as in other elementary school classes containing children of the same mental age. Simches and Bohn (1963), after reviewing more than 250 curriculum guides for the mentally retarded, concluded that most represent little more than a rephrasing or a reemphasis of the course of study used for normal children. Although this situation is sometimes criticized (Fuchigami, 1969), there is not necessarily anything wrong with teaching basically the same material to retarded children that is taught to everyone else, and since the learning characteristics of retarded children do not differ significantly from those of other children, there is no reason why methods effective with normal children would not be equally effective with the retarded. The main objection is that the special education curriculum is often more simplified and less challenging, and thus, the students are not being pushed to perform at their best possible level.

Perceptual-Motor Training

There is a group of special educators whose methods of teaching are in a sense qualitatively different from other approaches to teaching slow learning children. These are the intellectual descendants of Strauss and Lehtinen (1947) who did some of the seminal research on brain damage. These people deemphasize the teaching of the traditional tool subjects and place considerable stress on perceptual-motor training. The best known and most influential of these theorists today is Newell Kephart (1971). The original work was done in connection with brain injured children, but with the decline of interest in medical diagnoses in education, the method was extended to cover all slow-learning children.

The assumption behind the heavy emphasis on perceptual-motor training is that development must always follow an orderly course, with the differentiation of motor patterns preceding perceptual development, and perceptual development preceding conceptual learning. Many slow-learning children have experienced a disruption in this orderly course of development, either as a result of physical injury or because of some environmental deficiency. Because fundamental stages were not passed through normally, all subsequent stages are disrupted, and the child will have some sort of learning disability. The purpose of special education is to fill in this deficiency so that learning and development can proceed normally. Thus, in a very real sense, Kephart is trying to cure learning disabilities.

Kephart describes a large number of exercises that are specifically designed to remediate problems in development, and the implicit assumption is that as the child's perceptual and motor skills are improved through training, the learning difficulties will clear up because they were based on the faulty perceptual development. For example, he proposes specific training on a balance beam in order to facilitate the development of the concepts of laterality (left and right) and directionality. It is important that children learn these concepts not only in connection with the balance beam, but also in connection with other skills, such as reading and writing. Use of a trampoline develops the concepts of body image, balance, and rhythm. After children have mastered these groups motor skills, they can be trained on fine motor skills and the development of perceptual motor connections through the use of tracing or using a template to draw forms. Specific training of the eye muscles can be taught with a series of exercises in which the child fixates on various fixed and moving stimuli. Directionality concepts can be taught with a clock game in which eight points are drawn on a chalk board around the circumference of a circle, and the child is asked to draw lines with chalk from various points to the center. Other exercises to train perceptual skills include copying forms either by matching with sticks or with a pegboard or by doing puzzles.

A number of other theorists such as Ray Barsch (1965) and Gerald Getman (1966) have advocated similar techniques in which learning difficulties can be remediated through the systematic training of perceptual and motor skills. The most extreme advocates of this point of view are Doman and Delacato (Delacato, 1966) who have developed a very controversial technique called patterning. This theory is specifically directed toward brain injured children, and its goal is the reorganization of the nervous system through a series of exercises designed to take the child through all of the various developmental stages. For example, one of the exercises involves having four people move the child's limbs in a crawling pattern. The assumption behind this is that only by going through all of the various developmental stages can the child's nervous system become properly organized, and because crawling is a developmental stage, this exercise is necessary.

The Doman-Delacato method has achieved widespread notoriety because of extensive coverage in the popular press. Unfortunately, its professional acceptance has been less positive. In 1968, a number of prestigious organizations, including the American Academy for Cerebral Palsy, the American Academy of Physical Medicine and Rehabilitation, and the National Association for Retarded Children, adopted an official statement highly critical of the practice. Among the charges were unprofessional promotional methods such as suggesting that parents who refused to try patterning with their child were inadequate, undocumented claims of cure, and a regimen so demanding that it would place severe restrictions on the entire family. They cited a review of the effectiveness of the procedure (Robbins and Glass, 1969) that concluded that "the tenets are either unsupported or overwhelmingly contradicted when tested by theoretical, experimental, or logical evidence from the scientific literature. As a scientific hypothesis, the theory of neurological organization seems to be without merit" (Hallahan and Cruickshank, 1973, p. 95).

The perceptual motor training approach of Kephart, Getman, and Barsch has achieved considerable popular support among special educators of all types, but there is actually very little good experimental data indicating its effectiveness. A review of the effectiveness research by individuals relatively sympathetic to this viewpoint (Hallahan and Cruickshank, 1973) was forced to conclude that the vast majority of the research in this area was so poor that little could be learned from it, and the well-controlled research was as likely to find negative results (the treatment is ineffective) as it was to find positive effects. Another review by Goodman and Hammill (1973) came to the same conclusion.

Recent Innovations in Special Education: Clinical Teaching

A general dissatisfaction with the traditional approaches to special education has led to some important changes in the way that many mentally retarded children are being taught. The movement toward mainstreaming exceptional children has been accompanied by a much more individualized approach to teaching children with learning problems. This approach, which goes under several different names, clinical teaching (Smith, 1974), prescriptive teaching (Peter, 1972), or individually prescribed instruction or IPI (Scanlon, 1971), to name a few, is an innovative approach in two ways. First, it involves a much more thorough diagnosis of the child's problems that did earlier group teaching methods in which a detailed knowledge of each child's capabilities was not so important. The diagnostic process borrows heavily from some of the pioneering work on learning disabilities. The second innovation is the impact of behavioral psychology in that what is being taught is expressed in behavioral terms, what the child is actually able to do, rather than in the more traditional but vaguer terminology concerned with what the child knows or feels. Also, the material to be taught is usually broken down into its various components and taught in a hierarchy fashion, a process called task analysis.

The Diagnostic Process

Traditional diagnostic practices have been heavily criticized in recent years for a number of reasons, but one of the most important is the fact that the various labels that represented the end product of diagnosis implied little in the way of treatment. The knowledge that children are mentally retarded or neurologically impaired contributes little to their educational program. It may mean that the children are placed in some sort of special class, but one of the problems of special classes was that children were grouped by label rather than on the basis of educational needs. A class of children labeled EMR could contain almost as many different types of educational problems as there were children in the class. Diagnosis is only useful if different types of diagnoses imply different types of treatment, and all too often, this was not the case.

As a result, the new approach to the process of diagnosis places much less emphasis on simply labeling children. The aim is a much finer analysis of the child's functioning, determining in as much detail as possible how children learn, what children are able to do and not able to do in specific skill areas, and even their preferred mode of input, whether they function better with auditory, visual, or tactual stimuli for example. As a result, the kinds of formal tests used by educational diagnosticians, while they may produce an overall score that describes the child's general level of functioning, also analyze numerous subskills in order to pinpoint specific areas of weakness. One example of such a diagnostic test is the Illinois Test of Psycholinguistic Abilities described in Chapter 9. This test not only produces an overall score describing the child's general level of language ability, but it also produces 12 subscores describing performance in specific language areas in order that the diagnostician can specify with precision the exact areas of weakness. If a boy is referred to a remedial program because of poor language skills, it is of little use to the remedial teacher to know simply that although the child is nine years old, his language is more typical of a six year old. However, if the test reveals that his comprehension of language is nearly at the level of his chronological age but that he has unusual problems in, say, using grammatical inflections (Auditory-Vocal Automatic), this provides the therapist with enough information to begin to design a specific program for that child. Such an approach recognizes that intelligence, reading ability, and language skills are not unitary skills, but involve numerous different subprocesses, and that in many cases, a child is only having difficulty with one or two of these subprocesses. In other words, the concern is not only with the achievement level of the child, but also with the means by which the child reaches this level of achievement.

This approach to diagnosis has changed the type of formal tests now being published. Many educational tests are now criterion referenced rather than norm referenced. A norm-referenced test indicates how well a child is doing relative to other children. When an achievement test indicates that a child is reading at the third-grade level, this simply means that the child is reading as well as the average third grader. In other words, the child is being compared to other children. This is not particularly useful information for the teacher except in a very global way. Yet, until recently, most tests used in the schools, including all intelligence tests, were norm referenced. A criterion-referenced test, on the other hand, does not compare a child to other children, but instead compares the child only against himself or herself and against established criteria of what children ought to be able to do. Another way of saying this is that the test measures whether the child has achieved certain performance objectives. The type of learning implied by such an approach is called mastery learning because the aim is for all of the children to achieve all of the objectives, to master all of the material. In this way, it is not necessary for any child to ever fail, because although some children may learn various skills faster than others, all eventually master all of the material. With older methods of teaching, some children had to fail because when children are compared with each other, half the class must be below average.

This type of diagnosis also tends to use a lot of informal testing. Instead of relying strictly on standardized tests for a diagnosis, teachers may develop their own informal inventory of skills to test. For example, in order to make a reading diagnosis, the teacher may ask children to read aloud passages at several different levels of difficulty, and then the teacher will note carefully the various kinds of mistakes they make, whether they omit words, add extra words, misread words, use context cues to guess at new words, and so on as well as determining how well the children are able to comprehend what they read. In this way, the teacher is able to determine precisely which aspects of the reading process the child is having particular trouble with.

The following example from Smith (1974) may clarify this process. A certain child is having difficulty with arithmetic. The child's arithmetic performance is substantially lower than achievement in other areas. Arithmetic, like other subjects, is made up of numerous different subskills. The teacher first administers the Stanford Achievement Test, which distinguishes three components of arithmetic, computation, concepts, and applications. The child does well in the first two but is very weak in arithmetic applications. In other words, the child has difficulty using computational and conceptual skills to solve problems.

But solving problems is also a complex skill, and it is necessary to perform a finer analysis in order to determine the exact nature of the child's difficulty. Smith divides arithmetic problem solving into seven skills:

1. Recognizing that a problem has been posed and defining its dimensions, including what is being requested.

2. Analyzing the components of the problem and determining the sequence of steps that must be taken to arrive at a solution.

3. Translating the narrative components of the problem into a proper symbolic form that will lead to a solution.
4. Recalling facts, concepts, and notations that have possible pertinence to the solution of the problem.
5. Recalling whether the problem could be solved in more than one way, and if so, which strategy is the most effective.
6. Performing the required mathematical steps in proper sequence and with accuracy and efficiency.
7. Arriving at a conclusion that is based on the solution achieved from working the required mathematical steps.

In order to determine which of these steps the child is able to do and with which ones he or she is having trouble, the teacher would then give the child a number of problems to do and observe carefully as the child works them, interrupting periodically to determine exactly what the child is doing at any one time. For example, after the child has read the problem, the teacher might ask what the problem was asking for, and if the child had trouble answering, this could suggest that the difficulty was with skill number one above. The teacher might observe that the child can say what is being asked but has difficulty translating the information given in the problem into arithmetic notation, indicating difficulty with skill number three. In this way, the teacher or diagnostician is able to determine precisely where it is that the child is having difficulty and is able to focus his or her entire attention on that one area and not waste time going over skills that the child has already mastered.

Task Analysis

Once the child's problem has been diagnosed precisely, the next step is to teach the appropriate skills. The best way to do this is to perform a task analysis of the skills to be taught. A task analysis involves breaking a skill down into its component subskills and arranging these subskills in a hierarchy beginning with the most basic. It is best to express each skill in behavioral terms. That is, the language used in the task analysis should specify what the child can and cannot do rather than what the child does or does not know. Bloom et al. (1971) suggest that in writing instructional objectives, words such as the following are ambiguous and should be avoided: knowledge, comprehension, appreciation, grasps the significance of, works effectively, reads with ease, and uses basic skills. Far better are "point-atable" verbs such as to state, to recognize, to punctuate according to conventional rules, or to list the consequences of a course of action. For example, it is important for a child to be familiar with different consonant sounds and their relationship to the letters of the alphabet in order to be able to read. The competency "knows relationships between initial consonant sounds and letters" should be expressed in such a way that there can be no disagreement whether a given child has, in fact, mastered the competency. Wording such as "When shown each consonant, the child is able to say the appropriate sound with 95 percent accuracy" is unequivocal. Almost any teacher in the country would be able to agree on whether a given student has mastered this skill because it is worded so precisely.

The following is a list of instructional objectives to develop the skill of telling time, and it demonstrates such a task analysis.

Instructional Objectives: Time

3.2 The learner will demonstrate by both oral and written test that he can tell time by interpreting the clock to the nearest minute and the calendar to the exact day, month, and year. He will complete the criterion test with 90 percent accuracy.

- 3.2.1. The learner will demonstrate his ability to tell time on the hour and to write the hour shown on the clock. He will complete the criterion test with 90 percent accuracy.
  - 3.2.1.1. The learner will demonstrate his ability to read numerals to twelve.
  - 3.2.1.2. The learner will demonstrate his ability to read hours or numbers on clocks.
  - 3.2.1.3. The learner will demonstrate his ability to tell time on the hour.
- 3.2.2. The learner will demonstrate his ability to tell time to half-hour settings of the clock. He will complete a criterion test with 100 percent accuracy.
  - 3.2.2.1. The learner will demonstrate his ability to understand the :00 and :30 notation for time.
- 3.2.3. The learner will demonstrate his understanding of time to include the telling of time in multiples of five minutes and will demonstrate his understanding of passing time by completion of a criterion test with 90 percent accuracy.
  - 3.2.3.1. The learner will demonstrate his understanding of passing time.
  - 3.2.3.2. The learner will demonstrate his understanding of earlier than and later than in the time concept.
  - 3.2.3.3. The learner will demonstrate his ability to tell time in terms of multiples of five.

3.2.4. The learner will demonstrate his understanding of time by telling time in minutes and seconds. He will complete a criterion test with 90 percent accuracy.
    3.2.4.1. The learner will demonstrate his ability to recognize time to minutes and seconds.
    3.2.4.2. The learner will demonstrate his ability to set a clock to the minute and second.
3.2.5. The learner will demonstrate his ability to regroup hours, minutes, and seconds when adding and subtracting, by completing a criterion test with 90 percent accuracy.
3.2.6. The learner will demonstrate his ability to regroup hours to days and days to hours by completing a criterion test with 80 percent accuracy (Grieder et al., 1971, pp. 184–189).[1]

Clearly, this general approach to teaching is the current trend in education, not only for the mentally retarded, but also for children with learning disabilities, and even for normal children. Such an approach has a number of advantages. First, it is possible to provide individualized instruction for each child. Once the various programs have been written, each child is able to advance through each one at his or her own rate. A child who understands most of the material can advance rapidly, while a child who has difficulty may spend a good deal of time on one step, but everyone will eventually complete all of the learning. Such an approach lends itself particularly well to a resource room because the resource room teacher is able to make a thorough diagnosis of each child's learning problems and write individual prescriptions to be carried out either in the resource room or by the regular classroom teacher. It is not necessary to label children in order to provide different kinds of programming because a child's program does not depend on a diagnostic label.

Curriculum Considerations

Reading and the Mentally Retarded

Virtually all children diagnosed as mentally retarded have problems with reading. At best, retarded children can be expected to be reading at their mental age level, which for EMR children in elementary school is about two to four years below grade level. However, studies on reading in the retarded have found that most retarded children are reading considerably below even their mental age level, the average being about a year below for elementary

[1] From J. W. Grieder, et al. *Mathematics Design for Individually Paced Instruction*. Jacksonville, Fla.: Duval County School Board, 1971. Reprinted with permission of the author.

school pupils (Cegelka and Cegelka, 1970). This is a cause for serious concern because it means that most children diagnosed as EMR, even if they finish high school, will probably not have sufficient reading ability to understand a daily newspaper.

There are a number of different reasons why a child may not be reading up to grade level. Some children have perceptual problems and have difficulty distinguishing one letter from another. Others have unusual difficulty with auditory discrimination and cannot discriminate the various sounds in a word. Other children are word callers, they can read what is written, but they have difficulty comprehending what they read. There is general agreement that the reading problems encountered by retarded children are no different from problems encountered by other children who have difficulty with reading. There are no reading problems that are unique to the mentally retarded. This implies that the remedial process ought to be basically the same for all children with reading difficulties regardless of whether they are considered mentally retarded or not.

There are a number of issues surrounding the teaching of reading that have been and continue to be hotly debated. The fundamental issue concerns the basic way to teach reading. The two major camps on this issue are the whole-word method and the phonics approach. The former places initial stress on reading for meaning right from the start. This is the approach of the majority of basal readers. Once children are able to read a number of words by sight, then they are taught the relationship between individual letters and the sounds in the words. The phonics approach, on the other hand, starts out by teaching the alphabet code, the relationship between letters and sounds, and only later introduces reading for meaning. However, this is an oversimplification of the issue. Chall (1967), in a review of research covering basic reading methods, lists 10 different approaches to teaching reading. There are several different phonics approaches, some stressing synthetic phonics in which the child is encouraged to blend sounds together to make words, others stressing analytic phonics, in which the child starts with a word and then figures out the letter sound relationships. There are also a number of other fundamentally different approaches such as the Initial Teaching Alphabet (I.T.A.) in which children are first taught to read using an alphabet different from the normal English alphabet, which is supposedly better because there is always a one-to-one relationship between a letter and a sound. Another controversial approach is O. K. Moore's (1964) responsive environment, in which the child is seated at a specially programmed typewriter that is connected to a tape recorder. After an initial play period, the child must learn to press the key that matches the letter appearing in a window. The typewriter is programmed so that only the correct key can be pressed. Then the child advances to matching whole words. Moore advocates starting children on reading as young as possible.

Whenever there is a situation where there are a number of different ways to accomplish the same goal, it can be assumed that no one method is clearly superior, and this is certainly the case with reading. While there is some evidence that methods that emphasize the teaching of the alphabet code early are slightly superior for most children (Chall, 1967), there is now general agreement that there is no one best way to teach reading. Different children learn better with different methods.

To the extent that this is the case, the role of educational diagnosis becomes extremely important, and as a result, the methods of clinical teaching are probably more developed in the area of reading than in any other school subject. A number of good diagnostic tests have been developed in recent years with the specific aim of determining precisely what the nature of a child's reading problem is. Among these are the Gray Oral Reading Tests, the Sprache Diagnostic Reading Scales, and the Gates-McKillop Reading Diagnostic Tests. Similarly, there are a number of good clinical programs for teaching reading, emphasizing various methods. The weak link at the present time is in the relationship between a specific diagnosis and the determination of a specific method. While some approaches are relatively obvious, for example, a child who has unusual difficulty with auditory discriminations would probably learn better with an approach which deemphasized phonics, there are many patterns of skills for which one method or another is not clearly specified (Gillespie and Johnson, 1974). The reader who is interested in a more detailed discussion of clinical teaching methods of teaching reading to retarded children is referred to Smith (1974) or Gillespie and Johnson (1974).

Another area of controversy surrounding the process of teaching reading that is of particular interest to teachers of the retarded is the question of reading readiness. Many educators feel that reading should only be taught after children reach a mental age of about six because prior to this time, they will not have fully mastered the perceptual and cognitive skills necessary to read. If children are started on reading before they are ready, they may get discouraged and lose confidence in their abilities, and thus may never learn how to read because of the negative emotions associated with the reading process. It is the policy in many special education programs not to start to teach reading until the children are about nine years old for this reason. Such an approach has been harshly criticized by such people as Ginsburg (1972) and Baratz and Baratz (1970) who contend that the main reason why black children and children from poor families lag behind white middle-class children academically is because they are not taught to read as young as are white middle-class children. Poor children are given a test of reading readiness, on which they do poorly, and as a result, the first year or two of their education is spent not on teaching them to read, but on reading readiness exercises, which are supposed to prepare them to read. Evidence for this contention comes from the Goldstein et al. (1965) study described above in which slow children were randomly assigned to either special classes or regular classes. At the end of two years, the children who had been placed in regular classes were significantly better readers than were the children who had been assigned to special classes, and further investigation revealed that the reason for this difference was the fact that the special class had spent a good deal of time on readiness activities while the regular class had started right in teaching these children how to read. However, at the end of four years, there was no difference in reading ability between the two groups.

Activities to prepare children to read are widely used in many school systems, and while many of these activities are no doubt beneficial, the connection between readiness training and reading is occasionally tenuous. The principle focus of most readiness training is auditory and visual perception and discrimination, but sometimes, the material being taught is far removed from the reading process. For example, some programs teach children to discriminate between high- and low-pitched sounds or between various animal sounds, but research indicates that the perception of speech may be a qualitatively different process from the perception of nonlanguage sounds (Liberman et al., 1967), perhaps even occurring in different parts of the brain. Probably the most widely used program of training reading readiness is that developed by Frostig and Horne (1964), which provides training in visual perception. However, Frostig herself has never claimed that these materials will improve reading and most research on this question fails to demonstrate that the Frostig materials have a beneficial effect on the ability to read (Hammill and Wiederholt, 1973).

Speech and Language Training

Many EMR children have immature and inadequate language skills; their speech is somewhat repetitive and stereotyped and their vocabulary is limited. Many of these children have been exposed to what are considered to be poor speech patterns at home, and they speak in a ghetto dialect. Such children may have difficulty understanding what is said to them, and their articulation may be so poor that few people can understand them. Many such children are excessively shy and seldom or never speak out in class, and this behavior might lead the teacher to think that their language competence is less adequate than it actually is.

As a result, training in speech and language is an important component of virtually all EMR programs, at least at the elementary school level. Such training can be roughly divided into speech training and language training, the former focusing on articulation problems, stuttering, and the like, while the latter focuses on building vocabulary, training in proper grammatical usage, and encouraging these children to express their thoughts verbally.

Speech Training. The most common type of oral language disorder by far is a disorder of articulation in which the child either substitutes one sound for another (e.g., fumb for thumb) or omits a sound entirely (i cream for ice cream). Another type of articulation disorder is called oral inactivity in which the child is able to enunciate sounds correctly, but ordinarily tends to slur speech. There are numerous causes of articulation disorders. Mispronunciations are characteristic of the speech of younger children, and if a teacher is dealing with children with mental ages of seven or lower, many of the articulation problems simply result from immature speech. Most, but by no means all, children with articulation problems of this type can be expected to outgrow them. Other articulation problems are caused by structural problems such as a poor bite or poor tongue control (Anderson and Newby, 1973) or in some cases more serious problems such as a cleft palate. Another cause of articulation problems is that the child has been exposed to poor models. If a child's family speaks poorly, the child will learn to speak in the same fashion. Thus, in a sense, it is impossible to distinguish between an articulation disorder and a difference in dialect. Many of the speech differences of low-income black children used to be considered speech disorders, but now they are more likely to be considered as a different dialect.

Over half of the children in public school EMR classes have some sort of articulation problems (Wilson, 1966). Ideally, all children with speech problems should receive regular speech therapy from a trained speech therapist, but unfortunately, there are not nearly enough therapists to meet this need. Scofield (1972) concluded that only 11 percent of children in EMR classes in California were receiving any kind of speech therapy services. A child who is referred to a speech therapist may receive any one of a variety of different kinds of exercises depending on the problem. The most usual practice is drill on the specific sound or sounds with which the child has difficulty, but the child may also receive listening training or exercises to develop control of specific muscles or even vocabulary training.

Language Training. Language training can be further divided into instruction in grammar and more general types of enrichment to develop vocabulary and usage. Grammatical errors such as a lack of agreement between subject and verb (he don't know any better) and double negatives (they don't have no money) are fairly common among children in EMR classes. These problems usually result from poor speech usage within the child's family, and increasingly, they are being viewed as differences in dialect rather than as deficits in language. However, regardless of their cause, they ought to be corrected, and as a result, most EMR programs incorporate specific drill in proper grammatical usage.

The more serious types of language difficulty with the retarded are problems of vocabulary and a general lack of fluency. Both the expressive and receptive vocabularies of retarded children are more limited than those of their nonretarded peers, and this means that they have more difficulty understanding what is said to them and they have more difficulty putting their thoughts into words. As a result, their speech is more repetitive and less varied. This problem may be compounded by the fact that many mildly retarded children come from families where language is not used very much at home except to communicate basic feelings and wants, the restricted code discussed in Chapter 7. These children may have had little experience in trying to communicate ideas to other people or presenting logical arguments.

Oral language skills are particularly important to the mentally retarded because most retarded people are not able to rely on written language as a major source of information. Virtually all special classes and other programs for retarded children devote a good deal of time to developing oral language skills. The usual approach can be loosely labeled enrichment, simply exposing the children to more advanced types of language and vocabulary and encouraging the children to speak out and express their ideas as much as possible. In earlier times, the ideal student was one who never opened his or her mouth in class, but more current teaching methods, particularly in special classes, tend to encourage children to express their ideas.

A number of curricula and programs have been developed with the specific purpose of improving oral language skills. One program that is extensively used, particularly with retarded children, is the Peabody Language Development Kits (Smith and Dunn, 1967). There are a number of kits ranging in level from preschool up through third grade. Each is specifically designed to stimulate receptive and expressive language skills using a systematic program of activities that can be done with a group of children for roughly 30 minutes each day. Each kit contains materials designed to maintain the interest of the children, such as puppets, and each day's program is broken down into a number of different activities, also to keep interest level high. Examples of activities include Brainstorming (think of all the things that go with railroad, name all the animals you can), Vocabulary Building (she helps us learn, she is a __?__. I have eight arms and I like to stay on the bottom of the ocean. I am a __?__.), Storytelling (make up a story about a picture), Following Directions (close your eyes, stand on one foot), Imagination (let's imagine you are a giant. Where would you live? What would you eat?), and Relationships (which is larger, a 50 cent piece or a quarter?). The purpose of all of these exercises is to encourage the children to become more verbally fluent.

One vitally important reason for facilitating oral language skills is to prepare the child to learn to read and write. It is impossible for a child to learn to read unless he or she has first developed sufficient language skills.

Arithmetic and the Mentally Retarded

An understanding of the basic concepts of arithmetic is absolutely essential for independent living. Consider how difficult it would be to run your life if you were unable to add and subtract well enough to deal with money, tell time, or be able to understand basic measurement concepts such as foot, mile, or pound (centimeters, meters, or kilograms). As with reading, however, there is little that is unique about teaching arithmetic to retarded children, and it can generally be assumed that techniques that are successful in teaching arithmetic to normal elementary school children will be the best techniques to use with mildly retarded children of the same mental age. Unlike reading, however, there have been few attempts to develop specialized approaches to teach arithmetic, and far less debate surrounding the fundamental methods.

Research on the arithmetic achievement levels of mentally retarded children indicates that, on the average, their computational skills are roughly equivalent to their mental age. However, their performance on tests of arithmetic reasoning generally lags somewhat behind their mental age (Dunn, 1973). This is consistent with other findings that retarded children seem to have particular difficulty with abstract concepts, but are not unusually impaired in skills that require primarily rote learning. This means that EMR children can reasonably be expected to have mastered arithmetic skills to about the third- to fifth-grade level by the time they leave school. For the most part, this is sufficient for independent living. Most jobs, particularly the kinds of jobs that most retarded people apply for, do not require extensive knowledge of arithmetic beyond a basic understanding of counting.

Most arithmetic programs for the retarded do not differ in important ways from similar programs for normal children of equivalent mental level, with the possible exception of the fact that instruction is more concrete and there is greater emphasis on calculation rather than on theory. Thus, at the primary levels the emphasis is placed on instruction of basic concepts such as larger and smaller, more and less, longer and shorter, and so on. The concepts of number and amount are very important, and they are generally taught very concretely, as is the case with addition and subtraction. Once children understand these fundamental operations they are likely to receive specific instruction in time, money, measurement, and the like just as normal children do. Only at the secondary levels do mathematics programs for mildly retarded children differ significantly from what brighter children receive. There is a greater emphasis on the practical, applied aspects of mathematics such as how to balance a checkbook, how to determine which is the best buy, how to fill out simple tax forms, how to compute interest, and the like.

Personal, Social, and Vocational Skills

The day has long passed when schools were only expected to provide instruction in the three Rs, reading, 'riting, and 'rithmetic. As society becomes more complex and families become more fragmented, schools are devoting an increasingly large proportion of teaching time to units on health, social skills, career planning, consumer education, and other skills that are necessary for successful adjustment to the modern world.

Instruction in personal habits and social skills is particularly important for the mildly retarded for a number of reasons. In the first place, they are likely to come from homes that do not systematically teach this knowledge. While a more advantaged child will probably receive extensive training in good health practices, proper manners, grooming, and the like at home, the low SES families from which most EMR children come often do not systematically teach this knowledge, and thus, the responsibility lies with the schools. Second, research (see Chapter 17) indicates that the reason why most retarded people fail at jobs or fail to adjust to independent living is not because they don't possess the appropriate academic skills but because they have poor social and personal habits; they are too immature to get along with co-workers and supervisors or else they have peculiar mannerisms or habits that make employers reluctant to hire them. In a sense, higher standards of conformity are required of mentally retarded people than are demanded of other people. If college professors wear worn, badly fitting, unstylish clothes and walk around mumbling to themselves, they will probably be humored and their behavior will have little effect on their professional development. However, if people who have been labeled mentally retarded do the same thing, they may encounter difficulty in getting and keeping a job, renting an apartment, or the like, particularly if the other people with whom they must deal are skeptical about hiring or renting to retarded people to begin with.

Another reason why it is particularly important to teach proper personal and social skills to the retarded is that they have fewer opportunities to learn them on their own. Most adolescents acquire grooming, dating, and other social skills from friends, but as we have seen, many retarded people have few friends, and thus, this source of knowledge is closed to them. In addition, because their reading skills are generally poor, retarded people are unable to learn about proper health, grooming, and the like from books, magazines, and newspapers.

Health. Everyone, retarded or not, can benefit from instruction in basic health practices, and health education is a part of most curricula today. Health instruction usually includes systematic instruction in nutrition, proper care of teeth, basic first aid and safety, how to obtain medical care, the proper use of drugs, both legal and illegal, and other personal habits such as cleanliness, use of deodorant, and the like.

Perhaps the most controversial aspect of health education is sex education. Most people seem to have the view that interest in sex should be limited to those people who are young and normal, and such people are shocked to hear that a mentally retarded person or a person with some other handicap such as cerebral palsy plans to get married. For this reason, sex education for the retarded has only very recently become popular. However, statistics show that the marriage rate among the mildly retarded is only slightly below the national average, and it is probably true that many of those people who never marry are sexually active. Thus, sex education for the mentally retarded is absolutely essential. It is important that retarded people learn as much as possible, not only about the basic anatomy, physiology, and mechanics of sex, but also about birth control, venereal disease, masturbation, pregnancy, abortion, and various deviations from usual sexual practices such as homosexuality. Also included in any complete program of sex education would be a discussion of the various moral issues related to sex.

Home Management. The traditional home economics course has been a part of the school curriculum for girls for many years, and it is often a central focus of the high school curriculum for the retarded. However, there are some recent developments that have produced changes in the home economics course. The first is that educators have begun to recognize that boys ought to have a basic knowledge of how to cook, clean, do laundry, and otherwise run a household. Most boys will be living alone at some point in their lives, and they will need to take care of their own apartment and deal with cooking and cleaning. As a result, basic home management skills are increasingly being offered to boys as well as girls.

A second development is the addition of a unit on love, marriage, and child rearing. All too many people in our society, particularly teenagers, have a remarkably romanticized view of these issues, and they are only dimly aware of the difficulties and stresses that invariably arise in any marriage or long-term relationship. The purpose of such a unit is to make an attempt to instill more realistic attitudes in the students, making them aware of the possible pitfalls of early marriage and the difficulties involved in raising children. There is nothing that is unique about home management courses for the mentally retarded, and for the most part, there is no need for separate classes for them.

Consumer Education. Consumer education is a relatively new but rapidly growing area of instruction. Many mildly retarded people will be in lower income groups and thus ought to have a good knowledge of how to shop wisely and how to get the most value out of every dollar spent. A typical consumer education course should include the following: information on deceptive advertising and promotional techniques such as bait and switch, knowledge about installment buying and how much extra it will cost, how to select meats, fruits, and vegetables, how to do comparison shopping, proper budgeting techniques, how to rent an apartment, guarantees, how to check out a used car, how to buy auto insurance, the cost of running a car, how to deal with sales people, how to buy a house, homeowners insurance, and so on.

Government and the Law. Federal, state, and local governments have begun to provide so many different types of services that everyone needs to know how to deal with various government agencies, which services are available, and how to obtain good legal advice. This knowledge is particularly important to many retarded people because they are likely to require more government services than are other people. For example, at some time in their life, almost everyone, retarded or not, is likely to be eligible for one of the many government support programs such as welfare, food stamps, unemployment compensation, medicaid and medicare, legal aid, social security benefits, and the like. It is important that everyone know that these services are available, who is eligible for them, and how one can apply for them.

It is equally important that every citizen also have a fundamental understanding of how our government and legal system work. Thus, a basic civics unit is almost always a part of the EMR curriculum at the high school level. This generally includes a discussion of the various levels of government and their relation to each other, the role of some of the important government bodies, and every citizen's basic rights. Such courses frequently also have more practical aspects such as how to vote or what to do when you are arrested.

Vocational Training. Probably the single most important factor in determining whether a handicapped person will be able to live independently or not is whether that person is able to get and keep a job that will pay enough to meet basic needs. As a result, many people feel that vocational training is the most important aspect of the entire educational program for the mentally retarded. This is also perhaps the area of the curriculum where instruction for the mentally retarded differs most from that of the nonretarded students.

Particularly at the high school level, programs for the retarded are becoming increasingly oriented toward the specific goal of making sure that students will be employable after they graduate. Vocational education involves two aspects. The first is general vocational knowledge and attitudes, those skills that are not related to any one type of job or career but are desirable in almost any employment situation. Thus, retarded students are taught the importance of punctuality and dependability as well as how to get along with co-workers and supervisors. Also included here would be specific instruction in work-related knowledge such as payroll deductions, the role of labor unions, or the various ways that people are paid. The second aspect of vocational training involves training in how to do a specific job, such as how to be a janitor or how to run a sewing machine.

The ideal high school program for the mentally retarded is one that involves a good deal of actual work experience (Kolstoe and Frey, 1965). Many high schools now have some sort of work study programs in which students receive credit for working outside the school in jobs obtained by the vocational counselor. There are a number of benefits to such a program. In the first place, students are able to receive actual on the job experience working in a variety of different job situations. In this way, not only do they discover the advantages and disadvantages of different kinds of work, but they are also able to develop general work habits. If they are visited periodically by a vocational counselor, the students, the work supervisors, and the counselors can discuss how the job is going and make suggestions about ways that the students can improve their performances. A second advantage is that when the students are ready to leave school and start applying for a permanent job, they will not only have had the benefit of considerable work experience, but they will have also met many members of the community who might be able to help them find jobs. The want ad "Only those with experience need apply" does not pose as much of a barrier to a work-study student as it does to a graduate of a more traditional high school program.

What it Means to be Mentally Retarded

At some point in the educational career of every retarded child, there ought to be a discussion of what it means to be mentally retarded. Most retarded children have been teased about their stupidity, and they are often very confused about just what the term mentally retarded means. Such a discussion is often quite painful for the teacher. The most usual approach is to explain in some detail that people differ from each other and that some people are particularly slow at learning academic subjects. Being mentally retarded may mean that it will take them a little longer to understand certain things, but being mentally retarded is nothing to be ashamed of, and while they may be having trouble in school, most mentally retarded people have other things that they are good at. The teacher could then point to people in the group who had unusual talents.

The aim of such a discussion is to improve the children's self-esteem but at the same time to encourage them to recognize their limitations. Such a discussion is frequently incorporated into a unit on vocational opportunities and general future plans. It is important that individuals have an accurate perception of their strengths and weaknesses before making these important decisions, and an important part of this is an understanding of the mental retardation label.

Other Reading

This chapter has not been meant to be a thorough coverage of special education methods with the retarded but is merely intended to survey current issues and trends. There are a great many books available covering special education methods, curricula, and practices both for the mentally retarded child and for the handicapped child in general.

Two excellent survey texts covering educational practices for all types of exceptional children are Dunn's *Exceptional Children in the Schools* (1973) and Kirk's *Educating Exceptional Children* (1972). Both of these adopt the traditional approach of discussing each type of handicap separately, a chapter on the mildly retarded, a chapter on the hearing impaired, and so on. An alternative organization that has become popular within the past few years is not to consider each handicap separately but to discuss the instruction of all types of exceptional children together. Examples of this approach are *The Exceptional Child* by Smith and Neisworth (1975), *The Education of Exceptional Learners* by Hewett and Forness (1974), and *Teaching the Exceptional Child* by L'Abate and Curtis (1975), although the latter combines the two approaches. Smith (1974) is an important reference on the subject of individualized instruction and clinical teaching.

There are a number of books that are directly concerned with curriculum for the educable mentally retarded and have a great many more specific suggestions for day-to-day activities than do the above books. Among these are such books as *The Educable Mentally Retarded Child* by Waite (1971), *Teaching the Retarded* by Blake (1974), and *Forgotten Children—Techniques in Teaching the Mentally Retarded* by Greene (1972). Gillespie and Johnson's *Teaching Reading to the Mildly Retarded Child* (1973) is specifically concerned with reading problems of the mentally retarded, and Peterson's *Functional Mathematics for the Mentally Retarded* (1973) is specifically concerned with arithmetic. A number of books, such as Haring and

Phillips' *Analysis and Modification of Classroom Behavior* (1972), are specifically concerned with the use of behavior modification techniques in the classroom. The reader who is interested in mainstreaming should refer to Birch's *Mainstreaming: Educable Mentally Retarded Children in Regular Classes,* (1974) which describes a number of mainstreaming programs. Other books on mainstreaming include *Instructional Alternatives for Exceptional Children* by Deno (1974) and *Educating Exceptional Children in Regular Classes* by Love (1972).

Summary

In recent years, there has been a shift in the philosophy of special education for EMR children away from the self-contained special class and toward integrating EMR students into regular classes for as much of the day as possible, a process called mainstreaming. There are some clear advantages and some clear disadvantages to this movement. Among the disadvantages of integration are the following:

1. In a regular classroom, retarded children will fall continually farther behind their age mates, and in the higher grades much of what goes on in a regular classroom will be incomprehensible to them because of their limited basic skills.
2. In a self-contained special class, EMR children not only get more special attention because there are usually fewer students, but they can be exposed to methods and materials specifically designed for slower-learning students.
3. The quality of education in the regular classroom can be improved if the slower students, who often demand a disproportionate amount of the teacher's time, can be removed.
4. Since retarded children tend to be socially isolated anyway, there is little social damage done by removing them from a regular classroom, and they will not have to suffer the constant humiliations associated with being slower than the other students.

However, there are some equally compelling arguments against the self-contained special class and in favor of mainstreaming. Among these are the following:

1. Education is far more likely to be individualized and take account of differences between students today than was the case in the past, and, as a result, the regular classroom is better able to cope with the slower student.

2. There has been a realization that all retarded children do not learn in the same way, and thus, it makes little educational sense to place them all in the same classroom.
3. It is usually necessary to label children mentally retarded before they can be placed in a special class, and this label is stigmatizing and humiliating.
4. Once children are placed in a special class, less will be expected of them, and they are less likely to be challenged.
5. Special classes represent a form of racial segregation in some communities because a grossly disproportionate percentage of special class students are from racial minorities. However, a number of recent court decisions have made it illegal to place children in a special class on the basis of a test score if the test is racially biased, and thus, this problem is slowly being corrected.
6. If handicapped children are placed in regular classes, the other children will acquire a better understanding of the nature of various disabilities, and thus, they will be more tolerant of handicapped people.
7. Research in which the educational performance of retarded children in special classes was compared to retarded children in regular classes has failed to demonstrate that retarded children benefit academically from special class placement.

The principal alternative to the self-contained special class is the resource room. Under this arrangement, EMR children spend most of their school day in a regular classroom but goes to the resource room either every day or several times a week for special tutoring in areas in which they are most deficient. The resource room can be staffed either by a single teacher or by a number of experts representing various specialities. Another alternative arrangement is an itinerant teacher who does little actual teaching but consults with the regular classroom teachers on the particular problems presented by the EMR children.

A large number of different approaches to teaching EMR children have been proposed. Among the most important are the following:

1. The physiological method of Seguin—an educational program stressing the training of the senses and motor training.
2. Montessori's autoeducational system—a teaching method based on the assumption that education should be enjoyable and that children should choose for themselves those activities that are best for them.

3. Piaget's approach, which stresses that children learn by doing rather than by being lectured to and that children must discover logical relationships for themselves.
4. The unit method of Ingram—a teaching method emphasizing practical knowledge and the application of academic subjects to real life.
5. The modified traditional curriculum—although not advocated by most special education experts, in fact what probably happens in most special classes is that children receive a watered-down version of the regular curriculum.
6. Perceptual-motor training—an educational system emphasizing special perceptual and motor exercises to fill in gaps in normal development.

The most recent innovation in special education is an approach called clinical teaching in which the specific weaknesses of each child are determined through the use of diagnostic tests, and where individual programs are tailored to meet these needs. A related process is task analysis, the breaking of a complex skill down into its component subskills so that the subskills that the child has not yet mastered can be systematically taught.

Virtually all retarded children have difficulty with reading. However, the kinds of reading problems presented by retarded children are no different than the reading problems presented by nonretarded children who also happen to have difficulty learning how to read. There is considerable disagreement concerning the best way to teach reading, and there is a general consensus now that there is no one best way, but that different children can learn to read best with different approaches. Another area of controversy concerns the best time to start to teach reading. Many special education programs do not begin to teach the children how to read until they are eight or nine years old, and they spend the first two to three years in reading readiness activities. However, this approach has been criticized because it means that, at least for a while, the retarded children are poorer readers than they would be if they had had reading instruction starting at a younger age.

Many EMR children also have speech and language difficulties that require attention. The most common types of speech problems are articulation disorders, and these can often be corrected with speech therapy, although only a minority of children in EMR classes receive this service. A more serious kind of language difficulty is a limited vocabulary and a general lack of fluency, and a number of curricula have been developed to provide language enrichment. The most widely used of these are the Peabody Language Kits.

The arithmetic component of the EMR curriculum usually focuses on the practical and applied side, teaching skills such as how to use money, how to tell time, measurement, and so forth, as well as basic computational skills.

An important component of most EMR programs today is instruction in personal, social, and vocational skills. It is particularly important for the schools to provide instruction in these kinds of practical knowledge because most EMR children have few opportunities to learn this knowledge on their own. Thus, a complete EMR program ought to provide extensive coverage of health issues including sex education, home management, marriage and the family, consumer education, government and the law, vocational training, and what it means to be mentally retarded.

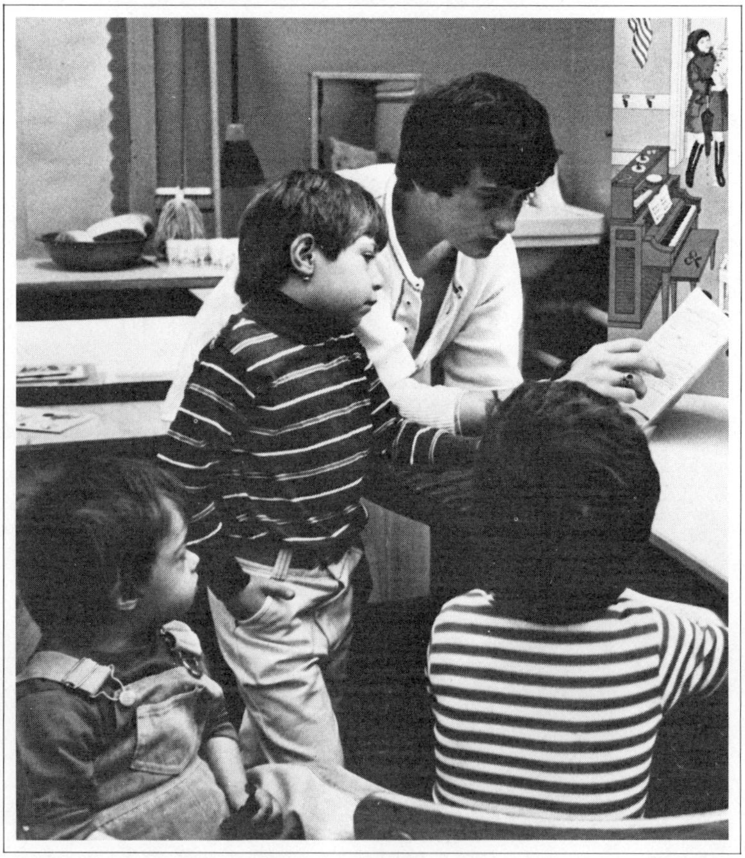

15

Education of the Moderately or Severely Retarded Child

Educational provisions for those children who are more than mildly retarded differ in some important ways from special education for mildly retarded children. Educators have traditionally referred to those children with IQs between 30 and 50 as trainable level children (TMRs) because their limited mental capacities preclude their learning formal academic subjects such as reading or arithmetic beyond a rudimentary level. Children with an IQ of less than 30 are sometimes referred to as custodial level because most of them cannot even be trained in basic self-care skills and thus, will require custodial care for their entire life. However, some people (e.g., Dunn, 1973) have objected to terms such as trainable and custodial because they are stigmatizing and they emphasize limitations rather than strengths.

Children with IQs of less than 50 comprise only a tiny minority of school age children. Typical estimates place the prevalence at about one in 400 children (Wirtz and Guenther, 1957). Unlike educable retarded children, the majority of these children have some sort of medical or organic cause for their diminished mental abilities. The largest single group is those children with Down's syndrome, but there are almost as many who have some sort of obvious brain damage, although, likely as not, the cause of this brain damage is unknown. Many children with IQs less than 50 are multiply handicapped, having some other significant disability such as cerebral palsy or visual handicap in addition to mental retardation.

Status of TMR Education

Because these children were considered ineducable, it has been traditional for schools to exclude them from any form of public school instruction. For example, in 1953, only 8 percent of the total number of moderately retarded children of school age were enrolled in public school programs. This figure has grown slowly since then, so that by 1963, 27 percent of trainable level children were enrolled, and, by 1973, more than half were enrolled (Dunn, 1973), but this is not a very admirable record for a nation that claims to have universal public education.

Parents of retarded children who had been excluded from school had three choices. They could institutionalize their child, they could send the child to a private school in the community where they would have to pay for the education, or they could keep the child at home and do nothing. None of these alternatives were very pleasant, and parents organizations began to pressure the schools to provide the education to which their children were entitled. A major breakthrough came in a 1971 Pennsylvania court suit (*Pennsylvania A.R.C.* v. *Commonwealth of Pennsylvania*). The essence of this ruling was that no child could be excluded from the public schools because of any handicap, either mental or physical. All children, regardless of their capabilities or limitations, are entitled to a full range of educational services appropriate to their needs. Since this decision, a number of other states have legislated a similar policy, often in order to avoid having such a policy forced on them by the courts. In 1975, Congress passed a major piece of legislation that encouraged all of the states to pass education-for-all legislation, and perhaps by the early 1980s, truly universal public education might be a reality in this country.

This rapid shift in policy has placed a considerable strain on many school districts. Moderately and severely retarded children are sufficiently different from normal children that any kind of mainstreaming except in a very limited fashion is not feasible, and thus it is necessary to establish self-contained segregated classes for these children. However, group teaching is largely ineffective with children with such severe limitations, they require a lot of individual attention in order to make any progress at all, but it is difficult to provide this because of a shortage of trained personnel who are able and willing to work with such children, and these new requirements are being forced on schools at the same time that they are facing unusual budget squeezes from other sources such as rising inflation, economic recession, and stronger teacher's unions. One approach that some school systems adopted was to simply provide grants to parents of moderately retarded children to enable them to send their child to a private school at public expense.

Teaching Methods in Trainable Level Classes

The Traditional Approach

The traditional approach to teaching trainable level children bears resemblance to the teaching approaches used in many nursery school and kindergarten programs. The emphasis was on group play, games, music, arts and crafts, language enrichment, physical education, and the like. Little attempt was made to individualize instruction or to provide a systematic, structured program geared to these children's particular needs. Dunn (1973) in reviewing the research on the effectiveness of traditional programs for trainable level students, found that the results were largely negative. There is little evidence that most special education programs were particularly effective in training self-care skills and skills of independent living. In fact, in some programs, there were no differences in abilities between children enrolled in school and similar children enrolled in no program at all (Cain and Levine, 1963). Follow-up studies of graduates of traditional programs for TMR children have found that virtually none of the graduates were able to live independently (Dunn, 1973).

Current Approaches to Teaching the Trainable Retarded: Behavior Modification

The major change in teaching lower functioning retarded children in recent years has been an increased emphasis on systematic, individualized instruction, generally from a behaviorist point of view. While the more traditional classroom was likely to provide generalized enrichment in a group setting, special education teachers are now more likely to provide a highly individualized program for each child in which the objectives are clearly specified in behavioral terms. This emphasis on individualized, competency-based instruction has permeated education at all levels, but its influence has been greatest for the training of extremely low-functioning children. With this type of child, it is very important to have a highly structured program in which each skill is specifically taught because the lower the mental capabilities of the individual, the less the individual can be relied on to learn simply by being exposed to material. Incidental learning skills, generalization abilities, and general concept formation skills are reduced in a trainable population, and as a result, such children must often be systematically taught what other children learn simply by observation or inference.

There are three important characteristics of the behavior modification approach to teaching low-functioning children. The first is that what is to be taught, the target behavior, is expressed in behavioral terms. A number of detailed curricula have now been published (e.g., Johnson and Warner, 1975; Fredericks et al., 1976; and Myers, Sinco, and Stalma, 1975), which consist of a large number of such behavioral objectives. One advantage of this approach is that it is quite easy to keep an accurate record of what children are able to do, what they are not able to do, and what kind of progress they are making toward the various goals that have been set for them.

A second characteristic of the behavioral approach is that positive reinforcement, both tangible such as food and intangible such as praise or a hug, are systematically used to teach children. In other words, instead of assuming that children will always be motivated on their own, their motivation is systematically directed toward their learning more advanced skills. Perhaps the most common way to dispense reinforcements is with tokens such as poker chips, check marks, gold stars, or anything that the children can turn in at a later time for a reward.

The third characteristic of the behavioral method is that the skills to be taught are systematically broken down into their various subskills and these subskills are taught sequentially. This not only facilitates learning, but it also provides an easy way to keep records and measure children's progress. Most of the rest of the chapter will consist of examples of such programs.

This behavior modification approach has been so much more successful than the more traditional group approach with the moderately, severely, and profoundly retarded that almost all training programs now employ these techniques, at least to some extent, and the typical TMR classroom is now likely to have extensive charts on the walls specifying the target behaviors determined individually for each child, the progress that each child is making toward these objectives, and the number of tokens that each child has accumulated. The following are some examples of the use of these techniques.

Toilet Training. For obvious reasons, teachers and parents of severely and profoundly retarded children are very concerned about toilet training such children, and a number of excellent systematic programs have been developed to accomplish this. Azrin and Foxx (1971) have described a technique that was originally used to toilet train profoundly retarded institutionalized adults. Each toilet on the ward was equipped with a moisture detector that played a tone when the subject eliminated in the toilet. The subjects were required to sit on the toilet for 20 minutes each day or until the tone sounded, in which case they were reinforced with candy and praise. During the rest of the day, the subjects wore an alarm device in their underpants that was triggered by moisture. As long as they remained dry, they received periodic reinforcement, but if they had an accident, they were cleaned up, then placed in a time-out room for one hour where they received no reinforcement. Thus, subjects were positively reinforced for eliminating in the toilet and reinforced for staying dry when not on the toilet. This program, in conjunction with a program that instructed these subjects to remove their pants appropriately, reduced the average number of toileting accidents on one ward from about 2 per resident per day to about .25 accidents per resident per day.

Putting on a Pair of Pants. Putting on a pair of pants may seem like an extremely simple behavior to most people, but it is sufficiently complicated to profoundly retarded adults or young moderately or severely retarded children that they may never learn how to do it on their own. However, this skill can be taught by breaking it down into a series of steps, and teaching each step individually. The following is a nine-step program developed by the author to train severely retarded children how to put on a pair of pants:

1. Pull the pants on over the children's feet up to their thighs and then guide their hands so that they grasp the top of their pants and pull them up the rest of the way.
2. The same procedure without guiding the children's hands. In other words, the children must pull their own pants up after they are put on up to their thighs.
3. Put the pants on only up to the ankles. Guide the children's hands so that they pull their pants up the rest of the way.
4. The same procedure without guiding the children's hands.
5. Put one leg through the appropriate opening. Guide the children's hands so that they put the other leg through the opening, then let them pull their pants up by themselves.
6. The same procedure without guiding the children's hands.
7. Hold the pants in the appropriate position and guide the children's hands and feet as necessary so that they put both feet into the appropriate openings. Then the children must pull the pants up all the way by themselves.
8. The same procedure without guiding the children.
9. Hand the children a pair of pants and permit them to put them on by themselves.

Children in such a program may have several trials each day until they master the last step. As with any program of this type, some steps might have to be varied somewhat to meet the needs of individual children, and different children might progress through the program at quite different rates. Some children might spend five or six trials a day for a week or more on one step, while others might progress through several steps in a single day. Ordinarily, children would receive a reinforcement of some sort such as a piece of candy or praise after each trial, as long as they were performing up to their best levels.

Notice that the steps are in reverse order. Instead of starting at the beginning of the process, step 1 teaches the final step and then each subsequent step works backward from there. This is a common practice in such programs, and the advantage of it is that the children are always reinforced for the same thing, in this case, pulling their pants up to their waists.

Training Language Skills. In many programs for lower-functioning retarded children, the single most important emphasis is on language training, and a number of excellent programs have been developed to teach various language skills. As is true with the other programs described in this section, the basic approach is to break the language learning task down into its component parts and then teach the various components systematically. However, it should be remembered that this approach is directly contrary to the normal language learning process, in which the child hears only whole sentences and must learn the rules of the language without the benefit of sequential instruction.

One of the best known operant programs of language training is that of Lovaas (1968). Using the principles of reinforcement and behavior shaping, he has developed a fairly complete program to teach basic vocabulary and syntax to children who are essentially nonverbal. Because this program is typical of many language training programs now being used around the country, it is described in detail. In general, the reinforcement used is food such as candy, but gradually, the child is switched from tangible to intangible reinforcers such as praise.

The first phase of the program involves the reinforcement of imitation behavior in the subject. Even this simple process requires four steps. In step 1, the child is reinforced for all vocalizations. During this stage, the child is also reinforced for fixating on the trainer's mouth. This procedure is continued until the child is averaging about one vocalization every five seconds and is attending to the trainer's mouth about half the time. In step 2, the trainer utters a sound such as "baby" periodically, and the child is reinforced only if he or she vocalizes within six seconds after the trainer's vocalization. During this step, the child is reinforced for any vocalization, even if it is not an imitation of what the trainer said. Step 3 is similar except that the child is only reinforced for matching the adult's vocalization; that is, the child actually has to imitate. This step is facilitated by the use of prompts. A prompt is a stimulus that will elicit the desired behavior with little training. For example, to facilitate the child uttering the sound "b," the trainer would hold the child's lips shut momentarily, then release the lips when the child exhaled. Once the child is imitating the "b" sound regularly, the prompt is faded out. Step 4 involves the introduction of a new sound so that the child has to discriminate between the two sounds and imitate the one that he or she hears. Subsequent steps involve the introduction of more new sounds.

Once the child is readily imitating the trainer, further language training is very much easier. The next phase of the program is called the establishment of an appropriate context for speech. In this phase, the child is taught to verbalize the names of common objects and behaviors. An object is placed in front of the child and the trainer says the name. The child imitates this and is reinforced. Gradually, the prompt is faded out; for example, the trainer might only say the first sound of the word. Once the child is able to name an object that is placed in front of him or her, the child is switched to a new object and the same procedure is repeated. Then the child is required to discriminate between the two. Then a third object is introduced and so on. When the child is able to reliably name six objects, the training procedure is changed, and the trainer asks the child to point to an object. The child is reinforced for pointing to the correct object rather than for verbalizing the name. This is training in receptive language. Notice that the Lovaas program teaches expressive language before receptive language, while in normal language learning, receptive language skills are usually well ahead of expressive language.

The third phase involves training in the use of common prepositions such as "on top of," "under," "beside," and "inside." An object that the child can already name, such as a penny, is placed inside a box, and the trainer says "Where is the penny?" If the child responds incorrectly, the trainer prompts by saying "The penny is inside the box." The child imitates this and is reinforced. Gradually the prompt is faded out. Various objects are used until the child can correctly use the preposition "inside." Other prepositions are taught in the same way. Then the child is asked to follow an instruction such as "Put the penny inside the box." Such a response may be guided by the trainer guiding the child's hand.

Similar procedures are used for training other constructions such as the proper use of pronouns and verbs. First the child is taught to verbalize the construction, then is taught to respond correctly to it. In both cases, prompts are used as needed.

One difficulty with this training program was that the children seldom or never used speech spontaneously. They would only speak in the training sessions. As a result, Lovaas had to specifically train them to use speech not only in training sessions, but in their day-to-day life as well. The people who worked with the children were instructed not to grant any privileges such as a glass of milk or permission to go outside unless the child verbalized the request. As in previous steps, first the child was given a prompt. For example, if the child wanted a glass of milk, the trainer would not give it until the child said the word "milk," but to help the child, the trainer would say the word and reinforce the child for imitating it. As in other steps, the prompt was faded out. Step by step, additional words were added such as "want milk," "I want milk," and so forth until the child could ask for a glass of milk with a whole sentence "I want a glass of milk."

Most other programs use similar principles. The crucial step in each of them is to get the child to imitate the model. Once this is accomplished, specific utterances can be taught. A number of such programs can be found in books edited by Sloane and MacAulay (1968) and by McLean, Yoder, and Schiefelbusch (1972). Snyder, Lovitt, and Smith (1975) provide a review of the use of operant techniques to train language.

Walking on a Balance Beam. Another important component of many TMR programs is training in gross motor skills, the sort of training that might be called physical education in more advanced classes. The following is an example of a 14-step program to train children to walk on a balance beam. As with similar programs, the child would receive a number of trials each day on the most advanced step that he or she was capable of and would receive systematic reinforcement for good performance. The only equipment necessary is a wide (about 10 inch) and a narrow (about 4 inch) balance beam.

1. Child stands on wide beam with help.
2. Child stands on wide beam alone.
3. Child stands on wide beam alone for 10 seconds.
4. Child takes 2 steps along wide beam with help.
5. Child takes 2 steps along wide beam alone.
6. Child takes 5 steps along wide beam alone.
7. Child takes 10 steps along wide beam alone.
8. Child stands on narrow beam with help.
9. Child stands on narrow beam alone.
10. Child stands on narrow beam alone for 10 seconds.
11. Child takes 2 steps on narrow beam with help.
12. Child takes 2 steps on narrow beam alone.
13. Child takes 5 steps on narrow beam alone.
14. Child takes 10 steps on narrow beam alone.

Curriculum Considerations for the Moderately, Severely, and Profoundly Retarded

The curriculum goals for the moderately and severely retarded differ in some important ways from those of EMR and nonretarded children. Trainable level children cannot reasonably be expected to ever learn to read much beyond the second-grade level, and as a result, while programs for the EMR tend to place a good deal of stress on reading, programs for moderately and severely retarded children usually spend little time on it. The main focus of TMR programs is on developing basic self-care skills and on language development and basic concept learning, the kinds of skills that many normal children do not need to be taught at all because they can learn them on their own.

A good rule of thumb is that a TMR child will be able to learn roughly the same skills that normal children of the same mental age are acquiring. Thus, the curriculum emphasis during the elementary school years is roughly similar to what the average nursery school child is learning. There is a heavy emphasis on language development, motor training, sensory training, and practical self-care skills. As the child grows older, it is possible to teach the child very basic reading and arithmetic skills, but the emphasis is usually on very practical reading and arithmetic, such as how to read "Men" and "Women" on the bathroom door or how to use money.

One of the best-known curricula for handicapped children is the Behavioral Characteristics Progression (BCP) developed by the Santa Cruz County (California) School District (1973). The BCP consists of a list of more than 2000 behavioral characteristics that can be used in both a descriptive manner to describe the child's present level of functioning and a prescriptive manner to set goals for the child. These behavioral characteristics are divided into 59 strands. Each strand contains up to 50 behaviors arranged in order from the most primary skills up through characteristics that are usually considered to be appropriate or acceptable adult behaviors. For example, the feeding/eating strand begins with such low level competencies as "Opens mouth when physically stimulated by spoon held by another," "Opens mouth voluntarily at the sight of food," and "removes semiliquid food from spoon with mouth when being fed—some rejection." The final three behavioral characteristics in this strand are "Carries own tray through serving line," "Serves self in cafeteria," and "Manages to eat different types of foods: liquids, crisp foods, slippery foods, sticky foods, chewy foods, foods with liquid and solids, foods requiring large bites and chewing."

The following is a partial list of the strands of the BCP, and it gives a good flavor of the range of different types of skills that are generally taught to more severely retarded children.

Feeding/eating
Drinking
Toileting
Grooming
Dressing
Undressing
Nasal hygiene
Oral hygiene
Self-identification
Sensory perception
Auditory perception
Visual motor
Gross motor
Prearticulation
Articulation
Language comprehension
Language development
Listening
Impulse control
Interpersonal relations
Responsible behaviors
Personal welfare (safety)
Self-confidence
Honesty
Social speech
Social eating
Attention span
Task completion
Reading
Practical math
Writing
Spelling
Reasoning
Music and rhythms
Arts and crafts
Prevocational skills
Kitchen skills
Homemaking skills
Outdoor skills

There are also special strands for those children with special sensory or physical disabilities such as manual language for the hearing impaired, wheelchair use, and mobility training for the visually impaired.

Other References

The above programs and lists of behavioral objectives represent only a small sample of the kinds of skills that are taught in most programs for TMR children. Children with Down's syndrome who go to school for 12 years are likely to have many hundreds of different skills taught to them during their educational career. The following books provide examples of curriculum guides for moderately, severely, and profoundly retarded children.

Alpern, G. D., & Boll, T. J. (Eds.) *Education and care of moderately and severely retarded children: with a curriculum and activities guide.* Seattle: Special Child Publications, 1971.

Fredericks, H. D. et al. *The teaching research curriculum for moderately and severely handicapped.* Springfield, Ill.: Charles C. Thomas, 1976.

Johnson, V. M., and Werner, R. A. *A step-by-step learning guide for retarded infants and children.* Syracuse: Syracuse University Press, 1975.

Molloy, J. S. (Ed.) *Trainable children: curriculum and procedures.* New York: John Day, 1972.

Myers, D. G., Sinco, M. E., & Stalma, E. S. *The right-to-education child: a curriculum for the severely and profoundly retarded.* Springfield, Ill.: Charles C. Thomas, 1974.

Waite, K. B. *The trainable mentally retarded child.* Springfield, Ill.: Charles C. Thomas, 1972.

Summary

The fastest growing area of special education today is the area of special training for children with IQs below 50, those children who have traditionally been referred to as trainable or custodial. Until recently, such children were routinely excluded from public schools, but several court decisions and recent legislation have affirmed the right of every child, even the most severely handicapped, to a full range of educational services.

Educational methods for these children often differ in important ways from those methods used with other children, and mainstreaming except in a very limited fashion is usually not feasible. The traditional approach to teaching these children has been relatively unstructured, with an emphasis on general enrichment. Because this approach was not particularly successful, there has been a shift in recent years toward an increasing emphasis on systematic, individualized instruction, generally from a behavioral point of view. In other words, what is to be taught is clearly specified in behavioral terms, reinforcements are dispensed systematically to maximize learning, and the various skills to be taught are systematically broken down into subskills, and these subskills are taught sequentially. Such methods have proved to be far more successful than traditional practices with low-functioning children.

The curriculum objectives for moderately, severely, and profoundly retarded children also differ in some important ways from the goals of higher-functioning children. There is less emphasis on academic skills and more stress placed on the activities of daily living, gross motor skills, self-care skills, basic language skills, and instruction in basic concepts. A good rule of thumb is that a TMR child will be able to learn roughly the same skills that a normal child of the same developmental level is acquiring.

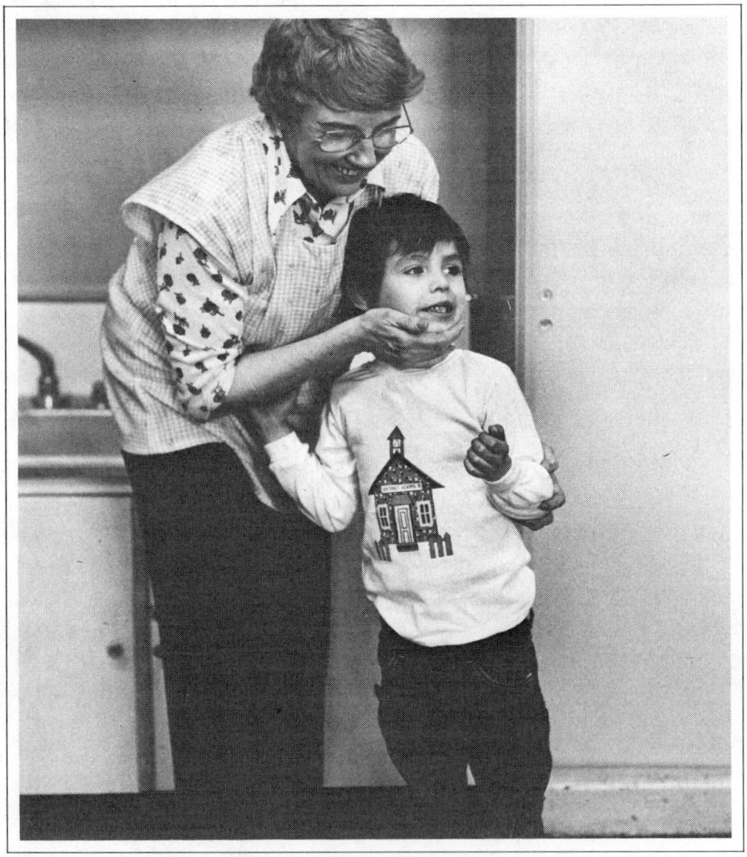

16

Preschool Programs for the Retarded

Prior to the 1960s, preschool programs for mentally retarded children or for children with other handicaps were virtually nonexistent. There were two reasons for this. The first was the generally held belief that the mentally retarded were largely unable to benefit from education or training, and the second was the belief that children of any mental level were unable to learn very much until they were five or six years old, and thus there was no need to begin education or training until that age. Even the best nursery schools for normal children at that time made little attempt to formally teach children anything. However, one of the most important conclusions that has come out of research with infants and preschoolers in the past few years is that they are far more competent than anyone suspected, being able to process certain types of high-level information shortly after birth, and that events in the first few years of life have important and possibly permanent effects on the child's social, emotional, and intellectual development. For example, research on disadvantaged children indicates that differences in mental abilities between low-income and middle-income children seem to appear some time in the second year of life, and that these differences are large by the time that the child reaches school age (White and Watts, 1974). Moreover, efforts at education and remediation after age five have been largely unsuccessful in reducing these differences. This is strong evidence that events in the first few years of a child's life may have a relatively permanent effect on the child's later course of growth.

As a result of such research, there has been a push in recent years to reach children born in potentially poor environments as young as possible in an attempt to prevent the often disastrous results that such an environment can produce. There is a similar movement toward providing special services for children diagnosed as handicapped during the preschool years in an attempt to minimize the effects of the handicap and to prevent the secondary disabilities such as emotional and behavior problems which frequently accompany such disabilities. An increasing number of people are beginning to propose that public education for all children begin at age three or four rather than at age five or six as is currently the case.

Screening and Case Finding

Mental retardation is often not formally diagnosed until the child is four or five years old, and some cases are not diagnosed until the child is well into elementary school. It is widely felt that by this age it is too late for any intervention to be truly effective, and that the best way to deal with the problem of functional retardation is to prevent it rather than to provide a massive dose of special education once it has been diagnosed. However, in order for this strategy to be effective, it is necessary to make a determination of which children are at high risk for becoming mentally retarded at some time in the future and to provide them with the necessary stimulation, training, and medical attention that they require but that their environment is not supplying.

As a step in this direction the federal government has mandated a program called the Early and Periodic Screening, Diagnosis, and Treatment Program (EPSDT). As its name implies, this program requires that all medicaid eligible children be given a medical checkup and screening on a periodic basis. Since the majority of children who are at risk for mental retardation are probably from families poor enough to receive medicaid, this program could provide the means of detecting most developmental disabilities early, when they are presumably more treatable.

At the present time, uniform assessment methods are not mandated (Rojcewicz and Aaronson, 1976), and a wide variety of different approaches are in use. Some people would like to define the at-risk population primarily in terms of medical criteria. For example, Parmelee et al. (1976) have developed a screening battery made up of fourteen items. Immediately after birth, in the neonatal period, five scores are determined: an obstetric complications score based on the presence or absence of optimal conditions during pregnancy, a postnatal factors score assessing the infant's health in the first month of life, a newborn neurological examination based on muscle tone, reflexes, and the like, a test of visual attention, and a sleep polygraph (assessment of sleep patterns is an indicator of the integration of the central nervous system). At three to four months, the infant is given four more tests, the sleep polygraph again, a pediatric examination to detect medical problems, the Gesell Developmental Examination (a widely used test of mental and motor development), and a test of visual attention. At eight or nine months the child is give five more tests, the pediatric exam and the Gesell Developmental Exam again, a test of hand manipulation and sensorimotor schemas, a test of exploratory behavior and preference for novelty, and a test of cognitive development. The authors report that no single score alone is adequate for making a determination that an infant is at risk, but that in combination, a reliable determination can be made.

The above test battery is fairly elaborate, and other screening programs tend to rely more on a single instrument which assesses general development. The most widely used test is the Denver Developmental Screening Test, which was described in Chapter 2. One difficulty with this approach is that prior to the age of about two, most such tests are poor predictors of later development except in cases of extremely slow development.

Still other programs tend to make the decision that a child is at risk for mental retardation primarily on the child's family background. Children in large black families who are in the lowest income levels and whose parents also have low intelligence have a greater than 50 percent chance of having a tested IQ in the retarded range during their school years (Heber, Dever, and Conry, 1968), and thus it makes good sense to consider children with such characteristics to be at risk.

Preschool Programs for Children at Risk for Mental Retardation

The first major effort to provide preschool programming to children who were considered to be at risk of becoming mentally retarded, or at least developmentally delayed, was the Head Start Program. The initial demonstration projects were funded by a 1965 federal act, which was a part of Lyndon Johnson's war on poverty. The expressed purpose of the Head Start programs was to provide compensatory education to children from low-income families in an effort to compensate for the presumably inadequate level of training and stimulation that these children were receiving at home, and thus bring them up to the level of middle-class children by the time that they started school. Head Start programs were run on a wide variety of different philosophies and models. Some were quite similar to the traditional nursery school, being relatively permissive and providing few structured learning situations but a good deal of general enrichment, such as field trips, games, and verbal stimulation. Others were just the opposite, providing a highly structured program that explicitly and formally set out to teach certain basic cognitive and verbal skills.

General Characteristics

There are a number of skills that almost all preschool programs emphasize. The most important of these is language skills. The preschool period is the time of the most rapid development of oral language skills, with many children increasing their spoken vocabulary at the rate of nearly two new words per day. There are numerous different techniques for increasing verbal abilities, mostly aimed at increasing vocabulary. For example, one Head Start Project used a process of verbal bombardment, with the teacher maintaining a steady stream of questions and comments (Perry Preschool Project, *It Works,* 1969). Other programs used games that encouraged oral language development, such as talking on the telephone or acting in little plays. Still other programs systematically taught language skills using operant conditioning techniques. For example, Baroff (1974) describes a 10-step procedure for teaching the word and the concept of "apple." The first step involves the teacher showing an apple to a child or to a group of children and saying "apple" as the teacher encourages the children to touch it. Then the teacher asks the child to make a two-choice discrimination, requesting the child to select which of two objects is an apple. The third step requires the child to select an apple from among a number of objects. The fourth, fifth, and sixth steps are similar to steps one to three except that they involve a picture of an apple rather than the real thing. The next three steps involve teaching the major functions of an apple, identifying its principal parts, and identifying its various attributes such as color and texture. The final step requires the child to actually say the word.

A second aspect of the curriculum in most preschool programs is the teaching of basic concepts. For example, it is not unusual for the basic spatial relationships such as on top of, beside, underneath, inside, and so forth to be systematically taught. This teaching involves not only teaching the word, but also the actual nature of the relationship must be taught to the child in many cases. In similar fashion, temporal relationships such as beginning and end or before and after might be taught. Almost any preschool program teaches colors to children who don't know them as well as concepts like same versus different and larger versus smaller.

Among the other skills that are taught more or less systematically in most preschool programs are gross and fine motor skills, perceptual abilities such as the ability to discriminate between the letters of the alphabet, basic number skills, social skills such as taking turns, sharing, and impulse control, listening skills and the ability to sit still, and whatever self-care skills are needed such as shoe tying, buttoning, and the like.

Another goal of many compensatory education programs is the development of a positive self-image and an expectancy of success. Usually, this is not taught systematically, but emerges as a result of teaching methods in which the children are seldom criticized and are seldom exposed to failure. One of the major problems both of mentally retarded children and of disadvantaged children is that they do not think highly of themselves, and they have been exposed to so many failure experiences that they expect to fail at new things. Thus, it is important for preschool programs to make an attempt to reverse this as young as possible or even to prevent such negative attitudes from developing in the first place.

Project Head Start and other compensatory education programs were not the overwhelming success that their supporters had hoped. Cicirelli (1969) reviewed the outcomes of various such projects and concluded that while some of the programs produced short-term gains in scores on IQ tests, within a year or so after the completion of the program, children who had been given this extensive enrichment were performing no better than similar children who had not received special attention and most of the programs had been unsuccessful in preventing academic failure.

However, some Head Start programs were far more successful than others, and current compensatory education programs are making an attempt to replicate the more successful features of these programs as well as continuing to try new methods. The reader who is interested in reading about some of the more successful programs is referred to a series of pamphlets published by the U.S. Office of Education called *It Works* (1969), which describes some of the better known and more successful programs.

Spicker (1971) reviewed the outcomes of a number of compensatory education programs in an attempt to determine what distinguished the more successful from the less successful type of program. He distinguished four basic curriculum models. The first was the traditional nursery school approach, which emphasized social and emotional development through unstructured free play, art, music, games, and the like. A second approach was the cognitive development model, which provided a much more highly structured teaching environment stressing basic cognitive skills such as oral language, memory, concept formation, and the like. The third was the perceptual-motor development model, of which the Montessori system is the best example. These programs emphasized sensory and perceptual training rather than cognitive or academic skills. The last approach was an academic skills curriculum in which specific academic skills such as language development, reading, and numbers were systematically taught in a highly structured program. Among his conclusions were the following:

1. Curriculum models that stress cognitive or academic skills development produce the largest IQ score increases.
2. The traditional nursery school approach is only effective with a program that contains specific goals, language development in particular, and is well supervised and highly structured.
3. Structured programs other than cognitively or academically oriented ones produce intellectual gains only if they incorporate strong oral language.
4. Those preschool programs that emphasize academic skills improve rote reading and arithmetic computation skills rather than improved comprehension and reasoning skills.
5. The emphasis in preschool programs should be on fine motor skills, memory, and oral language rather than on abstract or critical thinking or on creativity.
6. Home intervention is only important when no other school program is available.
7. All successful programs had a high ratio of adults to children.

The Milwaukee Project

One early stimulation project deserves special note because of its success. This is the Milwaukee Project, implemented by Heber and his associates (Heber and Garber, 1975). Unlike most other intervention programs that do not begin until the children are four or five years old, this project began working with infants at risk within the first six months after birth. The infants were placed in an education center for seven hours a day, five days a week where they received special training and stimulation. When the children were under 15 months old, the ratio of teachers to children was one to one; in other words, there was one teacher for each child. Even for older children, the teacher child ratio never exceeded one to four. In addition to the training that the children received at the school, their mothers were given special instruction in proper child-rearing techniques and in ways to facilitate the mental and physical development of their children.

The results of this program were nothing less than spectacular. The children selected for the program all came from the poorest sections of Milwaukee and all were black. In addition, the mothers of these children all had low intelligence. More than half of these children could normally be expected to have a tested IQ in the mentally retarded range by the time that they reached school age. However, the mean IQ of the children actually exceeded the average IQ of the community by a considerable amount, and the difference in IQ between the program children and a comparison group of children from a similar background who did not go through the program was 30 points. The program children exceeded the control group children by 18 months on language age as measured by the ITPA and were superior on numerous other tests of mental functioning.

There are a number of reasons why this project was so much more successful than other attempts to prevent cultural retardation. First, and perhaps most important, they reached the children when they were very young. Thus, the program is genuinely preventative, while most compensatory education programs attempt to cure a problem which already exists. Second, the Milwaukee Project was far more intensive than virtually any other compensatory education program. While the typical Head Start program worked with their children for a few hours a day for a few months, this project had the children all day for five years. Another measure of the intensity is the small ratio of teachers to children so that each child was receiving almost continual personal attention from an adult.

Preschool Programs for Handicapped Children

Head Start programs were aimed at children who, although they had not been formally diagnosed as mentally retarded, had a high risk of experiencing school failure and perhaps being diagnosed as retarded at a later time. A second type of preschool program is aimed at children who have already been determined to have a developmental disability of some sort. Thus, the aim of such programs is not to prevent developmental disabilities but to minimize the effect of the disability and to prevent the development of secondary emotional and behavioral disturbances. Actually the distinction between the two types of programs is not very important since the kinds of activities that go on in both are quite similar, and the distinction between the two is further blurred by recent federal legislation that mandated that the enrollments of Head Start programs contain at least 10 percent handicapped children.

The University of Washington Down's Syndrome Program

One of the most impressive of these programs is the Down's Syndrome Program at the University of Washington (Hayden and Haring, 1976), and it will be described in some detail as an example of an early stimulation program for handicapped children. The program is designed to serve children with Down's syndrome at any age under the first-grade level, but preferably the children should be enrolled as young as possible, and many children are enrolled when they are only a few weeks old. The goal of the program is to have the development of each child approximate normal development as closely as possible in each of the following skill areas: gross and fine motor, social, communication, cognitive, and self-help. The technique used is to develop a set of behavioral objectives for each child and then to write a specific program of sequential steps in order for the child to achieve each of the goals. These programs are continually assessed and precise records are kept so that improvements can be made. As is the case with other similar programs, parental involvement is encouraged so that they can carry through what is being taught in the classroom in the child's own home.

There are four levels of classes based on the age of the child. In the infant class, the parent and child visit the center once a week and the parents receive instructions in how to facilitate the motor and sensory development of their child. Goals are established for the child each week. Typical of the goals for an 18-month-old Down's syndrome child are that the child will, with 80 percent or better accuracy, be able to sit without support, stand for five minutes with support, make eye contact with people, reach, grasp, hold, and release objects on cue, drink from a cup, and so on.

The next level is called early preschool. During this time, the children attend 90-minute classes four days a week. The curriculum for this group emphasizes self-help skills such as dressing, washing, and toileting; work with manipulative materials such as crayons, blocks, and puzzles; language development; and continued emphasis on gross motor skills such as encouraging children to stand for a longer period of time and teaching them to move from one position to another. When the children are about three, they move to the advanced preschool class, which meets for two hours a day. This is basically an extension of the earlier class with a particular emphasis on language development. Among the behavioral objectives for this group are walking up and down stairs, riding a tricycle, recognizing colors, understanding number concepts up to 3, demonstrating an understanding of 10 action verbs, naming objects spontaneously, having clean and dry pants 80 percent or more of the time, and using the toilet with minimal assistance. The oldest group is the kindergarten section. Some of the behavioral objectives appropriate for this group are understanding calendar concepts, using appropriately in speech at least half of the nouns, verbs, and adjectives for which they have demonstrated receptive understanding, printing their first name, understanding number concepts from 1 to 5, and discriminating and naming letters.

Although there is no control group with which to make a formal comparison, it is apparent that this program has had a substantial impact on these children. Many of them are performing nearly up to their age norms, a rare feat for a child with Down's syndrome. Further evidence for its success comes from the observation that children who are not enrolled until they are older lag behind those children who have been in the program since infancy. The ultimate sign of success is that a number of the children are making the beginnings of learning how to read even though they are only five or six years old, truly a remarkable accomplishment for a child who would not normally be considered educable.

The Portage Project

Almost all preschool programs for the handicapped make an effort to involve the child's parents, and some programs use the parents as the child's principal teacher, with the professionals acting primarily in a consulting capacity. One of the best such programs is the Portage Project (Shearer and Shearer, 1976). This program is geared to provide preschool intervention to handicapped preschool children in an extremely rural Wisconsin region where transporting the children to and from school each day would be a major problem. There is no classroom program at all; all instruction is done by the child's own parents at home. A trained teacher or paraprofessional visits each home for 90 minutes each week and prescribes specific programs geared to the child's individual needs. Each child is given at least three behaviorally defined goals to be met each week. A set of 580 behaviors have been identified that can be taught, and a program has been developed to teach each one. The following is a sample of the kinds of behaviors that are taught to children functioning at the three to four year level: identifies big and little, completes six-piece puzzle, draws a square in imitation, matches three primary colors, identifies primary colors, counts to five in imitation, identifies boy and girl, and so on.

Each one of these competencies is accompanied by a number of activities that the parent can carry out at home. For example, there are six sequential activities to teach the skill "Identifies big and little."

1. Give the child 10 blocks of the same color, five large and five small, and have the child sort them by size.

2. Using two objects that differ only in size, ask the child to point to the big one or the little one. When the child can do this consistently, have the child name each one as he or she points.

3. Using small penny-sized candy bars and larger ones with the same wrapper, have the child name the big one and the little one, giving the child the candy as a reward.

4. Place cutout circles on the floor, some large and some small. At first have the child only step on the large circles, then only on the little circles. Then have the child tell the parent which circle to step on and indicate whether the parent was correct or not.
5. Place a reward on the circles and have the child name the size of the circle in order to get it.
6. Gradually reduce the size of the circles and repeat similar activities.

When the teacher makes the weekly visit to the home, he or she determines whether the goals were met, and then, in consultation with the parent, sets three goals for the upcoming week. The teacher then shows the parent the appropriate activities and makes sure that the parent knows what to do. The teacher also collects baseline data on the child so that the child's improvement over the course of the week can be determined. Throughout the week the parent fills out activities charts indicating what they did with the child each day and how the child performed. In the event that problems arise, the parent can call the teacher for advice.

The Portage Project staff has collected considerable data documenting the impact of the project on the children. For example, the average child in the program gained some 15 IQ points over an eight-month period (from 75 to 90). In the first year, an average of 128 prescriptions were written for each child, and 91 percent of these were met.

Summary

Recent research with infants and young children has indicated the importance of the first few years of life in determining the overall course of development of the child. As a result, preschool programs for children who are considered to be at risk for developing learning problems in the school years are proliferating. The assumption behind such programs is that it is easier to prevent developmental disabilities in the first place than it is to try to treat them once they have developed.

The first step is to identify children who are at risk for becoming mentally retarded or having other learning problems or disabilities later on. Some programs use primarily medical criteria, judging a child to be at risk if the child is underweight at birth or if there were other pregnancy complications or if the child has abnormal neurological signs. Other programs rely more on a developmental exam such as the Denver Developmental Screening Test to determine the at risk population. Still other programs define a child to be at risk if the child comes from a disadvantaged family.

Many of the early preschool programs for such children were funded by the Head Start Program. These projects used a variety of different teaching methods, some being relatively unstructured, others providing a good deal of structure. The early Head Start Programs were not as successful as their backers had hoped, since many of their graduates had academic problems once they started school. However, an analysis of the characteristics that distinguished the more successful from the less successful programs concluded that the more successful programs were those that were highly structured and that stressed cognitive and academic skills.

One early intervention project that deserves note is the Milwaukee Project, which provided low-income black children with an intensive training program outside the home starting shortly after birth. This program has been far more successful than most other compensatory programs because it began when the children were very young and because the program was very intensive.

Still other preschool programs are aimed primarily at children who have already been diagnosed as handicapped. Two examples are the Down's Syndrome Program at the University of Washington and the Portage Project in Wisconsin. The latter project is unique in that all of the teaching is done by the parents rather than by teachers.

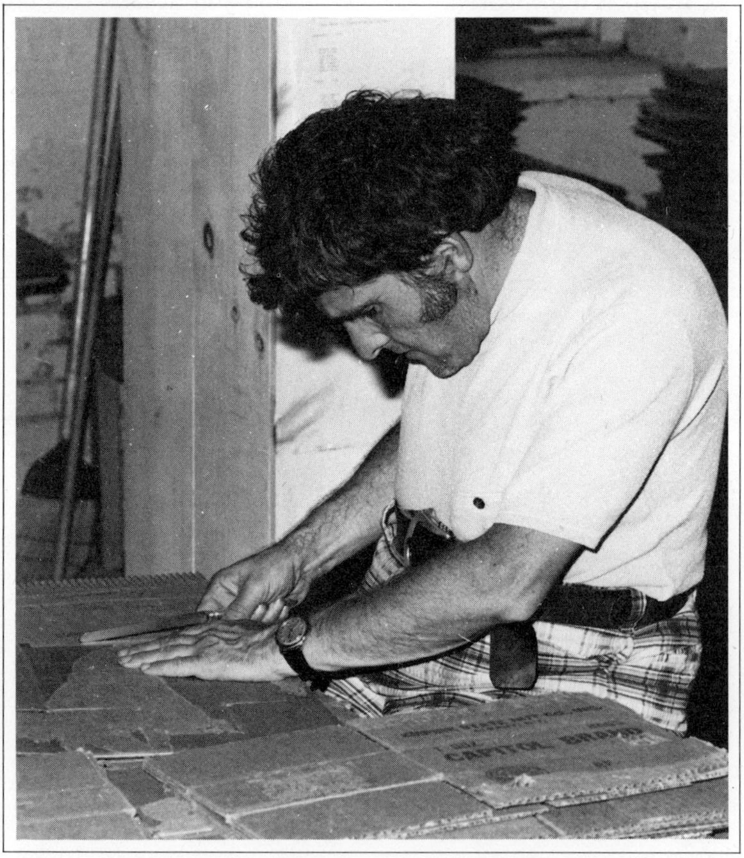
CAPITOL BRAND

17

The Mentally Retarded Adult

When most people hear the term mentally retarded, they think of children, apparently forgetting that these children grow up to become adults. Government social policy seems to have a similar bias, and, as a result, most programming for the retarded has provided services primarily for children rather than for adults. Until recently, there were only two alternatives available for mentally retarded adults; they could either be institutionalized, which entailed removing them from normal society almost entirely, or they could try to become a functional member of society with little or no support from social service agencies. There was no middle ground, no attempt to provide special programming or services for retarded adults within the community.

Fortunately, these deficiencies in programming are beginning to be met now. A major impetus for this increased community involvement in providing good services for the mentally retarded adult has been the recognition that the traditional residential institution was not the proper place for the vast majority of retarded people. Beginning in the early 1960s, government at all levels has begun to deemphasize the role of the residential institution in the programming for the retarded and placed new stress on small programs within each community. These services include sheltered workshops, vocational training programs, activity centers, recreation programs, and alternative living arrangements. However, the need for such services still outstrips the supply.

This chapter considers various types of programming for the mentally retarded adult in today's society. The first section reviews the research on what happens to retarded children when they become adults. The next section discusses the role of the residential institution as a part of the total management picture in the immediate past and in the present, and the last section considers community programming as an alternative to institutionalization, with particular emphasis on vocational rehabilitation.

The Status of the Mentally Retarded Adult

Follow-up Studies of the Educable Mentally Retarded

The label mentally retarded implies social incompetence, and it is widely assumed that almost all mentally retarded people will be dependent on others for most of their adult lives. However, researchers who have followed up on what happens to people who have graduated from special classes in the public schools or who have been released from residential institutions for the mentally retarded have consistently verified that this is not the case. In fact, a substantial majority of children who are considered mentally retarded grow up to lead independent, productive lives. They get married, hold jobs, buy homes, and are generally indistinguishable from other people in their community who come from similar backgrounds.

Although a large number of studies have verified this, only two will be described here, and the reader who is interested in pursuing this issue further is referred to Cobb (1972) for an excellent review. The classic study in this area was done by Charles (1953). He traced 151 people who had been in special classes for the mentally retarded during the 1930s. All had had an IQ of less than 70 while they were in school. At the time of the study, when the average age of the subjects was 42, the vast majority were living independently. Only six percent were institutionalized, including one in jail and two in mental hospitals. Of those who were still alive, 83 percent were employable and usually had employment. The majority were laborers, but some were higher on the occupational scale. One managed a cleaning establishment, another was a bookkeeper, and a third was a building contractor. Some 80 percent were or had been married, a figure only slightly below the national average, and over half owned or were buying their own home. Of those who were married, about 80 percent had one or more children, and the majority of these children were progressing normally in school. However, this study did find a significantly higher death rate and a somewhat higher rate of law violations than would be expected from the general population, although most of the legal infractions were minor.

A similar study by Kennedy (1966) followed a group of 256 people who had been diagnosed as morons (mildly retarded) during their school years. This study is particularly noteworthy because it used a control group, a group of nonretarded people of similar age, ethnic background, and socioeconomic status to the retarded people. Notice that the control group was not intended to be representative of the community as a whole.

In many ways, the group of mentally retarded subjects was remarkably similar to the control group in adult life. About the same percentage of each group had married (86 percent of the retarded and 92 percent of the controls), and the average number of children was virtually identical for the two groups. However, the children of the retarded subjects were more likely to show academic retardation than were the control group children. Approximately equal proportions of each group had received relief of some sort, and the same proportion of each group was employed and employable. Almost a third of the mentally retarded subjects were skilled workers of some sort. However, the average earnings of the control group were somewhat higher because a number of them had moved into managerial and professional occupations. The mentally retarded group showed a somewhat higher number of antisocial acts, although the overwhelming majority (88 percent) were law-abiding citizens.

The results of this type of research represent a consistent embarrassment to the mental retardation establishment because it suggests that many children who are considered mentally retarded by the schools, and indeed, many people who are in institutions for the mentally retarded, are capable of independent living, and thus, probably ought not to be considered mentally retarded. Recall that in order to be legally considered retarded, the individual must show an impairment in adaptive behavior, and clearly many of the retarded subjects in the Charles and the Kennedy studies were not impaired in adaptive behavior. This data has been instrumental in the recent trend toward labeling a smaller proportion of the population as mentally retarded (e.g., the dropping of the category of borderline retardation).

Predictors of Independent Living

While it is interesting to know that the majority of retarded adults are able to live independently, it is just as important to discover why some people are able to successfully adjust while others are unable to hold down a job and spend most of their lives dependent on other people or on social service agencies. It would be very useful for those people who work with the mentally retarded to be able to predict with reasonable accuracy whether a given individual will be likely to effect a successful adjustment or not. For example, institutions all over the nation are now in the process of releasing many of their long time residents, and it would be convenient if they had some reliable criteria to determine who is likely to successfully disappear into society and who is likely to require continued close supervision. Similarly, many vocational rehabilitation programs are mandated to only accept those clients who have a high probability of being successfully employed, and, thus, it is important for them to know what kinds of characteristics are conducive to vocational success.

Unfortunately, research into this question has been almost universally disappointing. The usual research technique is to compare a group of retarded people who have successfully adjusted with another group who have failed to adjust in order to determine what characteristics distinguish them, but this method has not proved to be very productive. Characteristics found to be important in one study are shown to be unimportant in another, and many characteristics that people feel ought to be good predictors of success have proved not to be. For example, it is reasonable to assume that IQ would correlate highly with successful adjustment of a retarded person, but Windle (1962), after reviewing more than 100 studies of the adjustment of retarded people released from institutions, concluded that there was no relationship between IQ and later social adjustment. There is no tendency for retarded people of higher IQ to be more successful than retarded people of lower IQ. This may appear to be a surprising finding, but it must be remembered that these studies are all dealing with a restricted range of intelligence, somewhere between IQ 50 and IQ 85. If a larger range of IQs were included, the expected relationship between intelligence and adjustment would almost certainly appear. However, it is clear that IQ by itself is not a very important predictor of adjustment, and Windle suggests that institutions place far too much emphasis on IQ when they are considering an individual for release.

Most vocational counselors and social workers who work with the retarded are convinced that what can loosely be called personality is far more important than intelligence in determing whether an individual will be successful in adjusting to independent living. A person who is emotionally mature and has a positive attitude toward working is likely to be successful regardless of IQ, while an immature, impulsive person will probably be continually getting into trouble regardless of that person's mental abilities. However, personality is often difficult to assess reliably, and there is not always full agreement concerning which aspects of personality are the most important for successful adjustment. Some studies have been able to produce lists of personality traits that seem to distinguish the successfully adjusted retarded person from the unsuccessful, but the relationship between these variables and adjustment is not large enough to be of much use. For example, Shafter (1957) found that the following characteristics distinguished the successful from the unsuccessful parolees from an institution at a statistically significant level: truthfulness, obedience, attention to detail, and less aggressiveness and quarrelsomeness during the individual's stay in the institution. However, the relationships, while statistically significant, were fairly small.

It is probably the case that as long as very gross measures of adjustment are used such as whether a retarded person who is released from an institution is returned or not, only slight relationships will be found between adjustment and personal characteristics. Adjustment is simply too complex to be determined by a small number of easily measurable personality traits. It is probably the case that an individual's adjustment is more dependent on the particular circumstances that he encounters than it is on his own particular characteristics. Jencks et al. (1972), after reviewing an enormous body of research on this issue (not with the mentally retarded but for the general population), concluded that prediction of success on the basis of capabilities or even family background could account for a relatively small proportion of the variance in income and status, and that a far larger percentage of the variance must be attributed to inherently unpredictable factors that could be labeled luck. In other words, trying to predict successful adjustment on the basis of personal characteristics is somewhat analogous to trying to develop a personality test that will predict winners of a state lottery.

This conclusion suggests that if we are interested in predicting the success of retarded people, we should pay less attention to the individual's personal characteristics and more to the characteristics of the environment. Not surprisingly, one environmental factor that has consistently been correlated with successful adjustment is the amount of support and supervision provided by family and friends. Studies dating as far back as 1919 (Fernald) have reported that those retarded individuals who are able to rely on their families for support and advice are likely to fare far better than those who do not have this advantage. An interesting variant of this was described by Edgerton (1967). He followed up a number of individuals who had been permanently released from an institution in order to determine how they were adjusting. Almost every successful person had acquired a benefactor, a normal individual who was able to help them with their many problems. This benefactor might have been a landlord, a neighbor, or an employer, but the fact that virtually every person who had been successfully rehabilitated had found a benefactor, and the frequency with which the benefactor came to their rescue indicates that this is an important ingredient in the successful adjustment of retarded people.

This finding has some implications for the planning of mental retardation services. When a retarded individual is being considered for release from an institution, it might be more beneficial to take into account the range of supportive services that are available in the community than it is to make the decision solely on the basis of the individual's capabilities.

Follow up Studies of the Trainable Mentally Retarded

There have been far fewer studies investigating what happens to moderately or severely retarded people after they leave school, but it is clear that the prognosis for these people ever achieving independence is far less bright. Stanfield (1973) followed up 120 graduates of public school programs for the moderately retarded. The IQ range was 30 to 50. This study was limited by the fact that the data were collected within three years after the subjects graduated, and it is possible that at least some of the subjects who were still dependent on their parents might be independent at some later time. However, at the time of the study, one one of the 120 was living alone. Several of them were in institutions or boarding homes, but an overwhelming 94 percent were still living with their parents. Not a single subject was self-supporting. Only 3 percent had any sort of competitive employment at all, and all of these were part time. About 40 percent were working in a sheltered workshop, but of these 48 subjects, 80 percent were earning less than $10 per week. An additional 11 percent attended an activity center, but 52 of the subjects (44 percent) had no program at all. They were simply hanging around the house. Their major activity was watching television, and virtually none had any kind of social or recreational life beyond participating in a recreation program for the retarded for a few hours each week. While almost all of the subjects could care for their basic needs, only 23 percent of the parents reported that they could leave home for extended periods of time, and 40 percent of the subjects never even left the front yard of their home unaccompanied.

An earlier study by Saenger (1957) on the same subject came to a basically similar conclusion. Like the Stanfield study, he found that virtually none of the moderately retarded subjects in his sample were living independently, and only 27 percent had jobs on a full- or part-time basis, including those working in sheltered circumstances. Their lives were characterized by loneliness, emptiness, and meaninglessness. The only positive note in this research was that virtually all of the subjects were able to take care of themselves and help around the house.

These two studies point out a real gap in programming for the retarded that is only beginning to be filled now, the need for meaningful activities for the more severely handicapped individual who can probably not hope to live independently. Many of these people are able to be productive workers in a sheltered situation, but even today, there are not enough positions in sheltered workshops to come close to filling the need, and there is still a tremendous need for other kinds of recreation and social activities for these people to relieve their emptiness and loneliness and to make them less of a burden on their families.

The Mentally Retarded and Employment

Probably the most important single factor determining whether handicapped individuals are able to live independently is whether they are able to obtain and hold a job that will pay enough to meet their needs. In fact, successful adjustment might almost be defined in terms of whether a person has a job or not. A paycheck is only one of the benefits of having a steady job. Work is important not only because it provides the individual with money to meet his material needs, but economists also talk about "psychological income" obtained from having a job, the status, the improvement in self-esteem from doing something meaningful and productive, the increased social contacts, the freedom from boredom, and so on. These benefits, while important to everyone, are particularly important to a handicapped person who is likely to be suffering from problems of low self-esteem and who is likely to have limited opportunities for social contacts and for developing other interests. The best way that retarded people can prove to themselves and to other people that they are "normal" is to have a job.

There are a number of generalizations that can be made concerning the employability of the mentally retarded. The first is that within the range of mildly retarded people, which includes about 85 percent of all those who are considered mentally retarded, there is no relationship between employability and IQ. This finding has been found in numerous studies (e.g., Kolstoe and Frey, 1965). This is consistent with the research on general social adjustment (Windle, 1962), which concluded that IQ was not a good predictor of adjustment. While this may surprise some people, it is consistent with a second generalization about work and the retarded. Retarded people seldom or never lose a job because they are unable to do the work (Gold, 1973). There are a great many jobs in this country that require no intellectual abilities at all, jobs such as stuffing envelopes or routine assembly skills or certain factory jobs that are highly repetitive, and mildly retarded people are able to perform most of these as well as anyone else. The reason why mentally retarded people lose their jobs is almost always because of some personality or behavior problems; they cannot get along with co-workers or with their boss or they are late or absent too frequently or they are unable to concentrate for long periods of time or they have peculiar mannerisms or are emotionally unstable. A third generalization is that there is no relationship between academic abilities and job success among the mentally retarded (Kolstoe and Frey, 1965). This is not surprising if one considers the types of jobs in which retarded people are usually found, simple laboring or service jobs that require little or no reading or calculating. A fourth generalization is that the very vast majority of mildly retarded people in this country are employable, meaning that they possess sufficient mental and physical abilities and have sufficient control over their emotions to be able to hold down some sort of regular job. Of course, this does not mean that everyone who is employable will have a job. Retarded people are just as subject to the whims of the economy as anyone else, and thus, when unemployment is high, many retarded people will be unable to find work even though they possess the necessary skills. Another unfortunate fact is that many employers still discriminate against retarded workers and are less likely to hire them. Most vocational rehabilitation counselors who work with the retarded agree that training the necessary skills in retarded clients is far easier than finding them a job after they have been trained.

It is difficult to make any generalizations about the kinds of jobs in which the retarded are likely to be found. Naturally, many of them take low-paying menial jobs such as kitchen work, maintenance, hospital work, or the most routine kinds of factory jobs, but the follow-up studies mentioned above reported that many retarded people are able to become skilled workers or even move into white-collar jobs. Probably the only type of work from which the retarded are virtually excluded are those occupations that require a good deal of education.

Becker (1976) surveyed job training programs for mentally retarded youths and gathered information on the various kinds of jobs in which retarded people were placed. The 1438 trainees were assigned to 185 different kinds of jobs. Table 17-1 lists those jobs to which at least one percent of the trainees were assigned. This list is instructive because it demonstrates the diversity of different jobs which are appropriate for retarded people. Since these people were trainees, presumably most of them would eventually move up the vocational ladder to higher level positions.

The Residential Institution

Society's traditional solution to the problem of individuals who are unable to take care of themselves has been to remove them from the community and place them in large public institutions on a long-term basis. These institutions are usually called state hospitals or state schools, but the term developmental center is becoming popular. They have always played an important role in the provision of services to the mentally retarded. In 1970, there were some 190 state residential facilities for the retarded in this country, at least one in every state except Nevada. At that time, these institutions housed about 186,700 residents (the term resident is generally preferred

Table 17-1 Job Training Assignments for 1438 Retarded Youths

Job Title	Number of Trainees Assigned
Janitor	156
Dishwasher	92
Bus boy/girl	80
Kitchen helper	59
Stock boy/girl	55
School cafeteria helper	52
Automobile washer	41
Motel maid	38
Waitress	37
Nurse's aide	34
Construction worker	25
Nursemaid	25
Dietary aide	24
Assembler	23
Short order cook	19
Bagger (grocery store)	19
Service station attendant	19
Pantrygirl/man	18
Office boy/girl	18
Groundskeeper	17
Child day care center worker	17
Cement mason helper	15
File clerk	15
Orderly (medical facility)	15
Materials handler	15

Adapted from Becker, 1976.

over such alternatives as inmate, patient, or student). An additional 30,000 mentally retarded people were housed in state mental hospitals, and an approximately equal number were in privately run residential facilities such as nursing homes (DHEW, 1972).

These institutions vary widely in size and in the quality and type of service which they provide. For example, in 1970, states such as California, Georgia, and Kansas spent more than $18 per resident per day in their public institutions, while states such as Alabama, Mississippi, and South Dakota spent less than $7 per day (DHEW, 1972). Some facilities provide little more than custodial care for most of their residents while other facilities provide a wide variety of services and are able to provide each resident with a relatively complete program appropriate to his needs.

The large, long-term residential institution has received such intense criticism both in professional journals and in the popular press that the traditional institution has few defenders, and there is a widespread movement to vastly reduce the role of such facilities in the provision of services. Many people even advocate phasing them out completely. One of the most important recommendations of the President's Panel on Mental Retardation (1962), the report which had such major impact on federal policy, was to base as many services as possible in the local communities rather than in the state institutions.

The Dehumanizing Climate of Residential Institutions

A word that is frequently used to describe these institutions is "dehumanizing"; the residents are treated either as objects to be warehoused or as animals to be caged up. They are removed from the mainstream of society against their will and are placed in cold, barren, dingy surroundings devoid of any normal human contact. All normal human rights are taken away from them. In many institutions, privacy is virtually nonexistent; until recently the residents slept in large wards with 30 or more beds, and even the bathrooms had no doors on the toilets so that the staff could keep an eye on them. Residents have little or no say in what happens to them, but all decisions concerning their lives are made by others. Not only do the residents of institutions have little say regarding what programs they would like to be in, but frequently, they are not even permitted to make trivial everyday decisions such as what to wear or whether to go to a movie or not. In many institutions, the residents are physically brutalized not only by other residents, but in some cases, even by the staff, who are usually more concerned with keeping order than with facilitating the development of the residents.

The following description by Burton Blatt (1970) captures some of the worst aspects of institutional life as he describes an excursion through several wards.

> *. . . almost immediately after I passed the threshold, an overwhelming stench enveloped me. It was the sickening, suffocating smell of feces and urine, decay, dirt, and filth, of such strength as to hang in the air and, I thought then and am still not dissuaded, solid enough to be cut or shoveled away. But, as things turned out, the odors were among the gentlest assaults on my sensibilities. I was soon to learn about the decaying humanity that caused them. . . .*
>
> *Several things strike a visitor to most institutions for the mentally retarded upon his arrival on the institution grounds. Sometimes there are fences, once in a while with barbed wire. Very frequently, the buildings impress him with their sheer massiveness and impenetrability. I have observed bars on windows and locks—many locks—on inside as well as outside doors. As I entered the dormitories and other buildings, I was*

impressed with the functional superiority of the new building, but, on the other hand, with the gross neglect in many of the older ones. I have observed gaping holes in ceilings of such vital areas as the main kitchen. In toilets, I frequently saw urinals ripped out, sinks broken, and the toilet bowls backed up. In every institution I visited, with the exception of the Seaside, I found incredible overcrowding. Beds are so arranged—side by side and head to head—that it is impossible, in some dormitories, to cross parts of the room without actually walking over beds; oftentimes the beds are without pillows. I have seen mattresses so sagged by the weight of the bodies that they were scraping the floor. . . .

Many dormitories for the severely and moderately retarded ambulatory residents have solitary confinement cells or, what is officially referred to and is jokingly called by many attendants, "therapeutic isolation". "Therapeutic isolation" means solitary confinement—in its most punitive and inhumane form. These cells are usually located on an upper floor, off to the side and away from the casual or official visitor's scrutiny. . . . Isolation cells are generally tiny rooms, approximately 7 feet by 7 feet, shielded from the outside with a very heavy metal door having either a fine strong screen or metal bars for observation of the "prisoner." Some cells have mattresses, other blankets, still others, bare floors. None that I had seen (and I found these cells in each institution visited) had either a bed, a wash stand or a toilet. What I did find in one cell was a 13 or 14 year old boy, nude, in the corner of a starkly bare room, lying on his own urine and feces. The boy had been in solitary confinement for several days for committing an institutional infraction, as I recall, directing abusive language to an attendant. Another child, in another institution, had been in solitary confinement for approximately 5 days for breaking windows. Another had been in isolation, through a long holiday weekend, because he had struck an attendant. Ironically, in the dormitory where the boy was being incarcerated, I saw another young man who had been "sent to bed early" because he had bitten off *the ear of a patient several hours previously. Apparently, it is infinitely more serious to strike an attendant (and it should not be understood that I condone this) than to bite off the ear of another resident. . . .*

I saw a great deal of restraint used with children. I observed many children whose hands were tied, legs bound, or waists secured. After a good deal of discussion with a number of attendants and supervisors in the four institutions, I was convinced that one of the major reasons for the frequent use of solitary confinement and physical restraint was the extraordinary shortage of staff in practically all of these dormitories. The attendant who requested the construction of two additional solitary confinement cells was, with one assistant, responsible for the supervision of an old multi-story dormitory, housing over a hundred severely retarded ambulatory residents. Almost in desperation, he asked me

"What can one do with those patients who do not conform? We must lock them up, or restrain them, or sedate them, or put fear into them.". . .

In each of the dormitories for severely retarded residents, there is what is called, euphemistically, the day room or recreation room. The odor in each of these rooms is overpowering, to the degree that after a visit to a dayroom, I had to send my clothes to the dry cleaners in order to have the stench removed (and, probably because of psychological reactions, whose odor I continued to smell months later whenever I wore certain clothes). The physical facilities often contributed to the visual horror as well as to the odor. Floors are sometimes made of wood and, as a result, excretions are rubbed into the cracks, thus providing a permanent aroma. Most dayrooms have a series of bleacherlike benches on which sit denuded residents, jammed together, without purposeful activity or communication or any kind of interaction. In each dayroom is an attendant or two, whose main function seems to be to "stand around" and, on occasion, hose down the floor, "driving" excretions into a sewer conveniently located in the center of the room.

I was invited into female as well as male dayrooms, in spite of the supervisor's knowledge that I, a male visitor, would be observing denuded females. In one such dormitory, with an overwhelming odor, I noticed feces on the wooden ceilings, and on the patients as well as the floors.

Early in the evening, sometimes at 5 o'clock, patients are put to bed. This is to equalize the workload among the different shifts. During the day, I saw many patients lying on their beds, apparently for long periods of time. This was their activity. During these observations, I thought a good deal about the perennial cry for attendants and volunteer workers who are more sympathetic and understanding of the institutionalized retarded residents. One of the things I realized was that attendants might be sympathetic, might interact more with patients, if institutional administrators made deliberate attempts to make patients cosmetically more appealing. For example, adult male residents should shave or be shaven more than once or twice a week. Dentures should be provided for any patient who needs them. It seems plausible to believe that it is much more possible to make residents more attractive and, therefore, more interesting to attendants than it is to attempt to convince attendants that they should enjoy the spectacle of unwashed, unkept, odoriferous, toothless old men and women. . . .

The living quarters for older men and women were, for the most part, gloomy and sterile. There were rows and rows of benches on which sat countless human beings, in silent rows, waiting for dinner call or bedtime. I saw resident after resident in "institutional garb." Sometimes, the women wore shrouds—inside out. I heard a good deal of laughter but saw little cheer. There were few things to be cheerful about. A great many of the men and women looked depressed and acted depressed. Even the television sets, in several of the dayrooms,

> *appeared to be co-conspirators in a crusade for gloom. These sets were not in working order, although, ironically, the residents continued to sit on their benches, in neat rows, looking at the blank tubes. I observed adult residents during recreation playing ring-around-the-rosy. Others, in the vocational training center, were playing Jacks. There were not always severely retarded patients. However, one got the feeling very quickly that this is the way they were being forced to behave. Or, as Hungerford said, ". . . in an institution, there is always tomorrow so that he who starts out a student ends up, by default, an inmate." Lastly, I viewed old women and very young girls in the same dormitories and old men and young boys as comrades in the dayroom. In the "normal" world, there is something appealing, even touching, about such friendships; in the institution, there is something opportunistic, sinister, and ludicrous. . . .*
>
> *The children's dormitories depressed me the most. Here, cribs were placed, as in the other dormitories, side by side and head to head. Very young children, one and two years of age, were lying in cribs without contact with any adult, without playthings, without apparent stimulation. In one dormitory that had over 100 infants and was connected to nine other dormitories that totalled 1,000 infants, I experienced my deepest sadness. As I entered, I heard a muffled sound emanating from the "blind" side of a doorway. A young child was calling, "Come, come play with me. Touch me." I walked to the door. On the other side were 40 or more unkempt infants crawling around a bare floor in a bare room. One of the children had managed to squeeze his hand under the doorway and push his face through the side of the latched door and was crying for attention. His moan begged me for some kind of human interaction (Blatt, 1970, pp. 13–18).*[1]

It is only fair to point out that this description is only characteristic of the worst facilities. Many institutions are making a sincere effort to provide a pleasant and livable environment for their residents, and the past few years have seen considerable progress in reducing the overcrowding and providing a more normal and human environment for these unfortunate people.

The general climate of a particular facility can be described in terms of four interacting components; the residents themselves, the direct care staff, the physical plant, and the programs available at the institution.

The Institutionalized Resident

Only a small percentage of the total population of mentally retarded people are ever institutionalized. It is no exaggeration to say that a large public institution houses a collection of the worst problem cases in the state, the people who are functioning at the lowest level, those who have the most physical

[1] From B. Blatt, *Exodus from pandmonium.* Boston: Allyn & Bacon, 1970. Copyright (©) 1970 by Allyn & Bacon. Reprinted with permission of the author.

deformities, those who have multiple handicaps such as both retardation and blindness or both retardation and cerebral palsy, and those people who present the most severe emotional, behavioral, and management problems.

Very few admissions to institutions today have IQs above 50, and the vast majority are severely and profoundly retarded. Many institutional residents are not toilet trained, and some are bed cases, functioning at so low a level that not only are they unable to walk, but they require total care to the extent of having to be spoon fed. For example, a survey of the characteristics of some 10,000 residents of California state facilities for the mentally retarded in 1974 produced the following results (California Department of Mental Hygiene, unpublished, cited in President's Committee on Mental Retardation, 1976a). Nearly half the institutional population, 49 percent, were profoundly retarded. An additional 29 percent were severely retarded and less than 8 percent of the residents were mildly retarded or above. About 45 percent of the population had had a history of epileptic seizures, 8 percent were totally blind, 5 percent were totally deaf, 17 percent were bedridden, and an additional 16 percent were confined to a wheelchair.

Many institutionalized residents have severe behavior problems, particularly the higher functioning residents. Some commonly assault other residents, others are hyperactive, others are self-destructive, engaging in such activities as chewing off their fingers or banging their head against the furniture. Some refuse to keep their clothes on, others are chronic stealers. Some are so totally withdrawn that they never respond at all. The presence of such behaviors requires that many of the residents be placed on some sort of tranquilizing medication, in some cases very heavy doses. One of the charges against institutions is that they restrain their residents in "chemical straitjackets," doping them up so heavily that they sit around barely conscious for most of the day. In cases where tranquilizers are ineffective, physical restraint must occasionally be used, and it is not unusual to see a resident who is tied hands and feet to a bed or a chair.

This section is in no way intended to imply that the victims of institutionalization are to be blamed for the sorry climate in many such facilities today. In many cases, this bizarre behavior has been caused by the resident being institutionalized. However, it is important to keep in mind that the amount of normalization possible in such a facility is constrained by the type of resident usually found there. Even the best facilities and training will only reduce but not eliminate these problems.

The Direct Care Staff

In 1970, the 190 public institutions for the retarded employed some 117,000 people. This figure represents one staff member for every 1.6 residents, a ratio that sounds very good. However, if one considers that many of these employees are administrators, secretaries, and the like who are not involved is the direct care of the residents and the fact that the institution must be staffed 24 hours a day, seven days a week, the ratio of direct care workers to residents at any given time is often very low, and it is not uncommon for one or two attendants to be the only staff supervising 40 or more residents for most of the day.

Over half of the employees of the typical institution are direct care workers, usually referred to as attendants, aides, or technicans, and these are the people who provide most of the actual services, the people who are in direct contact with the residents for most of the day. The aides are the backbone of the whole institutional system. They are usually responsible for the direct implementation of any new programs in the institution, and thus, any changes in procedure require their cooperation. Unfortunately, they are always the least trained and the lowest paid of all the employees. Their job has very little status; they have a great deal of responsibility but very little authority, and the work is not very glamorous. Not surprisingly, many institutions have difficulty attracting qualified people to be aides, and they have even more difficulty keeping those that they do attract. The turnover among the attendants in most institutions is tremendous, and the people who stay for a considerable length of time are not necessarily the best aides or the most dedicated, but the ones who would have difficulty finding other kinds of work.

Attendants have a tremendous variety of duties. They are responsible for the day-to-day custodial care of the residents; they must feed the ones who cannot feed themselves, they clean up and change the ones who are not toilet trained, they see that residents get up in the morning and go to bed at night, and they must keep a constant eye on all of the residents to assure that they do not get into trouble or harm themselves. In most institutions, they are also responsible for general housekeeping, making sure that the building stays as clean as possible. Finally, almost as an afterthought, the attendants are responsible for some of the training of the residents. Thus, the aide seems to have an impossible job. When there are only two or three people to supervise 40 severely retarded adults, some of whom are not toilet trained, others of whom are continual behavior problems, it is no wonder that they claim to have no time to provide proper training or individual attention to the residents.

Thormahlen (1965) observed and recorded the behavior of institutional attendants as they went about their daily routine. He was particularly interested in the extent to which they encouraged independent behavior in the ward residents. Only 12 percent of the total time was spent in behavior that seemed to promote independence on the part of the residents. Less than 2 percent of the aide's time was spent in formal teaching. However, more than a third of the aide's total time was spent in a manner that promoted dependency in the residents.

In another study, Warren and Mondy (1971) observed aide behavior in relation to the behavior of the ward residents. They were particularly concerned with the extent to which the attendants encouraged desirable behavior and discouraged undesirable behavior in institutionalized children. They found that an overwhelming majority of the behavior of the residents, both good behavior and bad behavior, was ignored by the staff. Only 16 percent of desirable child behavior was responded to in an encouraging way by the staff, and 82 percent of this desirable behavior was ignored. Similarly, aides ignored 79 percent of the undesirable behavior and actively discouraged this behavior only 11 percent of the time. In rare cases, they actually encouraged undesirable behavior.

Unfortunately, many aides, particularly those who have been working at their job for many years, have developed a very pessimistic and cynical attitude toward their job. They have become convinced that most of the residents are unable to learn anything, and they have seen enough different experimental and innovative programs come and go that they no longer have much faith in new training ventures. Any new program is bound to fail without the full cooperation of the aide staff. As a result, most institutions now provide some sort of in-service training for their staff that not only tries to alter some of these long ingrained attitudes, but also instructs the staff in specific training techniques such as behavior modification in order to improve their performance.

Institutional Architecture

Improving the attitudes of the staff will not by itself solve the problems faced by most institutions. Another major limitation to effective programming is the physical plant of the institution. Most institutions, particularly the older ones, were designed primarily for efficiency. The aim was to provide supervision for as many residents as possible with as small a staff as possible. As a result, the typical residence hall in most institutions consists of several large dormitory rooms with 30 or more beds and several day halls, large, barren rooms usually furnished with only a few chairs or benches and a television set. Many of the older buildings also have isolation rooms where disturbed residents could be isolated, but their use is gradually being phased out. It is usually impossible to provide much in the way of games or other kinds of amusements because they would be either lost or broken almost immediately. Thus, the lives of most of the residents consists of little more than sitting in the day room for most of the day. This sitting is only broken up by meals and by trips to the bathroom. Because of the chronic financial difficulties faced by most institutions, many buildings are often in a state of disrepair, with windows broken, holes in the walls, and broken furniture and fixtures. The environments in many of these buildings is so oppressive that it is little wonder that many of the residents become extremely withdrawn and unresponsive.

Such buildings are seldom being built anymore. The type of residence hall now in favor is the cottage, a much smaller, homelike building in which residents are housed two or three to a room. Such a building has a number of advantages. There is little question that much of the bizarre behavior that is so characteristic of institutionalized people is induced by the sterile architecture, and if residents are placed in a more normal, homelike atmosphere, they will begin to behave more like normal people. An additional advantage to such an arrangement is that it fosters a more familylike atmosphere between the staff and the residents. If there are three aides to supervise 40 residents, none of the aides is going to take much of an interest in any one resident, but if there is one aide to supervise 10 or 12 residents, the aide will become far more familiar with each resident and is more likely to take a personal interest in each one.

Programming

In theory, the advantage of a large residential institution is that it is possible to provide extremely specialized programming and therapy for severely retarded and multiply handicapped people, exactly the kind of programming that is least likely to be available in the community. In fact, the original purpose of such facilities was to act as a center of specialized services to the retarded. Unfortunately, in the past, many institutions were unable to provide an adequate program for each resident due to budget restrictions. However, lawsuits in recent years (e.g., *Wyatt* v. *Stickney,* 1972) have confirmed the right of all institutionalized individuals to a full treatment program appropriate to their needs. As soon as these decisions take full effect, institutions may again begin to assume their original role of being specialized training centers for the retarded, providing services not readily available elsewhere.

The most important function of an institution is its training function. Virtually all institutions have a school on the grounds in which the residents with the most potential, particularly the younger ones, can be exposed to special instruction. Today, there are relatively few institutional programs for the educable mentally retarded for the simple reason that there are very few institutionalized residents with an IQ above 50, but many institutions now have fine programs of instruction for the trainable level child. In many cases, institutions are able to provide more innovative and specialized instructional programs because the school is almost entirely devoted to the training of such a specialized population.

However, many institutionalized residents are unable to benefit from even the lowest levels of classroom instruction. These residents require training in the skills of daily living, such abilities as how to dress themselves, or in some cases, even how to feed themselves. Such training is usually carried out right in the individual's residence hall or cottage by the direct care staff. However, if this is to occur, the staff requires special instruction in training techniques and the time and motivation needed to carry out this training. It would seem that the motivation needed to provide self-care instruction to the residents would naturally be present in the staff because the time spent in toilet training residents or teaching residents to feed themselves would more than pay off in the long run. However, this is not the case. It is often easier to simply feed all the residents at meal time than it is to let them attempt to feed themselves, particularly if they cannot feed themselves very well and are slow and messy at it. Thus, an important function of in-service training programs is to motivate the staff to be teachers as well as attendants. Frequently, a team of teachers, psychologists, nurses, and the like will move from one ward to another, instructing the aides in better ways to help the residents.

Most institutions also provide some sort of vocational training for the higher functioning residents who are likely to eventually be released to the community. Thus, it is common to find a sheltered workshop of some sort on the grounds, and the more progressive institutions might also have an off grounds work program in which some residents are able to work for a part of the day in a competitive employment situation.

One aspect of institutional vocational training that has received extensive criticism is called peonage. Peonage refers to the common practice of having the residents perform much of the work of running the institution. It is customary in many placed to have jobs such as mopping floors, washing pots and pans, and changing soiled residents be performed by residents rather than by the staff. This practice is criticized primarily because these residents are not paid for their work. In a sense, this represents a form of slave labor because the residents have little or no say in their job placement or their hours and they are usually working for nothing. The practice of peonage has died out now for two reasons. First, there have been a number of lawsuits attacking the practice, and second, the number of residents who are able to do productive work is rapidly decreasing as the more capable residents are released to the community. An ideal arrangement, which is still only rarely adopted, would be for the institution to hire some of their former residents on a regular employment basis. This not only provides former residents with meaningful employment, but helps to reduce the high rate of turnover among the staff.

In addition to training and instruction, institutions are often able to provide a variety of specialized medical and medical related services that are not always readily available in every community. The mentally retarded, particularly those retarded people who are likely to be institutionalized, typically have many health problems that require frequent medical attention. For example, Down's syndrome children are likely to have congenital heart disorders, and many retarded children are likely to have epilepsy. Ideally, the institution should be able to provide good medical care for such problems because there is a medical staff constantly available, and this staff would be familiar with many of the problems often found among this population. However, one of the frequent charges against public institutions is that their professional staff, particularly the medical staff, is made up of poorly qualified people, partially because working with the mentally retarded is not very glamorous, and partially because institutions do not have the money to hire more qualified people.

In addition to general medical care, there are a number of ancillary medical services that institutions are usually prepared to offer. For example, many community dentists are reluctant to treat retarded children because they are frequently uncooperative. However, an institution can have a dental staff who is specially prepared and experienced in providing service to the retarded. The same is true of other types of therapists and providers of ancillary services, such as physical therapists, occupational therapists, speech therapists, psychologists, counselors, and social workers. In each case, it is possible to have a professional staff with special expertise in mental retardation who can provide the highly specialized services which this population requires.

However, it should not be assumed that all residents are receiving all of the services that they need. Most institutions have only a relatively small professional staff and can only provide service to a small minority of those who need it. For example, the vast majority of institutionalized residents have speech problems, but the speech therapists must decide which of the many residents would be most able to benefit from such therapy. State laws and judicial decisions will change this in the near future and require that institutions provide full services to everyone who needs them, but it is difficult to imagine how this can occur unless the states allocate a great deal more money for professional services, an occurrence that will probably not come about.

One of the major gaps in the programming for the retarded is adequate recreational activities. Many retarded people are unable to structure their leisure time well and need some sort of structured recreational program. This is a particularly severe problem with institutionalized individuals whose day-to-day lives are often extremely barren. Most institutions plan a wide variety of activities such as dances, movies, excursions, parties, sports activities such as bowling and swimming, organizations such as the Boy Scouts and Girl Scouts, all designed to relieve the boredom of institutional life. It is even possible to provide a good recreation program for the profoundly retarded. For example, a music teacher can visit various wards with simple rhythm instruments and have the residents keep time to records.

The Effects of Institutionalization

Not surprisingly, being placed in an institution seems to have detrimental effects on an individual both in terms of his general level of competence and in terms of his personality, attitudes, and general outlook. This is perhaps the most serious indictment of all, because rather than rehabilitating residents and preparing them for eventual independent living, apparently, most institutions have exactly the opposite effect, making their residents more dependent on others for their basic needs.

The best-known research on the effects of institutionalization is that which is concerned with its impact on the general intellectual development of young children. An institution, whether it be an orphanage, a mental hospital, or a residential facility for the mentally retarded, simply cannot provide the type of environment that fosters normal cognitive and emotional development. In order to develop to their maximum potential, children need lots of attention from adults, they need to be talked to a good deal, they need lots of stimulation and objects to play with, and most institutions provide none of these. As a result, placing young children in an institution may actually cause them to become more mentally retarded than they otherwise would have been. The classic study in this area was done by Skeels (1966). He found a number of children in a state orphanage who were under 18 months old and were already beginning to show signs of delayed mental development, although there was little in their past histories to suggest mental retardation. He selected 12 of them and placed them first on a ward with mildly retarded women, where they received a good deal of personal attention, and, eventually, most of these were placed in foster homes. He compared these to other children who remained in the unstimulating institution. These represented the control group. There was a marked difference in development between the two groups. The control group children almost all remained mentally retarded, with a median IQ of 60. Many remained in institutions for most of their lives, and even those who were released usually led a very marginal existence. However, the group who had been removed from the institution at a young age and given a program of stimulation and attention developed normally. Not only did they have IQs in the normal range, but many went on to relatively high-level occupations such as vocational counselor, nursing instructor, or real estate salesman. The implication of this research was that the control group subjects were made mentally retarded by the institution.

A number of researchers have compared institutionalized children to a presumably comparable group who were reared in their own homes. Frequently, this research is done with children with Down's syndrome, because it was common practice in the past to institutionalize many of these children at birth. A number of studies (Centerwall and Centerwall, 1960; Stedman and Eichorn, 1964) have verified that Down's syndrome children reared in their homes not only have higher IQs but also have considerably better developed self-help and social skills.

Institutions do not necessarily have to be so stifling. Mitchell and Smerglio (1970) found that a group of retarded children increased only 1.3 months in their social age over a 38-month period after they had been institutionalized, and this resulted in a drop in their average social quotient from 36 to 25. However, another group of institutionalized children gained 10.5 months in social age over the same period because they had been exposed to a special training program instead of the standard institutional treatment.

However, there are some other effects of institutionalization that are perhaps even more destructive than the impact on intelligence and competence. Being placed in an institution for any length of time seems to have very serious effects on an individual's spirit and outlook. Institutions, because of their chronic understaffing, are usually unable to permit their residents to be very independent. For example, it is often easier to simply line the residents up in the morning and dress each one than it is to permit them to try to dress themselves if their dressing skills are not very good. Similarly, it is a good deal easier to simply assign residents to various recreational activities than it is to ask them whether they are interested in participating or not. Because residents are not permitted to make even the simplest decisions on their own, they lose any initiative that they once had and become even more dependent on the institution. One of the difficulties that institutions face in releasing residents who have been institutionalized for many years is that they don't know how to make even low-level decisions for themselves such as what to wear or what to have for dinner. If they go to the beach, they wait to be told when to go into the water. If they are in a group home, they simply sit around until the house parent suggests that they take a walk or go some place. They are simply unable to take any responsibility for their own lives.

There are a number of ways in which institutions encourage the development of maladaptive, disruptive, and destructive behavior in their residents. Any normal person needs attention from other people, and in most institutions, the only way to get any attention from the staff is to do something disruptive. Aides have little time to pay attention to residents who are sitting quietly, but it is difficult to ignore residents who assault someone or residents who break windows or bang their heads against the furniture. Thus, residents are systematically reinforced for such behavior. In addition, all children learn certain behaviors by watching and imitating other people, a process called modeling, and institutions generally provide only the worst types of models. Many institutionalized residents have a long history of disruptive behavior, and it is not uncommon for a new resident who, prior to institutionalization, was relatively mild mannered to become aggressive and disruptive simply because the resident is surrounded by people engaging in these sorts of behaviors.

Trends in Institutionalization

The entire philosophy of the residential facility has changed drastically in the past 15 years. Throughout most of this century, the primary purpose of institutions was to provide custodial care for as many retarded people as possible at as low a cost as possible. It was considered desirable to remove retarded people from society in order to protect society from the criminal behavior and sexual misconduct that it was believed often accompanied retardation. While most institutions had a school on their grounds and provided various other rehabilitative services such as speech therapy or a sheltered workshop, because it was generally assumed that the retarded were unable to learn anything, most institution residents did not participate in these programs. The school could only provide instruction for a small minority of the most able residents, and the rest received no programming at all.

Beginning in the 1960s, however, institutional administrations and government funding agencies started to view the residential institution in a different light—the institution as a training center, not as a provider of custodial care. The main impetus behind this change in purpose was a change in the way that the mentally retarded were conceptualized, a switch from viewing the retarded as helpless, dependent, often dangerous individuals who were unable to learn anything to people who were able to improve their capabilities a good deal if they were exposed to the proper kind of instruction and rehabilitation.

The best reflection of this improvement in programming in residential institutions is the increase in financing and personnel that occurred during the decades of the 1960s and 1970s. In 1960, there was an average of 31.3 staff per 100 residents in public institutions for the retarded. By 1970, this figure had increased to 57.3 staff per 100 residents, a 54 percent increase. A substantial proportion of this increase was in professional personnel such as speech therapists, teachers, psychologists, physical therapists and the like rather than in aides. Every state in the nation increased its staff to resident ratio during this period (Roos, 1970). During this same period, expenditures increased even more rapidly. In 1960, the typical institution in this country was spending only $4.20 per resident per day (remember that because this is an average, half the institutions were spending less than this). By 1970, this figure had increased to $11.64 per day, still a small figure, but an increase of more than 150 percent over the decade. Now, in the late 1970s, New York State is spending nearly $50 per resident per day.

A number of the more innovative programs now being carried out in institutions have been financed through the federal government. One of the most widely known of these programs is the Foster Grandparent Program, in which retired senior citizens receive a small stipend to act as grandparents to individual children in the institution. These grandparents can provide a good deal of the specific training that these children need as well as taking care of some of the routine care, such as helping to dress or feed children who cannot do these things for themselves and giving the children a good deal more personal attention than they would otherwise receive from the busy staff. In addition to helping the child, this program also has the secondary benefit of providing many elderly people with a useful and meaningful activity.

However, increasing the quantity and quality of training and rehabilitation programs is only part of the solution. Most institutions are also making an effort to increase the quality of institutional life, in particular to make life in a residential facility more similar to life on the outside. This process is called normalization. One example of normalization is the construction of small cottages to replace the huge wards and dormitories. In a cottage, a small number of residents, perhaps 10 or 12, live in a familylike setting, two or three residents to a room rather than 40, and the staff acts more like parents and less like prison guards. Residents are permitted to select their own clothing rather than being forced to wear institutional garb. In most states, the institutional haircut, crewcuts for the males and pageboy cuts for the girls, have been phased out and residents are permitted to wear their hair any way they want within the limits of good hygiene. In the traditional institution, residents are strictly segregated by sex, not only in living arrangements, but also sometimes even in recreational activities. However, in more progressive facilities, men and women are permitted to interact together during work, leisure, and meals, and some facilities even have co-ed cottages. All of these changes have the specific aim of exposing institutionalized retarded people to a more normal life in preparation for their eventual return to the community.

A trend that is even more important than the normalization of the institution is the decreasing emphasis being placed on the institution in the overall programming picture. More and more people are beginning to consider the possibility of phasing out large residential institutions entirely, or at least drastically reducing their populations so that only the most severely handicapped will be institutionalized for any length of time. Since 1967, the total number of people in institutions in this country has begun to decrease, although the pace has been slow. In 1967 there were some 192,000 residents in public facilities for the mentally retarded, but in 1975 it was estimated that there were only 167,000 residents (PCMR, 1976). This reduction in population is being accomplished in several ways. First, many cases who would have been institutionalized a few years ago are now remaining in the community with their family or in a foster home. Second, and apparently more importantly, the average length of stay is being reduced. New admissions, rather than remaining institutionalized for the rest of their lives, are now returned to the community in a few years, and institutions are even having some success in returning many of their long-term residents to the community. Most of these people cannot be expected to live independently, but the quality of their life can be much improved if they can be appropriately placed in a group home or hostel or even in a nursing home rather than in an institution.

One of the major causes of dehumanizing conditions in institutions was their enormous size. It is difficult to provide a personalized program in an institution of 2000 people, just as students in large universities often complain about dehumanization. In recognition of this fact, the average size of public institutions has been dropping rather dramatically. In the decade of the 1960s, the total number of public institutions for the retarded nearly doubled (from 108 to 190), but the size of all of these newly constructed facilities was far smaller than those which had been constructed many years previously. As a result, the average number of residents per institution decreased from more than 1500 residents in 1960 to slightly under 1000 in 1970.

Alternatives to Institutions

Most states have now adopted a general policy of deinstitutionalization. They are aiming to decrease the total number of people in large residential institutions (not only the mentally retarded, but also the mentally ill) and to place as many of these people as possible back in the community. One danger of this policy is that institutions may simply dump their residents, send them out with no programming or supervision into a community with inadequate facilities, with the result that they are no better off than they were when they were institutionalized, and frequently, they are even worse off because at least in a state institution, there was someone to make sure that everyone had a bed to sleep in and enough to eat. Such a policy can be successfully implemented only if local communities are able to provide a comprehensive system of services that maximize the normalization of the life-style of every individual regardless of his handicap.

Living Arrangements

There are five alternative living arrangements for a mentally retarded adult, each with its advantages and disadvantages. The ideal living arrangement, the ultimate goal of almost any program providing service to the retarded, is for individuals to be able to live independently, obtaining their own apartment and living just like any other citizen in the community. This is the ultimate in normalization, and as we have seen, contrary to popular stereotypes about the mentally retarded, many mildly retarded and even some moderately retarded people are able to achieve this goal of total independence. Such an individual may occasionally require assistance from a parent, social worker, or other benefactor to handle such things as income taxes or insurance, but for the most part, these people are just like anyone else, and according to some definitions of mental retardation, they are not retarded; their retardation has been "cured."

However, there are some retarded people who, either because of the degree of the intellectual handicap or because of the presence of other disabilities such as cerebral palsy or emotional disturbance, are not able to achieve this ultimate goal. A second arrangement, almost as desirable, is for the retarded to live with their own families. This is probably the most common arrangement today for the moderately or severely retarded adult. Most families are able to provide a good environment for their retarded offspring, and certainly show a good deal more concern for their welfare than do most of the employees of state institutions. One important drawback of such an arrangement is that it may represent a major burden for the individuals' parents and the other members of their families. Particularly if the retarded person is unable to be left alone for extended periods of time, it is difficult for the rest of the family to go on trips or vacations or become involved in community activities as much as they would like to. A second drawback is that at least some homes are inadequate. This is one of the most frequent reasons why children are institutionalized in the first place. If the family is unable or unwilling to provide proper care and supervision, it becomes necessary to find an alternative.

The arrangement that has been most often hailed as the best living arrangement for those retarded people who cannot take care of themselves and who cannot live with their own families is the foster home, a private home where the retarded child lives. Either the retarded child is simply adopted by a family who will then raise it as their own, or, more often, the state will pay a family to care for one or more children in their own homes. The advantages of such an arrangement are obvious; a private home can certainly provide a more normal environment than can any other type of facility, and the retarded child is able to benefit from the individual attention provided by the family. However, foster homes are not always a satisfactory solution either. Many families are primarily interested in the money and provide very low quality care, in some cases, even lower than in a residential institution. Murphy, Rennee, and Luchins (1972) describe foster homes as the new back wards, and they cite some common abuses. There is frequently little or no interaction between the family and the retarded; the residents simply stay in their rooms all day while the family goes about its business. The family often makes no attempt to provide any sort of entertainment or recreation for the residents, and their lives are characterized by just as much regimentation as is found in an institution, and sometimes, even the quality of the food is poor because the family has no financial incentive to provide adequate nutrition. This does not imply that all foster homes are inadequate. Probably the majority are providing excellent care for these retarded children, but it is important to keep in mind that it is possible to abuse such a program.

Some mentally retarded people, particularly older ones or those who are very severely handicapped, have been placed in nursing homes, convalescent homes, or other extended care health facilities. Nursing homes are specifically designed to provide long-term care to the elderly or chronically ill individuals who cannot take care of themselves, and who frequently require some kind of nursing care. Thus, nursing homes are ideal living arrangements for at least some mentally retarded people. Not only do they obtain good physical care, but the better facilities also provide extensive recreational activities and other entertainment. However, nursing homes, like almost any other facilities, differ widely in quality, and many provide very poor quality care, as poor as is found in the worst back wards. Another disadvantage to nursing home care for the mentally retarded is that it is frequently very costly.

The final type of community residential arrangement for the retarded is the group home, sometimes referred to as a hostel or a halfway house if the placement is not viewed as permanent. There are a number of variations on this concept, but they all have in common the fact that a relatively small number of mentally retarded people, usually somewhere between 5 and 20, live together in a large house or small apartment building under the supervision of a small staff, often just a couple (houseparents) who help the residents with those activities which they cannot do for themselves. Some group homes are for children, others for adolescents, others for adults. Some are just for one sex or the other, but an increasing number are for both sexes.

One difficulty that is occasionally experienced in establishing a group home is the objection of the neighbors. They are afraid that having a group home for retarded people in the neighborhood will lower property values, and that the retarded people will be dangerous. There have been a number of very bitter legal battles over the placement of these homes, not just for the mentally retarded, but also for people who have been released from other institutions such as mental hospitals or prisons. Some communities have passed strict zoning ordinances in an attempt to block such facilities, but usually, these have been overturned.

The concerns of the neighbors are for the most part unfounded. While some mentally retarded people do get into minor legal difficulties or otherwise become a public nuisance, the vast majority do not, and very few retarded people are physically dangerous. Usually, every attempt is made to make the group home look as much as possible like every other home on the block. There is seldom a sign out front indicating the purpose of the building, and there is usually no indication to suggest that it is not a private residence. Thus, property values are not usually affected since a prospective buyer does not know that such a facility is in the neighborhood.

The advantage of a group home is that it can provide a reasonably normal life-style for its residents. Usually, they live 2 or 3 to a room rather than 40 as in some institutions, and they are living in a community rather than being segregated far from the mainstream. However, they can also be provided with whatever special care they may require. Because they are living with other people similar to themselves, most group homes are able to provide a wide range of social and recreational activities as well as counseling and instruction in activities of community adjustment. An additional benefit is that it provides companionship, a very important consideration in the often lonely lives of retarded people.

Vocational Rehabilitation

Community care means a good deal more than simply providing the retarded with a place to eat and sleep. Just like anyone else, the retarded need to have meaningful activities to give them a sense of purpose and a variety of leisure time activities and other recreation, as well as whatever instruction, training, and counseling is needed to increase their independence and improve their general level of functioning.

After their basic physical needs, food, clothing, shelter, and medical care have been provided for, the most important thing that the retarded need is a job. As we have seen, many retarded people are able to work in competitive employment if a position can be found for them, and a great many more are able to work in some sort of sheltered situation, a work environment specifically designed for the handicapped. Other retarded people are able to work if they can be given special skills and attitudes necessary for regular employment. Thus, one community program for the handicapped that has received widespread support for many years has been vocational rehabilitation. The aim of a vocational rehabilitation program is to restore functioning, train work skills, both general and specific, and change attitudes toward work in order to permit handicapped people to obtain competitive employment and become productive members of the community. The federal government has been providing funds for vocational rehabilitation since the 1920s and is the source of most rehabilitation money. The original rehabilitation programs were organized not from humanitarian motives but for economic ones; the community is better off if handicapped people are productive than if they are idle. As a result, rehabilitation programs only accepted those clients who had the best potential for eventual employment, and for many years, the mentally retarded were almost totally excluded because it was felt that they had little potential, despite the research data that were accumulating indicating that the majority of mentally retarded people were able to become productive members of the community even without the help of special training. It has only been since the 1950s that significant numbers of mentally retarded people have been trained in vocational skills through these programs.

The Sheltered Workshop

The principal type of facility involved in the vocational rehabilitation of the retarded is the sheltered workshop. A sheltered workshop is a work environment in which those people who are unable to obtain employment in industry because of a mental or physical handicap are able to work and earn money. Special allowances can be made for various types of handicaps. For example, jobs that are customarily done standing up can be redesigned to be done with the worker sitting down to benefit those people who are confined to a wheelchair. Another important difference between a sheltered workshop and a regular industrial situation is that the former is exempted from federal minimum wage laws. This is very important for people with limited abilities who could not perform a job fast enough to make it financially feasible to pay them the minimum wage. However, sheltered workshops are required to pay their workers for what they produce, based on prevailing wage patterns. That is, if a certain job pays $2.50 an hour in competitive employment, and the typical worker in that job is able to perform, say, 100 operations an hour, a person in a sheltered workshop who is only able to average 50 operations an hour on the same job must be paid at least $1.25 an hour.

A sheltered workshop serves a number of different and often conflicting purposes. The main goal of most workshops is to prepare handicapped clients for eventual competitive employment. This training process usually consists primarily of assigning clients to various different kinds of work situations in order to determine specifically what kinds of problems they are likely to encounter in employment and what kinds of work they seem to be particularly suited for. Perhaps more important than training specific work skills is the instruction in general work habits such as dependability, getting along with co-workers and with the supervisor, and the like. As we have seen, the vocational problems encountered by most retarded people are not based on an inability to do the job but are usually derived from emotional immaturity, poor attitudes, or poor social skills.

In conjunction with this goal, most workshops run other activities such as classrooms in which they teach basic social skills and job related knowledge such as how to fill out forms or how to behave on an interview. Another important function of most rehabilitation facilities is counseling. Virtually all workshops employ vocational counselors of some sort to help the clients to develop more positive attitudes about themselves and their abilities and a more positive and realistic attitude toward work.

A second function of many workshops is providing a relatively permanent place of employment for some clients who will never hope to work in competitive employment. This would include the more severely retarded, the multiply handicapped, or those people with sufficiently severe behavioral or emotional problems that competitive employment is unrealistic. For those people, a workshop is a place to go where they can earn at least a little money and where they can fill their needs to be productive. Although many rehabilitation facilities deemphasize their role as a terminal placement for their clients, this is nonetheless an important function, and the follow-up studies of the severely retarded described above emphasized the tremendous need for a place for these people to go to relieve loneliness and boredom and to provide some sort of meaning to their lives. Programs intended to be terminal work placements where many of the clients are only able to earn a few dollars a week are called work activity programs, to distinguish them from work training programs.

A third function of the workshop is its role in industry and commerce. In order for workshops to run, they have to get work that will pay the clients. The main source of this work is industrial subcontracting; local industries pay them to do various kinds of assembly work, packaging, sorting, or the like. Of course, it is necessary that this work meet certain quality standards and be accomplished by a certain deadline, and thus, many workshops find themselves in a conflict situation where they would like to train relatively unskilled workers on a job but are unable to because it would take too long or they may not meet quality standards for a while. The ideal contract is one that requires skills that must be taught, not skills that the client already has and would call for a variety of different kinds of work skills (Gold, 1973), but most workshops have enough difficulty getting jobs of any type so that they cannot afford to be very choosy. Work contracts are the most important ingredient in the success of a workshop, because without them there is not enough to keep the clients busy and not enough money to pay them. Because of the difficulty of obtaining enough different kinds of work, most workshops also try to start their own small businesses. There are a number of different types of trades which are feasible. For example, a workshop might have a ceramics plant and make various kinds of knickknacks to sell to local gift shops, or they might have a greenhouse in which they grow house plants to sell to the public. A particularly important type of business that many rehabilitation centers become involved in is either building maintenance or grounds maintenance services. These are useful because they directly train skills that the retarded clients are likely to be using later when they are in competitive employment.

A fourth function of a sheltered workshop is evaluation. One of the requirements for admission to most rehabilitation programs funded by the federal government is a potential for eventual competitive employment. However, even if this were not a legal requirement, it would be beneficial if the rehabilitation counselor were able to predict with some accuracy the vocational possibilities of a given client.

It is customary in most rehabilitation facilities to spend a considerable amount of time administering a complete battery of standardized tests to new clients prior to actually placing them in the workshop. The purpose of this assessment is to not only determine the clients' potential for eventual employment, but also to determine their specific weaknesses and strengths in order to determine what kind of training they may need and at what kinds of jobs they are most likely to be successful.

Undoubtedly, the most widely used type of test in this prevocational test battery is some sort of intelligence test. This is surprising, because research has consistently failed to support the notion that there is a high relationship between intelligence and employability, and within the IQ range of 50 to 80, the range in which most candidates for rehabilitation fall, there seems to be essentially no relationship at all. See Gold (1973) for a review of the use of intelligence tests in the vocational evaluation process.

A second type of test widely used in prevocational assessment is some sort of manual dexterity test. There are a number of well-standardized tests of fine motor coordination, all of which involve the subject performing a fine motor task under timed conditions. The most widely used test is probably the Purdue Pegboard, which requires the subjects to place small pegs in a pegboard as fast as they can. However, other similar tests such as the

O'Connor Finger Dexterity Test, the O'Connor Tweezer Dexterity Test, and the Minnesota Rate of Manipulation Test all correlate quite highly with the Purdue and with each other (Wagner and Hawver, 1965), indicating that they are measuring much the same skills. In general, these tests correlate more highly with later employability than do intelligence tests, perhaps because they are measuring skills more directly used in the kinds of jobs usually found in sheltered workshops.

A third type of assessment procedure is some sort of work sample. The clients are tried on various different types of jobs for brief periods of time to see how well they like and are able to do that kind of work and how well they are able to perform in work situations in general. These work samples might either be jobs borrowed from the workshop or else a contrived work situation in which a worklike task is developed but the client is not actually producing anything. For example, Tobias (1960) describes a work sample battery that included, among other tests, folding table cloths, sorting buttons, lacing display cards, assembling pistol key chains, assembling puzzles, packaging poker chips, and racking for electroplating. The correlation between the test battery and the hourly wage in the workshop (a measure of the productivity of the worker) was .52, indicating that the test had modest predictive validity. Unfortunately, Ladas (1961), using an almost identical test battery, failed to find any relationship between test performance and work performance. There have not been other extensive attempts to validate work sample tests, perhaps because they have such high face validity, that is, they appear to be measuring what they are supposed to measure. An additional problem with them is that to some extent each workshop develops their own tests for their own needs.

Two reviews of such evaluation procedures, Wolfensberger (1967a) and Gold (1973) have both been quite critical of their usefulness. The primary reason for this criticism is the low level of predictability obtained in most prevocational test batteries. There is simply not enough of a relationship between performance on standardized tests and individuals' later productivity, particularly after they have been exposed to training. Wolfensberger also points out the high cost of the assessment process, both in terms of money and in terms of the time involved. In many workshops, the assessment period may take as long as several weeks. He concluded that most such testing could be eliminated and it would be better to simply place incoming clients into the workshop immediately. The assumption behind this approach is that nothing predicts work performance like work itself. The work supervisors and vocational counselors would be able to get more valid information about the clients' general attitude toward work, their dependability, attention span, and other characteristics that are probably more predictive of long-term employment success than are the clients' abilities. An additional benefit for the clients is that they would be able to earn some money from the very first day without having to spend any time taking tests and doing make-work projects which pay nothing.

The Training Process. The actual training process in a workshop is often not very well defined. Clients are assigned to a work station, and a supervisor, who usually has had little training in mental retardation, simply shows the clients what at to do and then watches them to make certain that they are doing the job correctly. For many jobs, this procedure is sufficient. Some jobs are so simple that even a moderately or severely retarded person can learn them after several demonstrations and a short practice period. The main problem in most workshops is not teaching the clients to do the job, but maintaining their production at a high enough level; the problems are motivational and attitudinal and involve stamina and attention span rather than abilities. One of the main tools that workshops are using to overcome these problems is reinforcement techniques. In the traditional workshop, clients get paid every week based on their work performance. For many people, this is not a sufficient incentive to maintain a high rate of production. The reward is simply too far into the future. In addition, the more severely handicapped clients may only have a marginal understanding of money and may have no understanding at all of the relationship between the amount of money that they are given on Friday and the number of items that they packaged on Tuesday. Other clients may be more interested in socializing than in production and may spend much of their time talking with their neighbors or walking around the shop. Many of these problems can be eliminated if the workshop clients are reinforced more frequently and are made to understand the relationship between the reinforcement and how much work they have done. Various kinds of token techniques have proved to be particularly successful in reducing the frequency of such problems. Hunt and Zimmerman (1969) described such a program. Their subjects included 14 borderline mentally retarded adults who were working in an institutional sheltered workshop. Their job was to make scratch pads by counting out 75 sheets of paper, placing a cardboard backing on the counted sheets, placing them in a press, painting glue on one end, and wrapping them in brown paper. During a three-week baseline period, during which no reward techniques were used, production averaged about 15 per hour. During each of the next five weeks, clients had periods in which they were told that for each pad over their baseline rate that they produced, they would receive a bonus token that would entitle them to a purchase in the hospital canteen. During these bonus periods, production increased to nearly 21 pads per hour. Interestingly, the subjects maintained this high rate of production even after the bonus periods were eliminated. This study suggests that immediate reinforcement of high rates of production will improve the overall production rate considerably.

Sheltered workshops undoubtedly play an important role in community programming for the retarded, but it is important to keep their limitations in mind also. Like the special class and the residential institution, the sheltered workshop serves to segregate the handicapped from the nonhandicapped worker, thus perpetuating the devalued image of the handicapped. Also, they provide few positive role models of successful and effective workers, and often, very low productivity is tolerated as the norm. It would be preferable for sheltered work situations to be in regular factories and other normal work environments, but at the present time, this is seldom done.

Activity Centers

Another type of facility for the retarded is called an activity center, or sometimes a work activity center. This is an agency that provides a range of services to moderately or severely retarded adults who are unable to engage in productive work even in a sheltered setting, and for whom there is little hope of their being able to engage in competitive employment in the next few years. The study by Stanfield (1973), which followed up the graduates of a program for the trainable mentally retarded, indicated a tremendous need for such a facility because most trainable level people living in the community have little to do and spend almost all of their time at home watching television or in other equally unproductive activities. The need for these facilities has further increased by the release of many long-term institutionalized people to the community. In response to this need, the number of activity centers has increased rapidly, from only 94 activity centers nationwide in 1962 to 706 in 1971 (PCMR, 1972).

It is difficult to make generalizations about the nature of the activities that go on in activity centers because they are very diverse. Their general purpose is to provide general rehabilitation and recreation for people who are unable to work in a sheltered workshop. A major purpose of most activity centers is training in various self-care skills and skills of community adjustment. A recent government booklet on activity centers (PCMR, 1972) listed the following areas of instruction as the skills most frequently taught: grooming, useful home skills, communication, arts and crafts, community skills, academics, woodworking, travel training, music, and ceramics.

However, activity centers also perform a number of other functions. Many do some kind of industrial subcontracting similar to sheltered workshops, and one of the goals for many of the clients is eventual placement in a sheltered workshop. Recreation is another important function of these centers.

They provide the severely retarded with activities such as bowling, Ping-Pong, dancing, excursions to nearby places of interest, trips to watch spectator sports, and the like. They also provide a certain amount of relief for the parents. If a mother is able to send her retarded offspring to an activity center for much of the day, this will take a tremendous burden off her, and not only will the quality of her life be improved, but she will be far less likely to consider institutionalization if good services are provided in the community. Another implicit purpose of most of these centers is to structure the time of retarded adults who are unable to engage in productive work. The activity center provides the relief from boredom, the feeling of accomplishment, and the opportunity for social contacts that work provides for most other people.

Coordinating Community Services

One problem that arises when the burden of providing services is shifted from the institution to the community is that services are very likely to be fragmented, and it is necessary to develop some sort of superordinate agency to coordinate them. Many community services are provided by private agencies such as the local Association for Retarded Citizens or Goodwill Industries, others are provided by the local school districts, and still others are provided directly by various state agencies. Thus, it frequently happens that each agency provides certain types of services to certain types of clients, with no one knowing what the others are doing and no one to make sure that there were no duplications or gaps in services. In the past, it was common for some handicapped people to "fall between the cracks," to be inappropriate clients for any of the local agencies, with the result that they received no programming at all. This has always been the particular problem of multiply handicapped children, for example, children who were too disturbed to be accepted by a classroom for the mentally retarded, but because they were mentally retarded, programs for the emotionally disturbed would not accept them.

One of the provisions of a recent federal bill was to provide funds to each of the states to develop a statewide plan for the provision of services to the mentally retarded, and all of the states now have such a plan. These master plans are important not only because they point out specific gaps in the provision of services, but also because they prevent the proliferation of similar services and the general fragmentation that can so easily develop in a rapidly growing area. Many states have developed regional coordinating agencies to provide a continuum of care for each retarded person in a given catchment region. Such an agency is typically responsible for the initial diagnosis of mental retardation and any other developmental disabilities that may be present. Then it determines which types of programming and services that individuals need and implements this prescription, not usually by organizing programs themselves, but by insuring that the children are able to be enrolled in the appropriate program. As the individuals get older and are faced with different programming needs, they are referred back to the agency for a reevaluation and a new prescription. In this way, there is always one agency that has a complete record of all retarded persons in the community and knows what kind of services they are receiving. Thus, not only can they accurately assess the needs of that particular community, but the children are far less likely to be completely without a program because they have an advocate. If they discover that there are certain needs that are not presently being met by the various agencies, they can encourage the development of needed services either by providing money or by other means.

Summary

Research on what happens to children labeled mildly mentally retarded after they leave school has consistently found that the majority of these people are able to lead independent, productive lives. Most get married, many own their own homes, and they are able to get and hold a wide variety of different jobs, including some which require a good deal of skill. Unfortunately, research that has tried to determine what factors seem to discriminate the retardate who successfully adjusts as an adult from the one who consistently fails, has not resulted in many meaningful conclusions. In fact, it might well be true that whether retarded people are able to live independently depends more on the characteristics of the environment than it does on their own abilities.

Follow-up studies of trainable level children have painted a far less optimistic picture. Only a small percentage of those people with IQs below 50 are able to live independently or are even successful at obtaining and keeping competitive employment. Their biggest problem seems to be simply finding things to do to keep themselves occupied.

Probably the most important measure of successful adjustment is whether the individual has a job. Employment not only provides a paycheck, but also gives the retarded person a sense of being needed, provides relief from boredom, and represents an opportunity for social contacts. Most mildly retarded people are employable, although not all employable people will have jobs at any given time. The reason why most retarded people lose jobs is not because they cannot do the work, but because they have personality or social problems. There seems to be little relationship between employability and such measures as IQ or academic ability, but this is because retarded people normally only apply for the lowest-level jobs where these skills are not necessary.

Society's traditional solution to the problem of retarded people who could not live independently was to institutionalize them. However, the large state residential institution has received such intensive criticism that it now has few supporters. They have traditionally been extremely dehumanizing, depriving residents of any privacy and even the right to make everyday decisions about their lives. In addition, they are usually filthy, overcrowded, and understaffed.

The atmosphere of an institution is determined by four interacting components, the residents themselves, the direct care staff, the physical plant, and the programming and professional services. The residents of a large public institution are almost always severely or profoundly retarded and the majority present other problems besides being mentally retarded such as cerebral palsy, visual impairment, or severe behavior problems.

Over half the employees of most institutions are direct care workers, usually referred to as aides or attendants. These people often seem to have an impossible job, since they are usually responsible for taking care of a large number of people, some of whom are severely disturbed. Studies of aide behavior have shown that they spend little time actually interacting in a positive way with residents.

The architecture of many institutions also contributes to their oppressive atmosphere. Most older buildings are designed for maximum efficiency, with 40 or more residents living in a single large room. The more modern approach is to build cottages for a small number of residents where their lifestyle can more nearly approximate the normal.

In theory, the advantage of a large institution was that it could provide specialized programming for the retarded. While some institutions have fine educational and vocational programs for trainable and profoundly retarded people, all too many provided only minimal services. One aspect of vocational training that has received particular criticism is peonage, the use of the residents themselves to perform much of the routine maintenance, usually for no pay. Another criticism is that the professional staff of many institutions was weak.

Such a dehumanizing environment has a detrimental effect on anyone who spends any time in an institution. Research has documented that children raised in institutions have lower IQs than children raised in normal homes, and thus, in a sense, institutions are a cause of mental retardation. Also, because they are so regimented, institutions deprive their residents of any sense of independence or initiative. In addition, residents learn maladaptive behavior by watching other residents.

Fortunately, institutions are playing a much smaller role in the programming picture today than was the case a few years ago, and most states have an active deinstitutionalization program. This policy can only be effective if the local communities are able to provide good programming for the kinds of people who used to be institutionalized, and currently states are attempting to assure that this is the case.

The first component of community placement is living arrangements. There are five alternatives to institutions. The ideal situation is for the retarded to be able to live independently in their own apartments just as other people do. Another alternative is for the retarded to live with their own families, although often this places a tremendous burden on the parents, and sometimes the family environment is unsatisfactory. A third alternative is placing the child or adult with a foster family at state expense. This is usually a desirable arrangement, although some families abuse the policy and provide only minimal custodial care for the individual. A fourth alternative is a nursing home. This is an ideal arrangement for retarded people who have medical problems, particularly older ones. The fifth type of community residence is a group home or hostel, a facility housing a small number of retarded people, usually under the supervision of houseparents.

However, local communities must provide a good deal more in the way of services besides a place to live. Another important type of service is vocational training. This is most often provided in a sheltered workshop. Such workshops serve a variety of purposes. They train handicapped people in both general and specific vocational skills, they provide employment opportunities for them, they fulfill a role in industry, and they evaluate clients.

However, some people are so severely handicapped that they are unlikely to ever be able to work in competitive employment, and the best programming alternative for them is an activity center. Activity centers are expanding rapidly. They provide training in self-care and skills of community adjustment as well as giving the severely handicapped person a place to go each day.

One problem that arises when such services are provided in the community is that they are often fragmented because they are provided by a variety of different agencies. As a result, state planning agencies have developed to coordinate these services. Such an agency assures that there are no gaps in service, that each person who needs programming is admitted to the best program available, and that there is little duplication of services.

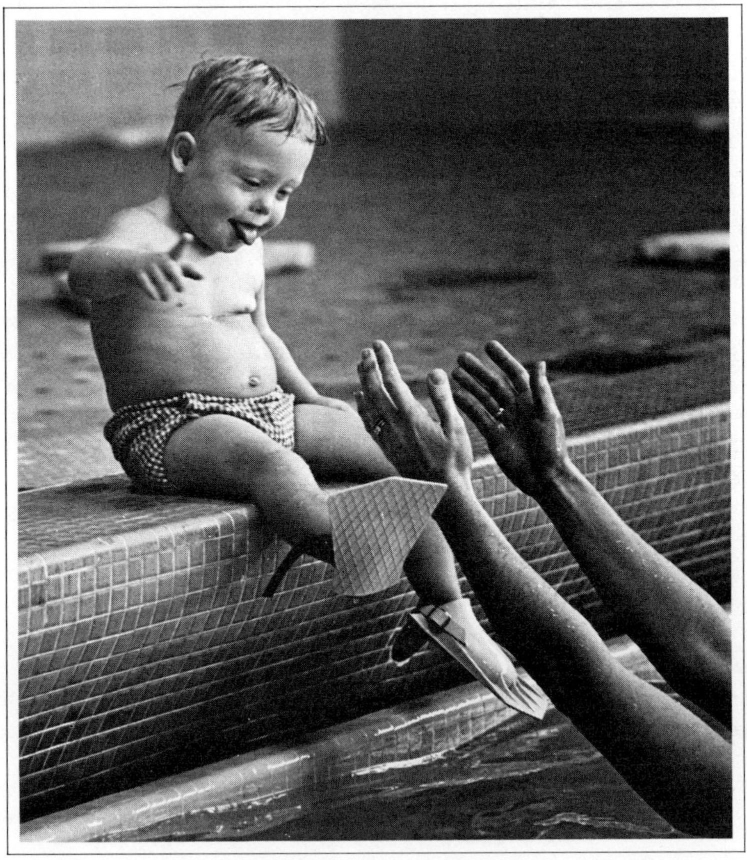

18

The Spirit of the Times

The proper study of any subject requires a sense of history. One of the single most important ideas that any student can learn is that what is thought to be true today was not believed to be true a few years ago and will probably be considered wrong a few years hence. Undoubtedly, someone reading this book in 30 years or so will find the language and the outlook somewhat quaint, just as we are amused by the strange vocabulary and concepts used in books about mental retardation 30 years ago. What is now considered an enlightened approach to providing services to the mentally retarded is likely to be seen as hopelessly narrow in a few years as more is learned about the nature of learning capacities and as the values of society change. For example, 30 years ago, many of the most progressive educators advocated placing handicapped children in special schools where they could be exposed to programming unique to their needs and where they would not be forced to compete with normal children. Today, most educational planners adopt exactly the opposite approach and attempt to integrate the handicapped into the educational mainstream as much as possible. In the 1950s, the IQ cutoff point that separated the mentally retarded from the nonretarded was raised to 85 by including the category of borderline retardation on the assumption that as society became more complex, a larger number of people would require special services and rehabilitation in order to live independently. In 1973, the cutoff point was reduced back to

70 in recognition of the fact that labeling people as retarded was usually more of a hindrance than a help even though the label entitled them to special services. Modern readers find archaic terminology such as idiot, moron, or feebleminded to be degrading and offensive, but it is likely that readers from future generations will find our present vocabulary equally quaint.

This chapter represents an attempt to characterize the present *zeitgeist* toward the mentally retarded. The 1960s and 1970s have witnessed an explosive growth in services for the retarded, but these have only come about as a result of a number of fundamental shifts in the attitudes of society toward the handicapped, and, in the long run, the quality of life of a retarded person is far more dependent on these general attitudes of society than it is on whatever specific programs happen to be in effect at any given time. These fundamental shifts suggest that the future of the mentally retarded people in this country is going to be a lot brighter than the past. The following is a list of 10 themes that are an attempt to capture the spirit of the times.

Ten Themes

1. *An emphasis on the similarities between retarded and nonretarded people rather than on their differences.* Whenever a group of people are given a special label and are selected out for special treatment, it is easy to think of them as being fundamentally different from other human beings. It is easy to justify placing retarded people in overcrowded, dehumanizing conditions if one thinks of them as being somewhat less than human, sort of a species apart. Good services for the retarded can come about only after people recognize that the retarded are basically just like anyone else, with the same kinds of emotions, feelings, and needs. The normalization principle, the attempt to make facilities for the retarded as similar to facilities for everyone else as possible, is a direct manifestation of this change in outlook.

An alternative way of expressing this is that there has been a shift away from thinking of a retarded person as a disabled person and toward thinking of the individual as a person with a disability. The former way of thinking implies that the retarded are totally helpless and requires assistance in everything they do, while the latter way of thinking implies that the retarded are essentially normal individuals who merely have unusual difficulty doing certain things.

2. *A recognition that retarded people can improve their level of functioning if they are given a proper opportunity.* One of the most consistent themes in the history of services to the retarded has been that their capabili-

ties have been underestimated. As long ago as 1919, Fernald followed up a group of retarded people who had been released from an institution, and was surprised to find that nearly half of them were able to live independently. Gold (1973) points out that the main reason why so few retarded people are ever let go from a job because they are unable to do the work is that they are so seldom given an opportunity to attempt any but the simplest types of work. Clearly, expectancy can have an important impact on performance. One of the reasons why people labeled mentally retarded have had less success than other people is that everyone, including the retarded people themselves, has assumed that they would not perform well. If the retarded are defined as nonlearners and are placed in a classroom where they are exposed to a watered-down curriculum, and everyone seems to assume that they will never be able to live independently, it is no surprise that they grow up into helpless, dependent individuals.

The developing technology of behavior modification has had a considerable impact on this change in expectancies. There have been repeated demonstrations that when the behavior to be taught is systematically broken down into its components and gradually shaped, it is possible to teach even severely and profoundly retarded people to perform skills far beyond what anyone believed possible. Changing expectations will not by themselves change performance, but without higher expectations, any attempt to improve the level of functioning of retarded people is destined to fail.

3. *A questioning of the concept of mental retardation.* Mental retardation is basically conceived of as a defect in intelligence, and the whole concept of intelligence has been under intense criticism for a good many years. The traditional conception of intelligence as a unitary ability that is largely constitutional and unchanging has completely given way to the idea that intelligence cannot be characterized by a single number because there are many essentially independent mental abilities. Similarly, it is almost universally recognized that one's level of mental functioning can be changed if his or her environment is altered.

This criticism has had an impact on the way that people conceive of mental retardation. Increasingly, it is recognized that mental retardation is not a condition that exists inside a person but results from an interaction between a given individual's unique cluster of abilities and the demands of the environment. Individuals who have particular difficulty with academic skills are likely to be considered retarded when they are in an environment such as a school where many academic demands are made on them, but are not likely to be labeled retarded after they leave school.

In the future, it is likely that the label of mentally retarded will be reserved only for those people who are so impaired that fully independent living is improbable. Many of the people who are now labeled mildly retarded will be released from the stigma of the retardation label. One result of this is the present widely cited prevalence figure that 3 percent of the total population is mentally retarded will have to be reduced.

Unfortunately, there are certain trends acting to increase the number of retarded people also. The number of programs providing services to the mentally retarded is proliferating rapidly, and, to some extent, such programs manufacture their own clients in order to continue to get funding. Nazzaro (1974) describes a clear example of this. The federal government, in an attempt to get Head Start Programs to enroll more handicapped children, required 10 percent of all spaces in Head Start Programs be reserved for handicapped children. In order to comply with this regulation, many programs arranged to have some of their children be labeled handicapped. Since many of these children would have been enrolled anyway, the main effect of this legislation was to have more children be labeled handicapped. If future legislation provides money to local school districts for education for the retarded, it will be to their advantage to label as many children retarded as possible in order to get this money.

4. *A deemphasis on labeling.* It is doubtful that labels will ever disappear, but there is recognition now of the fact that many of the labels that are in wide use today have little programmatic significance in the sense that they do not imply a specific type of treatment. The label mentally retarded is perhaps the best example of this. While labeling a child as mentally retarded may be an administrative convenience, it certainly does not benefit the child directly. The most important thing that a diagnosis of mental retardation contributes is the expectation that this child could not perform very much better than he or she has been performing. Because many retarded children learn in the same way that nonretarded children learn and have the same kinds of academic problems that many nonretarded children have, there is no need to make a diagnosis in most cases. If a child is having a reading problem, it is far more important to determine the precise nature of the problem and treat it than it is to give the child a general label such as mentally retarded or brain damaged.

5. *Increased individualization.* A trend that is closely related to the deemphasis on labeling is an increased recognition that each person, retarded or not, is an individual, with unique problems, unique needs, and unique goals. Any kind of label tends to disguise this fact and lumps a group of individuals together in some way. It is altogether too easy to provide just one type of program for all retarded people simply because they have all been given the same label. This trend is true not only with labels like mentally re-

tarded, but also for labels like third grader. Instead of forcing all third graders to use third-grade readers and third-grade arithmetic books, most schools are making an effort now to provide each child with a more individualized program.

The emphasis on individualization has altered the process of diagnosis. Ten years ago, the term diagnosis was essentially synonymous with the labeling process. A psychometrician's primary purpose in administering an intelligence test, for example, was to determine whether the child was retarded or not. Today, the term diagnosis is far more of a process to determine the individual needs of each case and to write individual prescriptions to fill these needs, independent of the specific diagnostic label. In this way, an individual program can be established for each child based on his or her own particular strengths and weaknesses rather than simply labeling a child as retarded and placing him or her in a classroom with all the other retarded children.

6. *Expansion of legal rights for the mentally retarded.* Until very recently, such basic restorative services as adequate medical care, an appropriate educational program, or access to counseling and vocational rehabilitation when needed were not recognized as basic human rights but as services to be provided only to individuals whose families could afford them or whose communities were wealthy enough to provide them. Beginning in about 1970, there was an abrupt change in this viewpoint, and a consensus is rapidly developing that such services are basic rights. The prime force behind this shift has been a series of law suits brought in behalf of various groups who had been deprived of these services. Freedman (1974) reports that between October 1971 and July 1973, at least 41 different court actions were initiated in federal, state, and local courts on behalf of mentally retarded people. Prior to that time, there were none. These suits have affirmed that all handicapped children are entitled to a full educational program, and that all institutionalized retarded people are entitled to a full range of services in order to make them as independent as possible. There is little doubt that within a few years, many rehabilitative services will be regarded as a basic right of every American who needs them.

Even more important has been the abolition of laws and legal practices that deprived mentally retarded people of rights accorded to others. For example, compulsory sterilization laws for retarded people were common a few years ago, and although they were never widely enforced, their very existence tended to confirm that retarded people were second-class citizens. Recent years have seen an increase in the number of mentally retarded people marrying. This practice was usually not explicitly outlawed, but guardians of the retarded often went to great lengths to discourage such marriages. Similarly, more and more retarded people are being encouraged to register and vote.

7. *An increased tolerance of deviance.* It is remarkable easy to convince oneself that one's own particular values, standards, and life-style are the best, and that people who differ from these standards are inferior. Such widespread ethnocentrism served to exclude many groups from full participation in American life because they differed from the white middle-class norm in some way. This was true not only of racial and cultural minorities, but also of other deviant groups such as the mentally and physically handicapped. Undoubtedly, one of the reasons why most institutions for the retarded are located far from population centers is that the retarded looked and acted differently from other people and their very differentness was repelling. One of the important shifts in cultural values during the recent decades has been an increased recognition that there are many possible alternative values and lifestyles and that the white middle-class norm is only one possible way to live one's life.

One can see numerous examples of this shift. The schools, once bastions of middle-class values, are now espousing a policy of cultural plurality, recognizing that the cultural background of every child has value and that all children should not be forced into the white middle-class mold. Black dialect, once considered an inferior way to speak, is now widely recognized as simply an alternative dialect of English. Another example is society's attitude toward homosexuality. A few years ago, any type of sexual deviance was considered a sign of a character defect and was treated as a crime. There was a gradual shift toward viewing homosexuality as a disease instead of as a moral transgression, and today homosexuality is increasingly being regarded merely as an alternative lifestyle.

Exactly the same kind of progression can be seen in the public's perception of the handicapped. Not so long ago, almost any kind of handicap was considered something to be ashamed of, and handicapped people were generally discouraged from participating in many activities. Handicapped children were routinely excluded from the public schools, and some communities actually had laws against deformed people displaying themselves in public. In recent years, the handicapped have "come out of the closet" and attempted to participate in life as fully as their limitations permit.

An alternative way of expressing this idea is that society is now making more of an attempt to shape itself to individual differences rather than trying to shape individuals to conform to society. A simple example of this principle is providing ramps for people in wheelchairs. Only a few years ago, a person in a wheelchair was virtually excluded from most public buildings because of architectural barriers. Yet it only takes a few minor changes in design such as the elimination of curbs or making doorways slightly wider to permit a handicapped individual to participate in a much wider range of activities.

Society is beginning to accommodate itself to the mentally retarded in the same way. By providing group homes, sheltered work situations, special recreation programs and the like, society is saying that there are many possible life styles, and if an individual cannot be molded to fit the norm, then communities will provide feasible alternatives.

8. *The recognition that some mental retardation arises out of conditions in society.* The traditional view of intelligence is that it is something constitutional and unchanging, determined by genetic background to a large extent. This viewpoint has been gradually eroded by the discovery that the conditions in which children are raised can have a considerable effect on their mental abilities. Children reared in circumstances of poverty where they do not receive adequate medical care and where they are seldom exposed to books or other intellectual stimulation are very likely to be retarded. At the same time, there has been a recognition of the fact that most poverty is not a result of defects in character but results from the structure of society. This is a very important shift because it suggests that society as a whole must take responsibility for its less fortunate citizens. As long as one could attribute poverty and mental retardation to characteristics inherent within the individual, then it is possible to ignore the suffering that so frequently accompanies them, but this suffering is far more difficult to ignore if it is perceived as arising out of conditions in society.

9. *An emphasis on prevention.* While mental retardation is no longer defined as an incurable condition, it is recognized that it is a good deal easier to prevent it than it is to cure it, once it has developed. One result of this has been the development of numerous programs with the specific purpose of preventing intellectual deficits and other developmental disabilities. One of the best preventive measures is providing pregnant mothers with proper nutrition and medical care to prevent birth complications such as prematurity. Social service agencies are making an effort to teach good child-rearing practices to mothers from disadvantaged backgrounds in order to prevent cultural retardation. Efforts are also being made toward the ultimate preventive technique, the elimination of poverty and ignorance, although achieving this goal probably lies far in the future.

In recognition of the fact that the earlier any developmental disability is detected, the more can be done for it, there is a trend toward establishing screening programs for children of progressively younger ages. These screening programs not only detect medical disorders such as PKU, but also future psychological difficulties and sensory impairments. Project Head Start had the specific goal of preventing the school failure that so frequently accompanies a disadvantaged background, and increasingly, such programs are taking not only four and five year olds but also two and three year olds. The Milwaukee Project, perhaps the most successful of all intervention programs, began its training essentially at birth.

Screening programs provide both primary and secondary prevention. Primary prevention refers to the prevention of the developmental disability in the first place, while secondary prevention refers to minimizing the symptoms of an already developed disorder and the prevention of the development of behavior problems or other complications arising from the primary condition. For example, if severe hearing impairment is detected at a young age, although usually nothing can be done to restore hearing, many of the severe language deficits that usually accompany hearing loss can be alleviated. The Down's Syndrome Project at the University of Washington cannot prevent Down's syndrome, but it can insure that each child is functioning at maximum potential.

To date, such preventive programs have made little progress in reducing the most common type of mental retardation, retardation caused by an inappropriate early environment. There have been a number of well-conceived programs such as Head Start, but these have had little impact in reducing the high rate of school failure among children of low SES families. The Milwaukee Project demonstrated that many of the problems associated with poor early environment could be overcome if the children are removed from their families for a considerable period of time each day starting essentially at birth, but a program of this type is not feasible on a large scale, not only because of its cost, but also because of the objections of leaders in the black community who resent so-called experts removing their children from their families and exposing them to a different culture.

One type of prevention that is still very controversial is euthanasia or mercy killing. Traditional moral values have prescribed that all human life must be preserved at all costs, and this has been the traditional orientation of the medical establishment and the legal system. However, there have recently been a number of breaks in this previously hard rule in the direction of placing more value on the quality of life rather than on extending life at all costs. This is seen in the liberalization of abortion laws, a recognition that it might be cruel to bring an unwanted child into the world; and in the right to die movement, the recognition that terminally ill people have a right to refuse treatment that will prolong their lives for a painful few weeks. Some medical personnel are now admitting that if a grossly deformed baby is born, the child might be quietly laid on the table in the hopes that he or she will not start to breathe, in contradiction to the usual medical practice of slapping a newborn to encourage breathing. It is doubtful that euthanasia will have much of an impact on the prevalence of mental retardation in the foreseeable future, but there is little question that this type of ethical question is going to be discussed more openly in the future.

10. *Planning and Coordination of Services.* In the past, one of the main difficulties with the delivery of services to the handicapped was a lack of coordination between various providers. The result was either a duplication of services or, more likely, gaps in services with the result that many handicapped people did not receive appropriate education or rehabilitation. All 50 states are now making an effort to alleviate this problem by setting up regional planning boards and other agencies to coordinate services.

One benefit of this coordinated planning is that a much wider variety of services have become available. In the past, there were often only two alternatives available to the handicapped, they could either be integrated into the mainstream of school or society where they received virtually no special services or they could be totally segregated from the mainstream as in a special class or an institution for the retarded. These planning boards and local school boards have tried to develop more "in-between" services. Schools are now experimenting with resource rooms and itinerant teachers to provide special services to the handicapped within the context of a regular school program. On the adult level, sheltered workshops, group homes, and recreational programs are springing up in many communities to provide special services within the mainstream of community life. Thus, the handicapped have a number of different alternatives available to them, and they can be placed in the least restrictive environment commensurate with their needs and capabilities.

The Future

Making accurate predictions about the future is always difficult. So many unforeseen events are continually occurring and interacting with one another that any prediction of social trends more than a few years into the future is bound to be wrong. The best predictive tool that we have available is the extrapolation of present trends; in other words, making predictions based on the assumption that society will continue to move in the direction that it has been moving for the past few years. Since programs and services for the mentally retarded have been expanding so rapidly in the past few years, it would be reasonable to assume that the future will be bright for the retarded in this country, with almost all retarded people integrated into the community or into regular public school classes and with many services available to them.

However, there are several variables in this equation that are very difficult to predict. Mental retardation programming is almost completely dependent on government spending for its support, and government spending is notoriously unpredictable. Taxpayers always seem to feel that their taxes are too high, and there are many other worthwhile programs competing for government dollars. The 1970s have seen the rapid rise in government services slowed almost to a halt, and unless government spending is again increased, it is unreasonable to expect much of an expansion of programs for the handicapped.

The welfare of the retarded is intimately tied in with the welfare of the nation as a whole. When the country is thriving, the mentally retarded are likely to be well off. One of the best things that can happen to the mentally retarded is a reduction in the general unemployment rate. During World War II, many retarded people were recruited into industrial and service jobs that, in more normal times, would have been closed to them, and many performed creditably despite a lack of training and experience. Certainly, some of the present vocational rehabilitation programs could be phased out if the labor market were such that anyone, even a handicapped person were able to find work. What many handicapped people need is not more training, but jobs. However, in an economy in which 6 to 8 percent of the labor force is unable to find work, it is not surprising that many retarded people have unusual difficulty getting and keeping a job, and this creates the illusion that they are unemployable and need more training.

Perhaps most important of all will be the future attitudes of the nation's citizens toward the disadvantaged of all types. The twentieth century has witnessed a gradual but decisive change in the way that America has viewed the unfortunate. The traditional outlook has been a "blame the victim" approach. Throughout the 1800s and the early part of this century, most people assumed that anyone who really wanted to be could make a success of himself or herself, and the only reason why someone was poor was some sort of defect in character. Thus, many people contended that poor people were basically lazy and deserved whatever happened to them. Proponents of this attitude are naturally opposed to most social welfare programs that have the goal of improving the lives of the less fortunate. Such attitudes are gradually changing toward the recognition that many people without jobs are just as anxious to work as anyone else, but they just don't have the education or the connections to get a decent job. This change in attitude has been reflected in the numerous social programs beginning with Roosevelt's New Deal and progressing through the New Frontier and Great Society programs of the 1960s. There are now hundreds of programs aimed at improving the quality of life of the nation's less fortunate people, everything from social security to medicaid to public housing to job training. Certainly, many of these programs have had problems and some must be considered failures, but if this attitude continues, there will be more experimental programs, more attempts to help the unfortunate. Some will no doubt fail and be criticized, but, eventually, ways will be found to include all Americans fully into the fabric of American society.

References

Abramowicz, H. K., & Richardson, S. A. Epidemiology of severe mental retardation in children: community studies. *American Journal of Mental Deficiency,* 1975, **80,** 18–39.

Achenbach, T. M. Comparison of Stanford-Binet performance of nonretarded and retarded persons matched for MA and sex. *American Journal of Mental Deficiency,* 1970, **74,** 488–494.

Adams, J. Adaptive behavior and measured intelligence in the classification of mental retardation. *American Journal of Mental Deficiency,* 1973, **78,** 77–81.

Alpern, G. D. & Boll, T. J. (Eds.) *Education and care of moderately and severely retarded children: with a curriculum and activities guide.* Seattle: Special Child Publications, 1971.

Alvin, J. The response of severely mentally retarded children to music. *American Journal of Mental Deficiency,* 1959, **63,** 988–996.

Anderson, V. A., & Newby, H. *Improving the child's speech.* (2nd ed.) New York: Oxford University Press, 1973.

Astin, A. W., & Ross, S. Glutamic acid and human intelligence. *Psychological Bulletin,* 1960, **57,** 429–434.

Atkinson, R. C., & Shiffrin, R. M. Human memory: A proposed system and its control processes. In K. W. Spence & J. T. Spence (Eds.), *The psychology of learning and motivation.* Vol. 2. New York: Academic Press, 1968.

Atwell, A. A., & Clabby, D. A. *The retarded child: Answers to questions parents ask.* Los Angeles: Western Psychological Services, 1971.

Axline, V. M. *Play therapy.* Boston: Houghton-Mifflin, 1947.

Axline, V. M. Some observations on play therapy. *Journal of Consulting Psychology,* 1948, **12,** 209–216.

Axline, V. M. Mental deficiency: Symptom or disease? *Journal of Consulting Psychology,* 1949, **13,** 313–327.

Azrin, N. H., & Foxx, R. M. A rapid method of toilet training the institutionalized retarded. *Journal of Applied Behavior Analysis,* 1971, **4,** 89–99.

Badt, M. Levels of abstraction in vocabulary definitions of mentally retarded school children. *American Journal of Mental Deficiency,* 1958, **63,** 241–246.

Baer, D. M., & Guess, D. Receptive training of adjective inflections in mental retardates. *Journal of Applied Behavior Analysis,* 1971, **4,** 129–139.

Bair, H. V., & Herold, W. Efficiency of chlorpromazine in hyperactive mentally retarded children. *American Medical Association Archives of Neurology and Psychiatry,* 1955, **74,** 363–364.

Baird, D. Social factors in obstetrics. *Lancet,* 1949, **1,** 1079–1083.

Baldwin, V. L. et al, *Isn't it Time he outgrew this? or a Training Program for parents of retarded children.* Springfield, Ill.: Charles C. Thomas, 1973.

Balthazar, E. E., & Stevens, H. A. *The emotionally disturbed mentally retarded: A historical and contemporary perspective.* Englewood Cliffs, N. J.: Prentice-Hall, 1975.

Baratz, S. S., & Baratz, J. C. Early childhood intervention: The social science base of institutional racism. *Harvard Educational Review,* 1970, **40,** 29–50.

Barrow, R. L., & Fabing, H. D. *Epilepsy and the law.* New York: Harper & Row, 1966.

Baroff, G. S. *Mental retardation: Nature, cause, and management.* Washington: Hemisphere Publishing Corp., 1974.

Barsch, R. *A movigenic curriculum.* Madison, Wis.: State Department of Public Instruction, 1965.

Barsch, R. H. *The parent of the handicapped child: The study of child-rearing practices.* Springfield, Ill.: Thomas, 1968.

Bateman, B., & Wetherell, J. Psycholinguistic aspects of mental retardation. *Mental Retardation,* 1965, **3**(2), 8–13.

Battle, E. S., & Rotter, J. B. Children's feelings of personal control as related to social class and ethnic group. *Journal of Personality,* 1963, **31,** 482–490.

Baumeister, A., Beedle, R., & Urquart, D. GSR conditioning in normals and retardates. *American Journal of Mental Deficiency,* 1964, **69,** 114–120.

Baumeister, A. A., & Forehand, R. Stereotyped acts. In N. R. Ellis (Ed.), *International review of research in mental retardation.* Vol. 6. New York: Academic Press, 1973.

Bayley, N. Consistency and variability in the growth of intelligence from birth to eighteen years. *Journal of Genetic Psychology,* 1949, **75,** 165–196.

Bayley, N. Comparison of mental and motor test scores for ages 1–15 months by sex, birth order, race, geographic location, and education of parents. *Child Development,* 1965, **36,** 379–411.

Bayley, N. *Manual for the Bayley Scales of Infant Development.* New York: Psychological Corporation, 1969.

Becker, R. L. Job training placement for retarded youth. *Mental Retardation,* 1976, **14**(3), 7–11.

Bee, H. L., Van Ergen, L. F., Streissguth, A. P., Nyman, B. A., & Leckie, M. S.

Social class differences in maternal teaching strategies and speech patterns. *Developmental Psychology,* 1969, **1,** 726–734.

Beier, D. C. Behavioral disturbances in the mentally retarded. In H. A. Stevens & R. Heber (Eds.), *Mental retardation: A review of research.* Chicago: University of Chicago Press, 1964.

Belmont, J. M. Long-term memory in mental retardation. In N. R. Ellis (Ed.), *International review of research in mental retardation.* Vol. 1. New York: Academic Press, 1966.

Belmont, J. M., & Butterfield, E. C. Learning strategies as determinants of memory deficiencies. *Cognitive Psychology,* 1971, **2,** 411–420.

Benda, C. E. *Down's syndrome: Mongolism and its management.* New York: Grune and Stratton, 1969.

Benda, C. E. Psychopathology of childhood. In L. Carmichael (Ed.), *Manual of child psychology* (2nd ed.). New York: Wiley, 1954.

Bereiter, C., & Engelmann, S. *Teaching disadvantaged children in the preschool.* Englewood Cliffs, N.J.: Prentice-Hall, 1966.

Bergin, A. E., & Garfield, S. L. (Eds.), *Handbook of psychotherapy and behavior change: An empirical analysis.* New York: Wiley, 1971.

Berko, J. The child's learning of English morphology. *Word,* 1958, **14,** 150–177.

Berkson, G., & Davenport, R. K. Stereotyped movements in mental defectives: I, Initial survey. *American Journal of Mental Deficiency,* 1962, **66,** 849–852.

Berkson, G., & Mason, W. Stereotyped behaviors of chimpanzees: Relation to general arousal and alternative activities. *Perceptual and Motor Skills,* 1964, **19,** 635–652.

Bernstein, B. Social class and linguistic development: A theory of social learning. In H. A. Halsey, J. Floud, & C. A. Anderson (Eds.), *Education, economy, and society.* New York: Free Press, 1961.

Bernstein, B. Social structure, language, and learning. In J. P. DeCecco (Ed.), *The psychology of language, thought, and instruction.* New York: Holt, Rinehart and Winston, 1967.

Bialer, I. Conceptualization of success and failure in mentally retarded and normal children. *Journal of Personality,* 1961, **29,** 303–320.

Bialer, I. Emotional disturbance and mental retardation: Etiologic and conceptual relationships. In F. Menolascino (Ed.), *Psychiatric approaches to mental retardation.* New York: Basic Books, 1970.

Bialer, I. Relationship of mental retardation to emotional disturbance and physical disability. In H. C. Haywood (Ed.), *Socio-cultural aspects of mental retardation.* New York: Appleton-Century-Crofts, 1970a.

Bickel, H., Girrard, J., & Hickmans, E. M. The influence of phenylalanine intake on the chemistry and behavior of phenylketonuric children. *Acta Paediatrica,* 1954, **43,** 64–77.

Birch, H. G., & Gussow, J. D. *Disadvantaged children: Health nutrition, and school failure.* New York: Grune and Stratton, 1970.

Birch, H. G., Richardson, S. A., Baird, D., Horobin, G., & Illsley, R. *Mental subnormality in the community.* Baltimore: Williams and Wilkins, 1970.

Birch, J. W. *Mainstreaming educable mentally retarded children in regular classes.* Reston, Virginia: Council for Exceptional Children, 1974.

Black, F. W. The word explosion in learning disabilities: A notation of literature trends, 1962–1972. *Journal of Learning Disabilities,* 1974, **7,** 323–324.

Blake, K. A. *Teaching the retarded.* Englewood Cliffs, N.J.: Prentice-Hall, 1974.

Blatt, B. *Exodus from pandemonium.* Boston: Allyn and Bacon, 1970.

Blodgett, H. H. *Mentally retarded children: What parents and others should know.* Minneapolis: University of Minnesota Press, 1971.

Bloom, B. J. *Stability and change in human characteritics.* New York: Wiley, 1964.

Bond, E. A. Tenth grade abilities and achievements. *Teachers College Contr. Educ.,* 1940, No. 813.

Borkowski, J. G., & Johnson, L. O. Mediation and the paired-associate learning of normals and retardates. *American Journal of Mental Deficiency,* 1968, **72,** 610–613.

Boshes, L. D., & Gibbs, F. A. *Epilepsy Handbook.* (2nd Ed.) Springfield, Ill.: Thomas, 1972.

Braginsky, B. M., and Braginsky, D. D. The mentally retarded: Society's Hansels and Gretels. *Psychology Today,* 1974, **7**(10), 18–21, 24–30.

Brainerd, C. J., & Allen, T. W. Experimental indications of the conservation of "first-order" quantitative invariants. *Psychological Bulletin,* 1971, **75,** 128–144.

Brazziel, W. F. A letter from the South. *Harvard Educational Review,* 1969, **39,** 200–208.

Brison, D. W., & Bereiter, C. Acquisition of conservation of substance in normal, retarded, and gifted children. In D. W. Brison and E. V. Sullivan (Eds.), *Recent research on the acquisition of conservation of substance,* Toronto: Ontario Institute for Studies in Education, 1967.

Brown, A. L. Context and recency cues in the recognition memory of retarded children and adolescents. *American Journal of Mental Deficiency,* 1972, **77,** 54–58.

Brown, A. L. Conservation of number and continuous quantity in normal, bright, and retarded children. *Child Development,* 1973, **44,** 376–379.

Brown, A. L. The role of strategic behavior in retardate memory. In N. R. Ellis (Ed.) *International review of research in mental retardation.* Vol. 7. New York: Academic Press, 1974.

Browning, P. L., & Keesey, M. Outcome studies on counseling with the retarded: A methodological critique. In Browning, P. L. (Ed.), *Mental retardation: Rehabilitation and Counseling.* Springfield, Ill.: Thomas, 1974.

Buck, J. N. The sage: An unusual mongoloid. In A. Burton & R. E. Harris (Eds.), *Clinical studies of personality.* New York: Harper & Row, 1955.

Buckley, F. Preliminary report on intelligence quotients scores of patients with Turner's syndrome: A replication study. *British Journal of Psychiatry,* 1971, **119,** 513–514.

Burger, A. L., & Blackman, L. S. Acquisition and retention of a mediational strategy for PA learning in EMR children. *American Journal of Mental Deficiency,* 1976, **80,** 529–534.

Burke, B. S., Beal, V. A., Kirkwood, S. B., & Stuart, H. C. The influence of nutrition during pregnancy upon the condition of the infant at birth. *Journal of Nutrition* 1943, **26,** 569–583.

Burt, C. Inheritance of general intelligence. *American Psychologist,* 1972, **27,** 175–190.

Butterfield, E. C., Wambold, C., & Belmont, J. M. On the theory and practice of improving short term memory. *American Journal of Mental Deficiency,* 1973, **77,** 654–669.

Butterfield, E. C., & Zigler, E. F. The effects of different verbal incentives on learning of mentally retarded and average chilren. Unpublished, 1961.

Cahalane, S. F. Phenylketonuria: Mass screening of newborns in Ireland. *Archives of Diseases in Children,* 1968, **43,** 141–144.

Cain, L. F., & Levine, S. Effects of community and institutional school programs on trainable mentally retarded children. *Council on Exceptional Children Research Monograph,* 1963, Series B, No. B-1. Arlington, Va.: *Council on Exceptional Children.*

Caldwell, B. M., Bradley, R. H., & Elardo, R. Early stimulation. In J. Wortis (Ed.), *Mental Retardation,* Vol. 7. New York: Grune and Stratton, 1975.

Cantor, G. N. A critique of Garfield and Wittson's reaction to the revised manual of terminology and classification. *American Journal of Mental Deficincy,* 1960, **64,** 954–956.

Cattell, P. *The measurement of intelligence of infants and young children.* New York: Psychological Corporation, 1947.

Cazden, C. B. *Child language and education.* New York: Holt, Rinehart and Winston, 1972.

Cegelka, J. A., and Cegelka, W. J. A review of research: Reading and the educable mentally retarded. *Exceptional Children,* 1970, **37,** 187–200.

Cegelka, W. J., & Tyler, J. L. The efficacy of special class placement for the mentally retarded in proper perspective. *Training School Bulletin,* 1970, **65,** 33–68.

Centerwall, S. A. and Centerwall, W. R. A study of children with mongolism reared in the home compared to those reared away from the home. *Pediatrics,* 1960, **25,** 678–685.

Chall, J. S. *Learning to read: The great debate.* New York: McGraw-Hill, 1967.

Charles, D. C. Ability and accomplishment of persons earlier judged mentally retarded. *Genetic Psychology Monographs,* 1953, **47,** 3–71.

Chase, H. P., & Martin, H. P. Undernutrition and child development. *New England Journal of Medicine,* 1970, **282,** 933–939.

Chess, S. Emotional problems in mentally retarded children. In F. J. Menolascino (Ed.), *Psychiatric approaches to mental retardation.* New York: Basic Books, 1970.

Chess, S., & Hassibi, M. Behavior deviations in mentally retarded children. *Journal of the American Academy of Child Psychiatry,* 1970, **9,**

Chisolm, J. J., & Kaplan, E. Lead poisoning in childhood. *Journal of Pediatrics,* 1968, **73,** 942–950.

Chomsky, N. *Aspects of a theory of syntax.* Cambridge, Mass.: M.I.T. Press, 1965.

Chow, B. F., Simonson, M., Hanson, H. M., & Roeder, L. M. Behavioral measurements in nutritional studies. *Conditional Reflex,* 1971, **6,** 36–40.

Cicirelli, V. *The impact of head start: An evaluation of the effects of head start on children's cognitive and affective development.* Springfield, Va. U. S. Dept. of Commerce Clearinghouse, 1969.

Cleary, T. A., Humphreys, L. G., Kendricks, S. A., & Wesman, A. Educational uses of tests with disadvantaged students. *American Psychologist,* 1975, **30,** 15–41.

Cobb, H. V. *The forecast of fulfillment.* New York: Teachers College Press, 1972.

Cole, M., & Bruner, J. S. Cultural differences and inferences about psychological processes. *American Psychologist,* 1971, **26,** 867–976.

Coleman, J. S. et al. *Equality of educational opportunity,* U. S. Department of Health, Education, and Welfare, 1966.

Cooper, L. Z., Ziring, P. R., Ockerse, A. B., Fedun, B. A., Kiely, B, & Krugman, S. Rubella: Clinical manifestations and management. *American Journal of Diseases of Children,* 1969, **118,** 18–29.

Corman, H. H. & Escalona, S. K. Stages of sensorimotor development: A replication study. *Merrill-Palmer Quarterly,* 1969, **15,** 351–361.

Costello, J. & Dickie, J. Leiter and Stanford-Binet IQs of preschool disadvantaged children. *Developmental Psychology,* 1970, **2,** 314.

Couveur, J., & Desmonts, G. Congenital and maternal toxoplasmosis. *Developmental Medicine and Child Neurology,* 1962, **4,** 519–530.

Cowley, J. J., & Griesel, R. D. The effect on growth and behavior of rehabilitating first and second generation low protein rats. *Animal Behavior,* 1966, **14,** 506.

Cravioto, J., DeLicardie, E. R., & Birch, H. G. Nutrition, growth, and neurointegrative development: An experimental and ecological study. *Pediatrics,* 1966, **38,** part 2, supplement, 319–372.

Crome, L., & Stern, J. *The pathology of mental retardation,* London: Churchill, 1967.

Cromwell, R. A social learning approach to mental retardation. In N. R. Ellis (Ed.), *Handbook of mental deficiency,* New York: McGraw-Hill, 1963.

Cruickshank, W. M. et al. *A teaching method for brain injured and hyperactive children.* Syracuse: Syracuse University Press, 1961.

Cummings, S. T., & Stock, D. Brief group therapy of mothers of retarded children outside of the specialty clinic setting. *American Journal of Mental Deficiency,* 1962, **66,** 739–748.

Dameron, S., & Lawrence, E. Development of intelligence of infants with mongolism. *Child Development,* 1963, **34,** 733–738.

Darwin, C. *The descent of Man.* (2nd ed.) Philadelphia: McKay, 1874.

Davenport, R. K., & Berkson, G. Stereotyped movements of mental defectives, II, Effects of novel objects. *American Journal of Mental Deficincy,* 1963, **67,** 879–882.

Davids, A., DeVault, S., & Talmadge, M. Anxiety, pregnancy, and childbirth abnormalities. *Journal of Consulting Psychology,* 1961, **25,** 74–77.

Davidson, R. E. Mediation and ability in paired associate learning. *Journal of Educational Psychology,* 1964, **55,** 352–356.

Davies, S. P. *The mentally retarded in society.* New York: Columbia University Press, 1959.

Davis, K. Final note on a case of extreme isolation. *American Journal of Sociology,* 1947, **57,** 432–457.

Delacato, C. H. *The diagnosis and treatment of speech and reading problems.* Springfield, Ill.: Thomas, 1963.

Deno, E. Special education as developmental capital. *Exceptional Children,* 1970, **37,** 229–237.

Deno, E. N. (Ed.) *Instructional alternatives for exceptional children.* Reston, Va.: Council for Exceptional Children, 1974.

Dentler, R. A., & Mackler, B. Ability and social status among normal and retarded children: A review of the literature. *Psychological Bulletin,* 1962, **59,** 273–283.

Department of Health, Education, and Welfare, *Children served in mental retardation clinics: Fiscal years 1970–1972.* U. S. Government Printing Office, 1973.

Deutsch, M. et al. *The disadvantaged child.* New York: Basic Books, 1967.

Deutsch, M., & Brown, B. Social influences in Negro-White intelligence differences. *Journal of Social Issues,* 1964, **20,** 24–35.

Dietary treatment of phenylketonuria, Editorial, *British Journal of Medicine,* 1968, **4,** 135.

Dicks-Mireaux, M. S. Mental development of infants with Down's syndrome. *American Journal of Mental Deficiency,* 1972, **77,** 26–43.

Dingman, H. F., & Tarjan, G. Mental retardation and the normal distribution curve. *American Journal of Mental Deficiency,* 1960, **64,** 991–994.

Doll, E. A. *Vineland Scale of Social Maturity,* Minneapolis: American Guidance Service, 1964.

Doll, E. A. The essentials of an inclusive concept of mental deficiency. *American Journal of Mental Deficiency,* 1941, **46,** 214–219.

Domino, G., Goldschmidt, M., & Kaplan, M. Personality traits among institutionalized mongoloid girls. *American Journal of Mental Deficiency,* 1964, **69,** 498–503.

Donovan, H. Organization of a speech program for mentally retarded children in the New York city public schools. *American Journal of Mental Deficiency,* 1957, **62,** 455–459.

Down, J. L. Observations on an ethnic classification of idiots. *London Hospital Reports,* 1866.

Drillien, C. M. *The growth and development of the prematurely born infant.* Baltimore: Williams and Wilkins, 1964.

Dunn, L. M. *Peabody Picture Vocabulary Test Manual.* Minneapolis: American Guidance Service, 1959.

Dunn, L. M. Special education for the mildly retarded—Is much of it justified? *Exceptional Children,* 1968, **35,** 5–22.

Dunn, L. M. (Ed.) *Exceptional children in the schools: Special education in transition.* New York: Holt, Rinehart and Winston, 1973.

Dyken, P., & Culley, W. Another propulation of phenylketonuria? Studies on atypical phenylketonurics. *Developmental Medicine and Child Neurology,* 1969, **11,** 718–729.

Eaton, J. W., & Weil, R. J. *Culture and mental disorders: A comparative study of the Hutterites and other populations.* Glencoe, Ill.: Free Press, 1955.

Edgerton, R. B. *The cloak of competence.* Berkeley, California: University of California Press, 1967.

Eells, K., Davis, A., Havighurst, R. J., Herrick, V. E., & Tyler, R. W. *Intelligence and cultural differences.* Chicago: University of Chicago Press, 1951.

Effron, M. L. Some experiences with screening for inborn errors of metabolism. In Crow, J. F., & Neel, J. V. (Eds.), *Proceedings of the Third International Congress of Human Genetics.* Baltimore: Johns Hopkins Press, 1967.

Elashoff, J. D., & Snow, R. E. *Pygmalion reconsidered.* Worthington, Ohio: Charles A. Jones Publishing Co., 1971.

Elkind, D. *Children and Adolescents.* New York: Oxford University Press, 1970.

Ellis, N. R. The stimulus trace and behavioral inadequacy. In N. R. Ellis (Ed.), *Handbook of mental deficiency.* New York: McGraw-Hill, 1963.

Ellis, N. R. A behavioral research strategy in mental retardation: Defense and critique. *American Journal of Mental Deficiency,* 1969, **73,** 557–566.

Ellis, N. R. Memory processes in retardates and normals. In N. R. Ellis (Ed.), *International review of research in mental retardation.* Vol. 4. New York: Academic Press, 1970.

Elmer, E., & Gregg, G. S. Developmental characteristics of abused children. *Pediatrics,* 1967, **40,** 596–602.

Erlenmeyer-Kimling, L., & Jarvik, L. F. Genetics and intelligence: A review. *Science,* 1963, **142,** 1477–1478.

Eysenck, H. J. *The effects of psychotherapy.* New York: International Science Press, 1966.

Fabia, J., & Drollette, M. Life tables up to age 10 for mongols with and without congenital heart defect. *Journal of Mental Deficiency Research,* 1970, **14,** 235–242.

Fantz, R. L. The origin of form perception. *Scientific American,* 1961, **204,** 66–72.

Farber, B. *Prevalence of exceptional children in Illinois in 1958.* Springfield, Ill.: Superintendent of Public Instruction, 1959, Circular-Census IA.

Farber, B. *Mental retardation: Its social context and social consequences.* Boston: Houghton Mifflin, 1968.

Farber, B. Effects of a severely retarded child on the family. In E. P. Trapp & p. Himelstein (Eds.), *Readings on the exceptional child.* (2nd Ed.) New York: Appleton-Century-Crofts, 1972.

Ferguson, R. G. A study of the problem of mental retardation in a large urban community. *American Journal of Orthopsychiatry,* 1957, **27,** 490–501.

Fisher, M. A., & Zeaman, D. Growth and decline of retardate intelligence. In N. R. Ellis, (Ed.), *International review of research in mental retardation.* Vol. 4. New York: Academic Press, 1970.

Fisher, M. A., & Zeaman, D. An attention-retention theory of retardate discrimination learning. In N. R. Ellis (Ed.), *International review of research in mental retardation.* Vol. 6. New York: Academic Press, 1973.

Fishler, K., Share, J., & Koch, R. Adaptation of Gesell developmental scales for evaluation of children with Down's syndrome. *American Journal of Mental Deficiency,* 1964, **68,** 642–646.

Flavell, J. H. *The developmental psychology of Jean Piaget.* Princeton, N.J.: Van Nostrand, 1963.

Flavell, J. H., Beach, D. R., & Chinsky, J. M. Spontaneous verbal rehearsal in a memory task as a function of age. *Child Development,* 1966, **37,** 283–299.

Floor, L., & Rosen, M. Investigating the phenomenon of helplessness in mentally retarded adults. *American Journal of Mental Deficiency,* 1975, **79,** 565–572.

Forehand, R., & Baumeister, A. A. The effect of auditory and visual stimulation on stereotyped rocking behavior and general activity of severe retardates. *Journal of Clinical Psychology,* 1970, **26,** 426–429.

Frankenburg, W. K., & Dodds, J. B. The Denver Developmental Screening Test. *Journal of Pediatrics,* 1967, **71,** 181–191.

Franks, D. J. Ethnic and social status characteristics of children in EMR and LD classes. *Exceptional Children,* 1971, **37,** 537–538.

Fredericks, H. D. et al. *The teaching research curriculum for moderately and severely handicapped.* Springfield, Ill.: Thomas, 1976.

Freeman, R. D. Psychopharmacology and the retarded child. In F. J. Menolascino (Ed.), *Psychiatric approaches to mental retardation.* New York: Basic Books, 1970.

Frostig, M., & Horne, D. *The Frostig program for the development of visual perception.* Chicago: Follett, 1964.

Fuchigami, R. Emerging curricula for the elementary level mentally retarded. *Mental Retardation,* 1969, **7,** 37–40.

Furth, H. G. *Thinking without language: Psychological implications of deafness.* New York: Free Press of Glencoe, 1966.

Gallagher, J. J. The special education contract for mildly handicapped children. *Exceptional Children,* 1972, **38,** 527–535.

Gardner, W. I. Mental retardation: A critical review of personality characteristics. In H. J. Prehm, L. A. Hammerlynck, and J. E. Crosson (Eds.), *Behavioral research in mental retardation.* Eugene, Ore.: University of Oregon Press, 1968.

Gardner, W. I. *Behavior modification in mental retardation.* Chicago: Aldine-Atherton, 1971.

Gardner, W. I. *Children with learning and behavior problems.* Boston: Allyn and Bacon, 1974.

Garfield, S. L., & Wittson, C. Some reactions to the revised "Manual on terminology and classification in mental retardation." *American Journal of Mental Deficiency,* 1960, **64,** 951–953.

Garrison, M., & Hammill, D. D. Who are the retarded? *Exceptional Children,* 1971, **38,** 13–20.

Gaudia, G. Race, social class, and age of achievement of conservation on Piaget's tasks. *Developmental Psychology,* 1972, **6,** 158–165.

Gay, G., & Abrahams, R. D. Does the pot melt, boil, or brew? Black children and white assessment procedures. *Journal of School Psychology,* 1973, **11,** 330–340.

Gerver, J. M., & Day, R. Intelligence quotients of children who have recovered from erythroblastosis fetalis. *Journal of Pediatrics,* 1950, **36,** 342–348.

Gillespie, P. H., & Johnson, L. *Teaching reading to the mildly retarded child.* Columbus, Ohio: Charles E. Merrill, 1973.

Ginsburg, H. *The myth of the deprived child.* Englewood Cliffs, N.J.: Prentice-Hall, 1972.

Ginsburg, H., & Opper, S. *Piaget's theory of intellectual development.* Englewood Cliffs, N.J.: Prentice-Hall, 1969.

Gittell, M. *New York City fact book.* New York: Institute for community studies, Queens College, 1971.

Goddard, H. H. *The Kallikak family.* New York: Macmillan, 1912.

Goffman, E. *Stigma: Notes on the management of spoiled identity.* Englewood Cliffs, N.J.: Prentice-Hall, 1963.

Gold, M. W. Research on the vocational habilitation of the retarded: The present, the future. In N. R. Ellis (Ed.), *International review of research in mental retardation.* Vol. 6, New York: Academic Press, 1973.

Golden, M., & Birns, B. Social class and cognitive development in infancy. *Merrill Palmer Quarterly of Behavior and Development,* 1968, **14,** 139–149.

Golden, M., Birns, B., Bridger, W., & Moss, A. Social class differentiation in cognitive development among black preschool children. *Child Development,* 1971, **42,** 37–45.

Goldstein, H., Moss, J., & Jordan, L. J. *The efficacy of special class training on the development of mentally retarded children.* Urbana, Ill.: University of Illinois Press, 1965.

Goldstein, K. *Aftereffects of brain injuries in war.* New York: Grune and Stratton, 1942.

Goodman, L., & Hammill, D. The effectiveness of the Kephart-Getman activities in developing perceptual-motor and cognitive skills. *Focus on Exceptional Children,* 1973, **4**(9), 1–9.

Goodman, M. B., Gruenberg, E. M., Downing, J., & Rogot, E. A prevalence study of mental retardation in a metropolitan area. *American Journal of Public Health,* 1956, **46,** 702–707.

Gorelick, M. C. *An assessment of vocational realism of high school and post high school educable mentally retarded adolescents.* Los Angeles: Exceptional Children's Foundation, 1966.

Gottlieb, J., & Budoff, M. Social acceptability of retarded children in nongraded schools differing in architecture. *American Journal of Mental Deficiency,* 1973, **78,** 15–19.

Graham, F. K., Ernhart, C. B., Thurston, D., & Craft, M. Development three years after perinatal anoxia and other potentially damaging newborn experiences. *Psychological Monographs,* 1962, **76,** Whole No. 522.

Graliker, B. V., Fishler, K., & Koch, R. Teenage reaction to a mentally retarded sibling. *American Journal of Mental Deficiency,* 1962, **66,** 838–843.

Green, A. H. Self-mutilation in schizophrenic children. *Archives of General Psychiatry,* 1967, **17,** 234–244.

Green, C., & Zigler, E. F. Social deprivation and the performance of retarded and normal children on a satiation type task. *Child Development,* 1962, **33,** 499–508.

Greene, R. *Forgotten children: Techniques in teaching the mentally retarded.* San Rafael, Cal.: Leswing Press, 1972.

Greulich, W. W., Thoms, H., & Twaddle, R. C. A study of pelvis type and its relationship to body build in white women. *Journal of the American Medical Association,* 1939, **112,** 485–492.

Grieder, J. W. et al. *Mathematics design for individually paced instruction.* Duval County School Board, Jacksonville, Fla., 1971.

Grossman, F. K. *Brothers and sisters of retarded children: An exploratory study.* Syracuse, N.Y.: Syracuse University Press, 1972.

Grossman, H. J. *Manual on terminology and classification in mental retardation, 1973 revision.* Washington, D.C.: American Association on Mental Deficiency, 1973.

Gruen, G. E., & Berg, B. Visual discrimination learning in familially retarded and normal children. *American Journal of Mental Deficiency,* 1973, **78,** 63–69.

Gruen, G. E., & Vore, D. A. Development of conservation in normal and retarded children. *Developmental Psychology,* 1972, **6,** 146–157.

Guess, D., Sailor, W., Rutherford, G., & Baer, D. M. An experimental analysis of linguistic development: The productive use of the plural morpheme. *Journal of Applied Behavior Analysis,* 1968, **1,** 225–235.

Guilford, J. P., & Hoepfner, R. *The analysis of intelligence.* New York: McGraw-Hill, 1971.

Guilford, J. P. *The nature of human intelligence.* New York: McGraw-Hill, 1967.

Guinee, V. F. Lead poisoning. *American Journal of Medicine,* 1972, **52,** 283–288.

Hallahan, D. P., & Cruickshank, W. M. *Psychoeducational foundations of learning disabilities.* Englewood Cliffs, N.J.: Prentice-Hall, 1973.

Hammill, D., & Wiederholt, J. L. *The resource room: Rationale and Implementation.* Philadelphia: Buttonwood Farms, 1972.

Hammill, D. D., & Wiederholt, J. L. Review of the Frosting Visual Perception Test and the related training program. In L. Mann and D. A. Sabatino (Eds.), *The first review of special education.* Vol. 1. Philadelphia: JSE Press, 1973.

Hanley, W. B., Partington, M. W., Rathbun, J. C., Amies, C. R., Webb, J. F., & Moore, J. E. The newborn phenylketonuria screening program in Ontario, Canada. *Canadian Medical Association Journal,* 1969, **101**(4), 185–190.

Haring, N. G., & Phillips, L. *Analysis and modification of classroom behavior.* Englewood Cliffs, N.J.: Prentice-Hall, 1972.

Harrell, R. F., Woodyard, E., & Gates, A. I., *The effects of mother's diets on the intelligence of offspring: A study of the influence of vitamin supplementation of the diets of pregnant and lactating mothers on the intelligence of their children.* New York: Teachers College Press, 1955.

Harter, S. Discrimination learning sets in children as a function of MA and IQ. *Journal of Experimental Child Psychology,* 1965, **2,** 31–43.

Hastings, D. Some psychiatric problems of mental deficiency. *American Journal of Mental Deficiency,* 1948, **52,** 260–262.

Havard, J. School problems and allergies. *Journal of Learning Disabilities,* 1973, **6,** 492–494.

Hayden, A. H. & Haring, N. G. Programs for Down's syndrome children at the University of Washington. In T. Tjossem (Ed.), *Intervention strategies for risk infants and young* children. Baltimore: University Park Press, 1976.

Heal, L. W. Research strategies and research goals in the scientific study of the mentally subnormal. *American Journal of Mental Deficiency,* 1970, **75,** 10–15.

Heal, L. W., & Johnson, J. T. Inhibition deficits in retardate learning and attention. In N. R. Ellis (Ed.), *International review of research in mental retardation.* Vol. 4. New York: Academic Press, 1970.

Hebb, D. O. Intelligence in man after large removal of cerebral tissue: Report of four left frontal lobe cases. *Journal of General Psychology,* 1939, **21,** 73–87.

Heber, R. Personality. In H. A. Stevens and R. Heber (Eds.), *Mental retardation: A review of research.* Chicago: University of Chicago Press, 1964.

Heber, R., Dever, R., & Conry, J. The influence of environmental and genetic variables on intellectual development. In H. J. Prehm, L. A. Hamerlynck, & J. E. Crosson (Eds.), *Behavioral research in mental retardation.* Eugene, Ore.: University of Oregon Press, 1968.

Heber, R., & Garber, H. The Milwaukee Project: A study of the use of family intervention to prevent cultural-familial retardation. In B. Z. Friedlander, G. M. Sterritt, and G. E. Kirk (Eds.), *Exceptional infant.* Vol. 3. New York: Brunner-Mazel, 1975.

Heiser, K. Psychotherapy in a residential school for mentally retarded children. *Training School Bulletin,* 1954, **50,** 211–218.

Herrnstein, R. J. IQ, *The Atlantic Monthly,* September 1971, 43–64.

Herrnstein, R. J. *IQ in the meritocracy.* Boston: Little Brown, 1973.

Hess, R. D., & Shipman, V. Early experience and socialization of cognitive modes in children. *Child development,* 1965, **36,** 869–886.

Hewett, F. M., & Forness, S. R. *Education of exceptional learners.* Boston: Allyn & Bacon, 1974.

Higgins, C., & Sivers, C. H. A comparison of Stanford-Binet and Colored Raven Progressive Matrices IQs in children of low socioeconomic status. *Journal of Consulting Psychology,* 1958, **22,** 465–468.

Hollingshead, A. B., & Redlich, R. C. *Social class and mental illness.* New York: Wiley, 1958.

Hollis, J. H. Body rocking: Effects of sound and reinforcement. *American Journal of Mental Deficiency,* 1971, **75,** 642–644.

Holmes, L. B., Mack, C., Moser, H. W., Pant, S. S., Halldorsson, S., & Matzilevich, B. *Mental retardation: An atlas of diseases with associated physical abnormalities.* New York: Macmillan, 1972.

Holt, K. S. Home care of severely retarded children. *Pediatrics,* 1958, **22,** 744–755.

Honzik, M. P., McFarlane, J. W., & Allen, L. The stability of mental test performance between two and eighteen years. *Journal of Experimental Education,* 1948, **17,** 309–324.

Hook, E. B., & Kim, D. Prevalence of XYY and XXY karotypes in 337 nonretarded young offenders. *New England Journal of Medicine,* 1970, **283,** 410–411.

Hopkins, T., Bice, H. V., & Colton, K. *Evaluation and education of the cerebral palsied child.* Washington, D.C.: International Council for Exceptional Children, 1954.

Horrobin, J. M., & Rynders, J. E. *To give an edge: A guide for new parents of Down's syndrome children.* Minneapolis: The Colwell Press, 1975.

Horton, D. L., & Kjeldergaard, P. M. An experimental analysis of associative factors in mediated generalization. *Psychological Monographs,* 1961, **75,** No. 11.

House, B. J., & Zeaman, D. Reversal and nonreversal shifts in discrimination learning of retardates. *Journal of Experimental Psychology,* 1962, **63,** 444–451.

Howard, J. W. (Ed.) *A report of the committee to study the education of handicapped children.* Trenton, N.J.: Department of Education, 1954.

Hudson, F. P. Phenylketonuria. *Proceedings of the Royal Society of Medicine,* 1967, **60,** 1152–1155.

Huessy, H. R. Study of the prevalence and therapy of the choreatiform syndrome or hyperkinesis in rural Vermont. *Acta Paedopsychiat.* 1967, **34,** 130–135.

Hunt, J. G., & Zimmerman, J. Stimulating productivity in a simulated sheltered workshop setting. *American Journal of Mental Deficiency,* 1969, **74,** 43–49.

Hunt, N. *The world of Nigel Hunt,* New York: Garrett, 1967.

Illingsworth, R. S. Convulsions in mentally retarded children with and without cerebral palsy: Their frequency and age incidence. *Journal of Mental Deficiency Research,* 1959, **3,** 88–93.

Ingram, C. *Education of the slow learning child.* Yonkers: World Book Co., 1935.

Inhelder, B. *The diagnosis of reasoning in the mentally retarded.* New York, John Day Co., 1968.

Jaffe, T. R. Attitudes of adolescents toward the mentally retarded. *American Journal of Mental Deficiency,* 1966, **70,** 907–912.

Jastak, J. F., McPhee, H. M., & Whitemen, M. *Mental retardation: Its nature and incidence.* Newark, Del.: University of Delaware Press, 1963.

Jencks, C., Smith, M., Acland, H., Bane, M., Cohen, D., Gintis, H., Heyns, B., & Michelson, S. *Inequality: A reassessment of the effect of family and schooling in America.* New York: Basic Books, 1972.

Jensen, A. R. How much can we boost IQ and scholastic acheivement. *Harvard Educational Review,* 1969, **39,** 1–123.

Jensen, A. R. A theory of primary and secondary mental retardation. In N. R. Ellis (Ed.), *International review of research in mental retardation.* Vol. 4. New York: Academic Press, 1970.

Jensen, A. R. *Educability and group differences.* New York: Harper & Row, 1973.

Jensen, A. R., & Rohwer, W. D. The effect of verbal mediation on the learning and retention of paired-associates by retarded adults. *American Journal of Mental Deficiency,* 1963, **68,** 80–84.

Johnson, G. O. A study of the social position of mentally retarded children in the regular grades. *American Journal of Mental Deficiency,* 1950, **55,** 60–89.

Johnson, J. T., & Olley, J. G. Behavioral comparisons of mongoloid and nonmongoloid retarded persons: A review. *American Journal of Mental Deficiency,* 1971, **75,** 546–559.

Johnson, R. C. Behavioral characteristics of phenylketonurics and matched controls. *American Journal of Mental Deficiency,* 1969, **74,** 17–19.

Johnson, V. M., & Werner, R. A. *A step-by-step learning guide for retarded infants and children.* Syracuse, N.Y.: Syracuse University Press, 1975.

Jones, K. L., Smith, D. W., Ulleland, C. N., & Streissguth, A. P. Patterns of malformation in offspring of chronic alcoholic mothers. *Lancet,* 1973, **i,** 1267–1271.

Jones, R. L. Labels and stigma in special education. *Exceptional children,* 1972, **38,** 553–564.

Journal of Learning Disabilities, News, 1974, **7,** 283.

Kahn, J. V. Training EMR and intellectually average adolescents of low and middle

SES for formal thought. *American Journal of Mental Deficiency,* 1974, **79,** 397–403.

Kanner, L. Early infantile autism. *Journal of Pediatrics,* 1944, **25,** 211–217.

Kanner, L. *Child Psychiatry* (3rd Ed.). Springfield, Ill.: Thomas, 1957.

Kanner, L. *A history of the care and study of the mentally retarded.* Springfield, Ill.: Thomas, 1964.

Kaufman, M. E. Group psychotherapy in preparation for return of mental defectives from institution to community. *Mental Retardation,* 1963, **1**(5), 276–280.

Keane, V. E. The incidence of speech and language problems in the mentally retarded. *Mental Retardation,* 1972, **10**(2), 3–5.

Kempe, C. H., Silverman, F. N., Steele, B. F., Droegmueller, W., & Silver, H. K. The battered child syndrome, *Journal of the American Medical Association,* 1962, **181,** 17–21.

Kempton, W., Bass, M. S., & Gordon, S. *Love, sex, and birth control for the mentally retarded: A guide for parents.* Philadelphia: Planned Parenthood Association, 1973.

Kennedy, C., & Ramirez, L. S. Brain damage as a cause of behavioral disturbance in children. In H. G. Birch (Ed.), *Brain damage in children: The biological and social aspects.* Baltimore: Williams and Wilkins, 1964.

Kennedy, R. J. R. *A Connecticut community revisited.* Report on Project No. 655. Jan. 1966. Office of Vocational Rehabilitation, Washington, D.C.

Kennedy, W. A., VanDeRiet, V., & White, J. C. A normative sample of intelligence and achievement of Negro elementary school children in the southeastern United States. *Monographs of the Society for Research in Child Development,* 1963, **28,** No. 6.

Kephart, N. C. *The slow learner in the classroom.* (2nd Ed.) Columbus, Ohio: Merrill, 1971.

Kessler, S., & Moos, R. H. The XYY karotype and criminality: A review. *Journal of Pediatric Research.* 1970, **7,** 153–170.

Kirk, S. A. Experiments in the early training of the mentally retarded. *American Journal of Mental Deficiency,* 1952, **56,** 692–700.

Kirk, S. A. *Educating exceptional children.* 2nd. Ed. Boston: Houghton Mifflin, 1972.

Kirk, S. A., & Bateman, B. Diagnosis and remediation of learning disabilities. *Exceptional Children,* 1972, **29,** 73–80.

Kirk, S. A., & Weiner, B. B. The Onondaga census—Fact or artifact. *Exceptional children,* 1959, **25,** 226–231.

Klaus, R., & Gray, S. The early training project for disadvantaged children: A report after five years. *Monographs of the Society for Research in Child Development,* 1968, **33,** No. 120.

Klugh, H. E., & Janssen, R. Discrimination learning by retardates and normals: method of presentation and verbalization. *American Journal of Mental Deficiency,* 1966, **70,** 903–906.

Knobloch, H., Rider, R., Harper, P., & Pasamanick, B. Neuropsychiatric sequelae of prematurity: A longitudinal study. *Journal of the American Medical Association,* 1956, **161,** 581–585.

Knox, W. E. An evaluation of the treatment of phenylketonuria with diets low in phenylalanine. *Pediatrics,* 1960, **26,** 1–11.

Kolstoe, O. P. *Teaching educable mentally retarded children.* New York: Harper & Row, 1970.

Kolstoe, O. P. Programs for the mildly retarded: A reply to the critics. *Exceptional Children,* 1972, **39,** 51–56.

Kolstoe, O. P., & Frey, R. M. *A high school work study program for the mentally subnormal student.* Carbondale, Ill.: Southern Illinois University Press, 1965.

Kosc, L. Developmental dyscalculia. *Journal of Learning Disabilities,* 1974, **7,** 164–177.

Kramm, E. R. *Families of mongoloid children.* Washington, D.C.: U.S. Government Printing Office, 1963.

Krush, T. P. The search for the golden key. *Bulletin of the Menninger Clinic,* 1964, **28,** 77–82.

L'Abate, L., & Curtis, L. T. *Teaching the exceptional child.* Philadelphia: W. B. Saunders Co., 1975.

Labov, W. The logic of nonstandard English. In F. Williams, (Ed.), *Language and Poverty,* Chicago, Markham Press, 1970.

Ladas, P. G. Worksample learning rates of the mentally retarded trainee as indicators of production in a work training center. *Personnel and Guidance Journal,* 1961, **39,** 396–402.

Lee, E. S. Negro intelligence and selective migration: A Philadelphia test of the Klineberg hypothesis. *American Sociological Review,* 1951, **16,** 227–233.

Leland, H., & Smith, D. E. *Play therapy with mentally subnormal children.* New York: Grune and Stratton, 1965.

Lenneberg, E. H. The natural history of language. In F. Smith and G. A. Miller (Eds.), *The genesis of language.* Cambridge, Mass.: M.I.T. Press, 1966.

Lenneberg, E. H. *Biological foundations of language.* New York: Wiley, 1967.

Lenneberg, E. H. Nichols, I. A., & Rosenberger, E. F. Primitive stages of language development in mongolism. *Disorders of Communication.* Vol. XLII. Baltimore: Williams & Wilkins, 1964.

Lesser, G. S., Fifer, G., & Clark, D. H. Mental abilities of children from different social class and cultural groups. *Monographs of the Society for Research in Child Development.* 1965, **30**(4).

Levinson, E. J. *Retarded children in Maine: A survey and analysis.* Orono, Maine: University of Maine Press, 1962.

Levitt, H., & Kaufman, M. E. Sound induced drive and stereotyped behavior in mental defectives. *American Journal of Mental Deficiency,* 1965, **69,** 729–735.

Levy, D. M. On the problem of movement restraint. *American Journal of Orthopsychiatry,* 1944, **14,** 644–671.

Liberman, A. M., Cooper, F. S., Shankweiler, D. P., & Studdert-Kennedy, M. Perception of the speech code. *Psychological Review,* 1967, **74,** 431–461.

Lipman, R. S. Learning: Verbal, perceptual-motor, and classical conditioning. In N. R. Ellis (Ed.), *Handbook of Mental Deficiency.* New York: McGraw-Hill, 1963.

Lipman, R. S. Results of a survey on psychotropic drug usage in institutions for the mentally retarded. Paper presented at the meeting of the American Association on Mental Deficiency, Denver, 1967.

Lister, C. M. The development of a concept of weight conservation in E. S. N. children. *British Journal of Educational Psychology,* 1969, **39,** 245–252.

Lister, C. M. The development of a concept of volume conservation in E. S. N. children. *British Journal of Educational Psychology,* 1970, **40,** 55–64.

Lobb, H., & Childs, R. Verbal control and intradimensional transfer of discrimination learning in mentally retarded vs. intellectually average subjects. *American Journal of Mental Deficiency,* 1973, **78,** 182–192.

Lobb, H., & Stogdill, D. Low IQ deficit in intradimensional shift despite overtraining and verbal feedback. *American Journal of Mental Deficiency,* 1975, **79,** 455–461.

Lovaas, I. A program for the establishment of speech in psychotic children. In H. N. Sloane & B. D. MacAulay (Eds.), *Operant procedures in remedial speech and language training.* Boston: Houghton Mifflin, 1968.

Lovaas, I. *Behavior Modification: Teaching language to psychotic children.* Englewood Cliffs, N.J.: Prentice-Hall, 1969 (Film).

Lovaas, I. After you hit a child, you can't just get up and leave him: You are hooked to that kid. *Psychology Today,* January 1974, 76.

Lovaas, I., & Simmons, J. Q. Manipulation of self-destruction in three retarded children. *Journal of Applied Behavior Analysis,* 1969, **2,** 143–157.

Love, H. D. *Educating exceptional children in regular classes.* Springfield, Ill.: Thomas, 1972.

Lozar, B., Wepman, J. M., & Hass, W. Lexical usage of mentally retarded and nonretarded children. *American Journal of Mental Deficiency,* 1972, **76,** 334–339.

Ludins-Katz, F. Creative arts expression of the mentally retarded. In E. Katz (Ed.). *Mental health services for the mentally retarded.* Springfield, Ill.: Thomas, 1972.

Luria, A. R. Psychological studies of mental deficiency in the Soviet Union. In N. R. Ellis (Ed.), *Handbook of mental deficiency,* New York: McGraw-Hill, 1963.

Lyle, J. G. The effect of an institution environment on the verbal development of imbecile children: I, Verbal intelligence. *Journal of Mental Deficiency Research,* 1959, **3,** 122–128.

Lyle, J. G. The effect of an institution environment upon the verbal development of imbecile children: II. Speech and language. *Journal of Mental Deficiency Research,* 1960, **4,** 1–13.

MacMillan, D. L. Motivational differences: Cultural familial retardates vs. normal subjects on expectancy for failure. *American Journal of Mental Defiency,* 1969, **74,** 254–258.

MacMillan, D. L., Jones, R. L., & Aloia, G. F. The mentally retarded label: A theoretical analysis and review of research. *American Journal of Mental Deficiency,* 1974, **79,** 241–261.

MacMillan, D. L., & Keogh, B. K. Normal and retarded children's expectancy fo failure. *Developmental Psychology,* 1971, **4,** 343–348.

Maloney, S. C. Observations concerning counseling with parents of mentally retarded children. *American Journal of Mental Deficiency,* 1958, **63,** 81–86.

Malott, R. W. *Contingency management in education and other equally exciting places.* Kalamazoo, Mich.: Behaviordelia, 1972.

Martin, A. S. The effect of the novelty-familiarity dimension on discrimination learning by retardates. Unpublished doctoral dissertation, University of Connecticut, 1970.

Martin, C. J., Boersma, F. J., & Bulgarella, R. Verbalization of associative strategies by normal and retarded children. *Journal of General Psychology,* 1968, **78,** 209–218.

Martin, H. P. Microcephaly and mental retardation. *American Journal of Diseases of Children,* 1970, **119,** 128–131.

Martyn, M. M., Sheehan, J., & Slutz, K. Incidence of stuttering and other speech disorders among the retarded. *American Journal of Mental Deficiency,* 1969, **74,** 206–211.

Marwits, S. J., & Stenner, A. J. Hyperkinesis: Delineation of two patterns, *Exceptional Children,* 1972, **38,** 401–406.

May, J. G. Moral, ethical, and legal considerations in behavior modification. In W. D. Gentry (Ed.), *Applied Behavior Modification.* St. Louis: Mosby, 1975.

McArthur, C. C. Review of the Rorschach. In O. K. Buros (Ed.), *The Seventh Mental Measurements Yearbook.* Vol. 1. Highland Park, N.J.: Gryphon Press, 1972.

McCracken, G. H., Shinefeld, H. R., Cobb, K., Rausen, A. R., Dische, M. R., & Eichenwald, H. F. Congenital cytomegalic inclusion disease. *American Journal of Diseases of Children,* 1969, **117,** 522–539.

McNeill, D. Developmental psycholinguistics. In E. Smith and G. A. Miller (Eds.) *The genesis of language.* Cambridge, Mass.: M.I.T. Press, 1966.

McGanity, W. J., Bridgeforth, E. B., Martin, M. P., Nebill, J. A., & Darby, W. J. The Vanderbilt cooperative study of maternal and infant nutrition, VIII: Some nutritional implications. *Journal of the American Dietetic Association,* 1955, **31,** 582.

McLean, J. E., Yoder, D. E., & Schiefelbusch, R. L. (Eds.) *Language intervention with the retarded.* Baltimore: University Park Press, 1972.

McManis, D. Conservation of mass, weight, and volume by normal and retarded children. *American Journal of Mental Deficiency,* 1969, **73,** 762–767.

McNemar, Q. *The revision of the Stanford-Binet Scale.* Boston: Houghton Mifflin, 1942.

Menkes, M. M., Rowe, J. S., & Menkes, J. H. A twenty-five year follow up study on the hyperactive child with minimal brain dysfunction. *Pediatrics,* 1967, **39,** 393–399.

Menolascino, F. J. Infantile autism: Descriptive and diagnostic relationships to mental retardation. In F. J. Menolascino (Ed.), *Psychiatric approaches to mental retardation.* New York: Basic Books, 1970.

Mercer, J. R. *Labeling the mentally retarded.* Berkeley: University of California Press, 1973.

Mercer, J. R., Butler, E. W., & Dingman, H. F. The relationship between social developmental performance and mental ability. *American Journal of Mental Deficiency,* 1964, **69,** 195–205.

Meyen, E. L. *Developing units of instruction for the mentally retarded and other children with learning problems.* Dubuque, Iowa: W. C. Brown, 1972.

Michaels, R. H., & Mellin, G. W. Prospective experience with maternal rubella and associated congenital malformations. *Pediatrics,* 1960, **26,** 200–209.

Milgram, N. A., & Furth, H. G. Position reversal versus dimension reversal in normal and retarded children. *Child Development,* 1964, **35,** 701–708.

Milgram, N. A., & Reidel, W. Verbal context and visual compound in paired associate learning of mental retardates. *American Journal of Mental Deficiency,* 1969, **73,** 755–761.

Milkovich, L., & van den Berg, B. J. Effects of prenatal meprobamate and chlordiazepoxide hydrochloride on human embryonic and fetal development. *New England Journal of Medicine,* 1974, **291,** 1268–1271.

Mitchell, A. C., & Smerglio, V. Growth in social competence in institutionalized mentally retarded children. *American Journal of Mental Deficiency,* 1970, **74,** 666–673.

Molloy, J. S. *Trainable children: Curriculum and procedures.* (Rev. ed.) New York: John Day, 1972.

Moore, O. K. Autotelic responsive environments and exceptional children. In J. Hellmuth (Ed.), *The special child in century 21.* Seattle, Washington: Special Child Publications, 1964.

MR Source Book. Department of Health, Education and Welfare, Washington D.C.: U.S. Government Printing Office, 1972.

Mueller, M. W., & Weaver, S. J. Psycholinguistic abilities of institutionalized and noninstitutionalized trainable mental retardates. *American Journal of Mental Deficiency,* 1964, **68,** 775–783.

Murphy, D. P. The outcome of 625 pregnancies in women subject to pelvic radium-roentgen irradiation. *American Journal of Obstetrics and Gynocology,* 1929, **18,** 179–187.

Murphy, H. B., Pennee, B., & Luchins, D. Foster homes: the new back wards? *Canada's Mental Health,* 1972, Suppl. No. 71.

Myers, D. G., Sinco, M. E., & Stalma, E. S. *The right-to-education child: A curriculum for the severely and profoundly mentally retarded.* Springfield, Ill.: Thomas, 1975.

Nadler, H. L., Inouye, T., & Hsia, D. Y. Classical galactosemia. In D. Y. Hsia (Ed.), *Galactosemia,* Springfield, Illinois; Thomas, 1969.

Natkamura, H. An inquiry into systematic differences in the abilities of institutionalized adult mongoloids. *American Journal of Mental Deficiency,* 1965, **69,** 661–665.

Nazzaro, J. Head start for the handicapped—What's been accomplished? *Exceptional Children,* 1974, **41,** 103–106.

Neisser, U. *Cognitive psychology.* New York: Appleton—Century—Crofts, 1967.

Neisworth, J. T., & Smith, R. M. *Modifying retarded behavior.* Boston: Houghton Mifflin, 1973.

Nelson, M. M., & Forfar, J. O. Cogenital abnormalities at birth: Their association in the same patient. *Developmental Medicine and Child Neurology,* 1969, **11,** 3–16.

Newfield, M. U., & Schlanger, B. B. The acquisition of English morphology by normal and educable mentally retarded children. *Journal of Speech and Hearing Research,* 1968, **11,** 693–706.

O'Grady, D. J., Berry, H. K., & Sutherland, B. S. Cognitive development in early treated phenylketonuria. *American Journal of Diseases of Children,* 1971, **121,** 20–23.

Olshansky, S. Chronic sorrow: A response to having a mentally defective child. *Social Casework,* 1962, **43,** 191–194.

Olshansky, S., Johnson, G., & Sternfield, L. Attitudes of some G.P.s toward institutionalizing mentally retarded children. In *Institutionalizing mentally retarded children: Attitudes of some physicians.* Washington, D.C.: U.S. Government Printing Office, 1964.

Olshansky, S., & Kettell, M. Attitudes of some interns and first year residents toward the institutionalization of mentally retarded children. *Training School Bulletin,* 1963, **59,** 116–120.

Osborne, R. T., Unequal educational opportunity. *Psychological Reports,* 1973, **33,** 412.

Papania, N. A qualitative analysis of the vocabulary responses of institutionalized mentally retarded children. *Journal of Clinical Psychology,* 1954, **10,** 361–365.

Parmelee, A. H., Sigman, M., Kopp, C. B., & Haber, A. Diagnosis of the infant at high risk for mental, motor, and sensory handicap. In T. D. Tjossem (Ed.), *Intervention strategies for high risk infants and young children.* Baltimore: University Park Press, 1976.

Pasamanick, B., & Knobloch, H. Retrospective studies on the epidemiology of reproductive casualty: Old and new. *Merrill-Palmer Quarterly of Behavior and Development,* 1966, **12,** 7–26.

Pavlov, I. P. *Conditioned Reflexes.* London: Oxford Univ. Press, 1927.

Payne, R., & Murray, C. Principals' attitudes toward integration of the handicapped. *Exceptional Children,* 1974, **41,** 123–125.

Pearson, G. H. J. The psychopathology of mental defect. *Nervous Child,* 1942, **2,** 9–20.

Penrose, L. S., & Smith, G. F. *Down's anomaly.* Boston: Little Brown, 1966.

Peter, L. J. *Prescriptive teaching system, Vol. 1. Individual instruction.* New York: McGraw-Hill, 1972.

Peterson, D. L. *Functional mathematics for the mentally retarded.* Columbus, Ohio: Merrill, 1973.

Phillips, I. Psychopathology and mental retardation. *American Journal of Psychiatry,* 1967, **124,** 29–35.

Phillips, J. L. *The origins of intellect: Piaget's theory.* (2nd ed.) San Francisco: W. H. Freeman Co., 1975.

Piaget, J. *The Psychology of Intelligence,* New York: Harcourt Brace, 1950.

Piaget, J. *The origins of intelligence in children.* New York: International University Press, 1952.

Plummer, G. Anomalies occuring in children exposed in utero to the atomic blast in Hiroshima. Pediatrics, 1952, **10,** 687.

Polani, P. E. Autosomal imbalance and its syndromes, excluding Down's. *British Medical Bulletin,* 1969, **25,** 81–93.

Premack, D. Reinforcement theory. In D. Levine (Ed.), *Nebraska Symposium on Motivation.* Lincoln, Neb.: University of Nebraska Press, 1965.

President's Committee on Mental Retardation. *The six hour retarded child.* Washington, D.C.: U.S. Government Printing Office, 1970.

President's Committee on Mental Retardation, *Mental Retardation: Trends in State Service,* Washington, D.C.: U.S. Government Printing Office, 1976.

President's Committee on Mental Retardation, *Mental Retardation, The Known and the Unknown.* Washington, D.C.: U.S. Government Printing Office, 1976a.

President's Panel on Mental Retardation. *A proposed program for national action to combat mental retardation.* Washington, D.C.: U.S. Government Printing Office, 1962.

Quay, L. C. Language dialect, age, and intelligence test performance in disadvantaged Black children. *Child Development,* 1974, **45,** 463–468.

Reitan, R. M. A research program on the psychological effects of brain leisons in human beings. In N. R. Ellis, (Ed.), *International review of research in mental retardation.* Vol. 1. New York: Academic Press, 1966.

Repp, A. C., & Dietz, S. M. Reducing aggressive and self-injurious behavior of institutionalized retarded children through reinforcement of other behaviors. *Journal of Applied Behavior Analysis,* 1974, **7,** 313–325.

Rider, R. V., Tayback, M., & Knobloch, H. Associations between premature birth and socioeconomic status. *American Journal of Public Health,* 1955, **45,** 1022–1028.

Rimland, B. *Infantile Autism,* New York: Appleton—Century—Crofts, 1964.

Ring, E. M., & Palermo, D. S. Paired associate learning of retarded and normal children. *American Journal of Mental Deficiency,* 1961, **66,** 100–107.

Ringelheim, D. The effects of failure on verbal expectancies in male defectives. *Abstracts of Peabody Studies in Mental Retardation,* 1960, **1,** No. 14.

Rist, R. C. Student social class and teacher expectations: The self-fulfilling prophecy in ghetto education. *Harvard Educational Review,* 1970, **40,** 411–451.

Robbins, M., & Glass, G. V. The Doman-Delacato rationale: A critical analysis: In J. Hellmuth (Ed.), *Educational Therapy.* Vol. II. Seattle, Special Child Publications, 1969.

Robinson, H. B., & Robinson, N. M. *The mentally retarded child.* New York: McGraw-Hill, 1965.

Robinson, N. M., & Robinson, H. B. *The mentally retarded child.* (2nd ed.) New York: McGraw-Hill, 1976.

Rogers, C. R. *Client centered therapy.* Boston: Houghton Mifflin, 1951.

Rohwer, W. D., & Lynch, S. Retardation, school strata, and learning proficiency. *American Journal of Mental Deficiency,* 1968, **73,** 91–96.

Rojcewicz., S. J., & Aaronson, M. Mental health and the Medicaid screening program. In T. D. Tjossem (Ed.), *Intervention strategies for high risk infants and young children.* Baltimore: University Park Press, 1976.

Roos, P. Psychological counseling with parents of retarded children. *Mental Retardation,* 1963, **1,** 345–350.

Rosenthal, R., & Jacobson, L. *Pygmalion in the classroom.* New York: Holt, Rinehart and Winston, 1968.

Ross, A. O. Conceptual issues in the evaluation of brain damage. In J. L. Khanna (Ed.), *Brain damage and mental retardation.* Springfield, Ill.: Thomas, 1968.

Rotter, J. B. *Social learning and clinical psychology.* Englewood Cliffs, N.J.: Prentice-Hall, 1954.

Rubin, R. A., Krus, P., & Balow, B. Factors in special class placement. *Exceptional Children,* 1973, **39,** 525–531.

Saenger, G. *The adjustment of severely retarded adults in the community.* Albany, N.Y.: Interdepartmental health resources board, 1957.

Salapatek, P., & Kessen, W. Visual scanning of triangles by the human newborn. *Journal of Experimental Child Psychology,* 1966, **3,** 113–122.

Salzinger, K., Feldman, R. S., & Portnoy, S. Training parents of brain-injured children in the use of operant conditioning procedures. *Behavior Therapy,* 1970, **1,** 4–32.

Santrock, J. W. Relationship of type and onset of father absence to cognitive development. *Child Development,* 1972, **43,** 455–469.

Sarason, S. B., & Doris, J. *Psychological problems in mental deficiency.* (4th ed.) New York: Harper & Row, 1969.

Sattler, J. M. Racial experimenter effects in experimentation, testing, interviewing, and psychotherapy. *Psychological Bulletin,* 1970, **73,** 137–160.

Sattler, J. M. *Assessment of children's intelligence.* Philadelphia: Saunders, 1974.

Scanlon, R. G. *Individually prescribed instruction: A system of individualized instruction.* Philadelphia: Research for Better Schools, 1971.

Schiefelbusch, R. L. (Ed.) *Language of the mentally retarded.* Baltimore: University Park Press, 1972.

Schiefelbusch, R. L., Copeland, R. H., & Smith, J. O. *Language and mental retardation.* New York: Holt, Rinehart and Winston, 1967.

Schipper, M. T. The child with mongolism in the home. *Pediatrics,* 1959, **24,** 132–144.

Schlanger, B. B., & Gottsleben, R. H. Analysis of speech defects among the institutionalized mentally retarded. *Journal of Speech and Hearing Disorders.* 1957, **22,** 98–103.

Schonnel, F. J., & Watts, B. H. A first survey of the effects of a subnormal child on the family unit. *American Journal of Mental Deficiency,* 1956, **61,** 210–219.

Schwarz, R. H., & Flanigan, P. J. Evaluation of examiner bias in intelligence testing. *American Journal of Mental Deficiency,* 1971, **76,** 262–265.

Schwebel, M., & Raph, J. (Eds.) *Piaget in the classroom.* New York: Basic Books, 1973.

Scofield, P. Oral language for the educable mentally retarded. In M. V. Jones (Ed.), *Language development: The key to learning.* Springfield, Ill.: Thomas, 1972.

Seguin, E. *The moral treatment, hygiene, and education of idiots and other backward children.* Paris: Balliere, 1846.

Seguin, E. *Idiocy and its treatment by the physiological method.* Albany, N.Y.: Brandow, 1866.

Schaffer, J. W. A specific cognitive deficit observed in gonadal aplasia (Turner's syndrome). *Journal of Clinical Psychology,* 1962, **8,** 403–406.

Shafter, A. J. Criteria for selecting institutionalized mental defectives for vocational placement. *American Journal of Mental Deficiency,* 1957, **61,** 599–616.

Sheare, J. B. Social acceptance of EMR adolescents in integrated programs. *American Journal of Mental Deficiency,* 1974, **78,** 678–682.

Shearer, D. E. & Shearer, M. S. The Portage Project: A model for early childhood intervention. In T. D. Tjossem (Ed.), *Intervention strategies for high risk infants and young children.* Baltimore: University Park Press, 1976.

Shepard, R. N. Recognition memory for words, sentences, and pictures. *Journal of Verbal Learning and Verbal Behavior.* 1967, **6,** 156–163.

Shepp, B. E., & Turrisi, F. D. Learning and transfer of mediating responses in discriminative learning. In N. R. Ellis (Ed.), *International review of research in mental retardation.* Vol. 2. New York: Academic Press, 1966.

Shuey, A. M. *The testing of Negro intelligence.* New York: Social Science Press, 1966.

Shumaker, J., & Sherman, J. A. Training generative verb usage by imitation and reinforcement procedures. *Journal of Applied Behavior Analysis,* 1970, **3,** 273–287.

Silverstein, A. B. The measurement of intelligence. In N. R. Ellis (Ed.). *International review of research in mental retardation.* Vol. 4. New York: Academic Press, 1970.

Silverstein, A. B., Brownlee, L., Hubbell, M. & McLain, R. E. Comparison of two sets of Piagetian scales with severely and profoundly retarded children. *American Journal of Mental Deficiency,* 1975, **80,** 292–297.

Simches, G., & Bohn, R. Issues in curriculum research and responsibility. *Mental Retardation,* 1963, **1,** 84–87.

Skeels, H. M. Adult status of children with contrasting early life experiences. *Monographs of the Society for Research in Child Development,* 1966, **31,** No. 3.

Skinner, B. F. *Behavior of organisms: An experimental analysis.* New York: Appleton—Century—Crofts, 1938.

Skinner, B. F. *About behaviorism.* New York: Knopf, 1974.

Slivkin, S. E., & Bernstein, N. R. Group approaches to treating retarded adolescents. In F. J. Menolascino (Ed.), *Psychiatric approaches to mental retardation.* New York: Basic Books, 1970.

Sloane, H. N., & MacAulay, B. D. *Operant procedures in remedial speech and language training.* Boston: Houghton Mifflin, 1968.

Smith, D. W., Blizzard, R. M., & Wilkins, L. The mental prognosis in hypothyroidism of infancy and childhood. *Pediatrics,* 1957, **19,** 1011–1020.

Smith, D. W., & Wilson, A. A. *The child with Down's syndrome (mongolism).* Philadelphia: Saunders, 1973.

Smith, G. F. Clinical aspects of genetics in mental retardation. In R. M. Allen, A. D. Cortazzo, & R. P. Toister (Eds.), *The role of genetics in mental retardation.* Coral Gables, Fla.: University of Miami Press, 1971.

Smith, R. M. *Clinical teaching: Methods of instruction for the retarded.* (2nd ed.) New York: McGraw-Hill, 1974.

Smith, R. M., & Neisworth, J. T. *The exceptional child: A functional approach.* New York: McGraw-Hill, 1975.

Snyder, L. K., Lovitt, T. C., & Smith, J. O. Language training for the severely retarded: Five years of behavior analysis research. *Exceptional Children,* 1975, **42,** 7–16.

Solnit, A. J. & Stark, M. H. Mourning and the birth of a defective child. *Psychoanalytic Study of the Child,* 1961, **16,** 523–537.

Somerville, J. W., Warnberg, L. S., & Bost, D. E. Effects of cubicle versus increased stimulation on task performance by first grade males perceived as distractible and nondistractible. *Journal of Special Education,* 1973, **7,** 169–186.

Spearman, C. *The abilities of man,* New York: Macmillan, 1927.

Spicker, H. H. Intellectual development through early childhood education. *Exceptional Children,* 1971, **37,** 629–640.

Spitz, H. H. The role of input organization in the learning and memory of mental retardates. In N. R. Ellis (Ed.), *International review of research in mental retardation.* Vol. 2. New York: Academic Press, 1966.

Sprague, R. L., & Werry, J. S. Methodology of psychopharmacological studies with the retarded. In N. R. Ellis (Ed.). *International review of research in mental retardation.* Vol. 5. New York: Academic Press, 1971.

Spreen, O. Language functions in mental retardation: A review: I. Language development, types of retardation, and intelligence level. *American Journal of Mental Deficiency,* 1965, **69,** 482—494.

Stamm, J. Behavioral counseling with the mentally retarded. In Browning, P. L. (Ed.), *Mental retardation: Rehabilitation and counseling.* Springfield, Ill.: Thomas, 1974.

Stanfield, J. S. Graduation: What happens to the retarded child when he grows up? *Exceptional Children,* 1973, **39,** 548–552.

Statistical Abstract of the United States. Washington, D.C.: U.S. Government Printing Office, 1975.

Stedman, D. J., & Eichorn, D. H. A comparison of the growth of institutionalized and home reared mongoloids during infancy and early childhood. *American Journal of Mental Deficiency,* 1964, **69,** 391–401.

Stephens, J. M. *The process of schooling.* New York: Holt, Rinehart and Winston, 1967.

Stephens, W. B. Symposium: Developmental gains in the reasoning, moral judgment, and moral conduct of retarded and nonretarded persons. *American Journal of Mental Deficiency,* 1974, **79,** 113–115.

Stephens, W. B., & McLaughlin, J. A. Two year gains in reasoning by retarded and nonretarded persons. *American Journal of Mental Deficiency,* 1974, **79,** 116–126.

Stephens, M. W., & Deyls, P. External control expectancies among disadvantaged children at preschool age. *Child Development,* 1973, **44,** 670–674.

Stern, L. W. *The psychological method of testing intelligence.* Tr. by G. M. Whipple, *Educational Psychology Monographs,* 1914, No. 13.

Sternlicht, M. Psychotherapeutic procedures with the retarded. In N. R. Ellis (Ed.), *International review of research in mental retardation.* Vol. 2. New York: Academic Press, 1966.

Sternlicht, M., & Deutsch, M. R. *Personality development and social behavior in the mentally retarded.* Lexington, Mass.: D. C. Heath, 1972.

Stewart, M., Ferris, A., Pitts, N., & Craig, A. G. The hyperactive child syndrome. *American Journal of Orthopsychiatry,* 1966, **36,** 861–867.

Stewart, N. A.G.C.T. scores of army personnel grouped by occupation. *Occupations,* 1947, **26,** 5–41.

Stoch, M. B., & Smythe, P. M. Does undernutrition during infancy inhibit brain growth and subsequent intellectual development. *Archives of Diseases of Children,* 1963, **38,** 546–552.

Stoddard, G. D. *The meaning of intelligence,* New York: Macmillan, 1943.

Stodolsky, S. S., & Lesser, G. Learning patterns in the disadvantaged. *Harvard Educational Review,* 1967, **37,** 546–593.

Stone, N. D. Family factors in willingness to place the mongoloid child. *American Journal of Mental Deficiency,* 1967, **72,** 16–20.

Strauss, A. A., & Lehtinen, L. E. *Psychopathology and education of the brain-injured child.* New York: Grune and Stratton, 1947.

Tarnopol, L. *Learning disabilities: Introduction to educational and medical management.* Springfield, Ill.: Thomas, 1969.

Taylor, A. I. Autosomal trisomy syndromes: A detailed study of 27 cases of Edward's syndrome and 27 cases of Patau's syndrome. *Journal of Medical Genetics,* 1968, **5,** 227–252.

Telford, C. W., & Sawrey, J. M. *The exceptional individual.* Englewood Cliffs, N.J.: Prentice-Hall, 1972.

Thomson, A. M. Historical perspectives of nutrition, reproduction, and growth. In N. S. Scrimshaw & J. E. Gordon (Eds.), *Malnutrition, learning and behavior.* Cambridge, Mass.: M.I.T. Press, 1968.

Thormahlen, P. W. A study of the ward training of trainable mentally retarded children in a state institution. *California Mental Health Research Monographs,* 1965, No. 5.

Thorne, F. C. Counseling and psychotherapy with mental defectives. *American Journal of Mental Deficiency,* 1948, **52,** 263–271.

Throne, F. M., Schulman, J. L., & Kaspar, J. C. Reliability and validity of the Wechsler Intelligence Scale for Children for a group of mentally retarded boys. *American Journal of Mental Deficiency,* 1962, **67,** 455–457.

Throne, J. M. A radical behaviorist approach to diagnosis in mental retardation. *Mental Retardation,* 1970, **8,**(3), 2–5.

Tizard, J., & Grad, J. *The mentally handicapped and their families: A social survey.* London: Oxford University Press, 1961.

Tobias, J. Evaluation of vocational potential of mentally retarded young adults. *Training School Bulletin,* 1960, **56,** 122–135.

Tredgold, A. F. *A textbook of mental deficiency.* (6th ed.) Baltimore: Wood, 1937.

Turnure, J. E. Types of verbal elaboration in the paired associate performance of educable mentally retarded children. *American Journal of Mental Deficiency,* 1971, **76,** 306–312.

Turnure, J. E., & Zigler, E. Outerdirectedness in the problem solving of normal and retarded children. *Journal of Abnormal and Social Psychology,* 1964, **69,** 427–436.

Tyson, F. Music therapy in the rehabilitation of the retarded child. *Newsletter of the Musicians' Fund,* 1957, **3,** 1–4.

Ullman, D. G. Breadth of attention and retention in mentally retarded and intellectually average children. *American Journal of Mental Deficiency,* 1974, **78,** 640–648.

United States Bureau of the Census. *The social and economic status of the Black population in the U.S.* Current Population Reports, Series P-23, No. 48, 1973.

Uzgiris, I. C., & Hunt, J. M. *Assessment in infancy: Ordinal scales of psychological development.* Urbana, Ill.: University of Illinois Press, 1975.

Vandenberg, S. G. The nature and nurture of intelligence. In D. C. Glass (Ed.), *Genetics.* New York: Rockefeller University Press and the Russell Sage Foundation, 1968.

Wagner, E. E., & Hawver, D. A. Correlates between psychological tests and sheltered workshop performance for severely retarded adults. *American Journal of Mental Deficiency,* 1965, **69,** 685–691.

Waite, K. B. *The educable mentally retarded child: Guidance and curriculum.* Springfield, Ill.: Thomas, 1971.

Waite, K. B. *The trainable mentally retarded child.* Springfield, Ill.: Thomas, 1972.

Walker, S. Drugging the American child: We're too cavalier about hyperactivity. *Psychology Today,* December 1974, **8**(7), 43–48.

Warren, S. A., & Mondy, L. To what behaviors do attending adults respond? *American Journal of Mental Deficiency,* 1971, **75,** 449–455.

Waskowitz, C. H. The parents of retarded children speak for themselves. *Journal of Pediatrics,* 1959, **54,** 319–329.

Webster, T. G. Unique aspects of emotional development in mentally retarded children. In F. J. Menolascino (Ed.), *Psychiatric approaches to mental retardation.* New York: Basic Books, 1970.

Wechsler, D. *The measurement of adult intelligence,* 3rd Ed. Baltimore: Williams & Wilkins, 1944.

Wechsler, D. *Wechsler Adult Intelligence Scale Manual.* New York: Psychological Corporation, 1955.

Wechsler, D. *Manual for the Wechsler Preschool and Primary Scale of Intelligence,* New York: Psychological Corporation, 1967.

Wechsler, D. *Wechsler Intelligence Scale for Children—Revised.* New York: Psychological Corporation, 1974.

Weismann, A. *The germ-plasm: A theory of heredity.* New York: Scribner, 1892.

Weigl, V. Functional music—A therapeutic tool in working with the mentally retarded. *American Journal of Mental Deficiency,* 1959, **63,** 672–678.

Wender, P. H. *Minimal brain dysfunction in children.* New York: Wiley, 1971.

Wesman, A. G. Intelligent testing. *American Psychologist,* 1968, **23,** 267–274.

White, B. L., & Watts, J. C. *Experience and environment: Major influences on the development of the young child.* Englewood Cliffs, N.J.: Prentice-Hall, 1973.

Whorf, B. L. *Language, thought, and reality: The selected writings of Benjamin Lee Whorf,* J. B. Carroll (Ed.) Cambridge, Mass.: M.I.T. Press, 1956.

Wiegerink, R., & Simeonsson, R. J. Public schools. In J. Wortis (Ed.), *Mental retardation.* Vol. 7. New York: Brunner/Mazel, 1975.

Wiener, G., Rider, R. V., Opell, W. C., & Harper, P. A. Correlates of low birth weight: psychological status at eight to ten years of age. *Pediatric Research,* 1968, **2,** 110–118.

Williams, D. L., & Jaffa, E. B. *Ice cream, poker chips, and very goods: A behavior modification manual for parents.* McLean, Va.: School for Contemporary Education, 1971.

Wilson, F. B. Efficacy of speech therapy with educable mentally retarded children. *Journal of Speech and Hearing Research,* 1966, **9,** 423–433.

Wilton, K. M., & Boersma, F. J. Conservation research with the mentally retarded. In N. R. Ellis (Ed.), *International review of research in mental retardation.* Vol. 7. New York: Academic Press, 1974.

Wilton, K. M., & Boersma, F. J. *Eye movements, surprise reactions, and cognitive developments.* Rotterdam: University of Rotterdam Press, 1974a.

Windle, C. Prognosis of mental subnormals. *American Journal of Mental Deficiency,* 1962, **66,** Monogr. supplement.

Winick, M. Fetal malnutrition and growth processes. *Hospital Practice,* 1970, **5,** 33–41.

Wirtz, M. A., & Guenter, R. The incidence of trainable level handicapped children. *Exceptional Children,* 1957, **23,** 171–175.

Wishik, S. M. Handicapped children in Georgia: A study of prevalence, needs, and resources. *American Journal of Public Health,* 1956, **46,** 195–203.

Wolf, M. M., Risley, T., & Mees, H. Application of operant conditioning procedures to the behavior problems of an autistic child. *Behavior Research and Therapy,* 1964, **1,** 305–312.

Wolfensberger, W. Counseling the parents of the retarded. In A. A. Baumeister (Ed.), *Mental retardation: Appraisal, education, and rehabilitation.* Chicago: Aldine, 1967.

Wolfensberger, W. Vocational preparation and occupation. In A. A. Baumeister (Ed.), *Mental retardation: Appraisal, education, and rehabilitation.* Chicago: Aldine, 1967a.

Woodward, M. The behaviour of idiots interpreted by Piaget's theory of sensorimotor development. *British Journal of Educational Psychology,* 1959, **29,** 60–71.

Woody, R. H., & Billy J. T. Counseling and psychotherapy for the mentally retarded: A survey of opinions and practices. *Mental Retardation,* 1966, **4**(6), 20–23.

Wortis, H. Parent counseling. In J. Wortis (Ed.), *Mental Retardation.* Vol. 4. New York: Grune and Stratton, 1972.

Wyoming Mental Abilities Survey, 1957–1958. Cheyenne, Wyo.: State Department of Education, 1959.

Yando, R., & Zigler, E. Outerdirectedness in the problem solving of institutionalized and noninstitutionalized normal and retarded children. *Developmental Psychology,* 1971, **4,** 277–288.

Zeaman, D., & House, B. J. Approach and avoidance in the discrimination learning of retardates. *Child Development,* 1962, **33,** 355–372.

Zeaman, D., & House, B. J. The role of attention in retardate discrimination learning. In N. R. Ellis (Ed.), *Handbook of mental deficiency,* New York: McGraw-Hill, 1963.

Zeaman, D., & House, B. J. The relation of IQ and learning. In R. M. Gagne (Ed.), *Learning and individual differences.* Columbus, Ohio: Merrill, 1966.

Zigler, E. F. Social deprivation and rigidity in the performance of feebleminded children. *Journal of Abnormal and Social Psychology,* 1961, **62,** 413–421.

Zigler, E. F. Mental retardation: Current issues and approaches. In L. W. Hoffman and M. L. Hoffman (Eds.), *Review of child development research.* Vol. 2. New York: Russell Sage Foundation, 1966.

Zigler, E. F. Research on personality structure in the retardate. In N. R. Ellis (Ed.), *International review of research in mental retardation.* Vol. 1. New York: Academic Press, 1966.

Zigler, E. F. Familial mental retardation: A continuing dilemma. *Science,* 1967, **155,** 292–298.

Zigler, E. F. Developmental vs. difference theories and the problem of motivation. *American Journal of Mental Deficiency,* 1969, **73,** 536–555.

Zigler, E. F. The retarded child as a whole person. In D. K. Routh (Ed.), *The experimental psychology of mental retardation.* Chicago: Aldine, 1973.

Zigler, E. F. Why retarded children do not perform up to the level of their ability. In R. M. Allen, A. D. Cortazzo, and R. P. Toister (Eds.), *Theories of cognitive development: Implications for the mentally retarded.* Coral Gables, Fla.: University of Miami Press, 1973a.

Zigler, E. F., & Butterfield, E. C. Motivational aspects of changes in IQ test performance of culturally deprived nursery school children. *Child Development,* 1968, **39,** 1–14.

Zigler, E. F., & DeLabry, J. Concept switching in middle class, lower class, and retarded children. *Journal of Abnormal and Social Psychology,* 1962, **65,** 267–273.

Zigler, E. F., Hodgden, L., & Stevenson, H. W. The effect of support and nonsupport on the performance of normal and feebleminded children. *Journal of Personality,* 1958, **26,** 106–122.

Zwerling, I. Initial counseling of parents with mentally retarded children. *Journal of Pediatrics,* 1954, **44,** 469–479.

Index